Natural Products for Skin Diseases: A Treasure Trove for Dermatologic Therapy

Edited by

Heba Abd El-Sattar El-Nashar
Department of Pharmacognosy
Faculty of Pharmacy
Ain Shams University
Cairo
Egypt

Mohamed El-Shazly
Department of Pharmacognosy
Faculty of Pharmacy
Ain Shams University
Cairo
Egypt

&

Nouran Mohammed Fahmy
Department of Pharmacognosy
Faculty of Pharmacy
Ain Shams University
Cairo
Egypt

Natural Products for Skin Diseases: A Treasure Trove for Dermatologic Therapy

Editors: Heba Abd El-Sattar El-Nashar, Mohamed El-Shazly & Nouran Mohammed Fahmy

ISBN (Online): 978-981-5179-66-8

ISBN (Print): 978-981-5179-67-5

ISBN (Paperback): 978-981-5179-68-2

need for a court order if at any point you breach any terms of this License Agreement. In no event will any delay or failure by Bentham Science Publishers in enforcing your compliance with this License Agreement constitute a waiver of any of its rights.

3. You acknowledge that you have read this License Agreement, and agree to be bound by its terms and conditions. To the extent that any other terms and conditions presented on any website of Bentham Science Publishers conflict with, or are inconsistent with, the terms and conditions set out in this License Agreement, you acknowledge that the terms and conditions set out in this License Agreement shall prevail.

Bentham Science Publishers Pte. Ltd.
80 Robinson Road #02-00
Singapore 068898
Singapore
Email: subscriptions@benthamscience.net

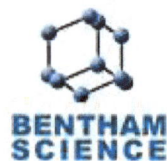

CONTENTS

FOREWORD

In a world where modern medicine continues to advance at an unprecedented pace, it is easy to overlook the timeless wisdom that nature has to offer. Plants, with their vast array of bioactive compounds, have been used for centuries by various cultures to address a myriad of health issues. Among their many applications, the treatment of skin diseases stands out as an area where these botanical wonders have consistently proven their efficacy.

In this comprehensive volume, we embark on a journey to explore the remarkable potential of plants in treating skin diseases. Assembled within these pages are the collective efforts of esteemed researchers, each contributing their expertise to shed light on different facets of this fascinating subject.

Chapter 1 opens our exploration, focusing on the essential topic of protecting our skin from harmful radiation. The authors guide us through the ways in which natural compounds can act as a shield against the damaging effects of the sun and other environmental factors.

Moving on, Chapter 2 delves into the challenging domain of burns, presenting insights into the potential of natural products to address these complex cases. By unraveling the secrets of traditional remedies, the authors offer a fresh perspective on tackling this persistent medical concern.

Chapter 3 takes us on a historical journey through the treatment of wounds, revealing the enduring efficacy of natural remedies. In a world increasingly reliant on synthetic pharmaceuticals, this chapter serves as a reminder of the healing potential rooted in our botanical heritage.

The significance of skin pigmentary anomalies cannot be understated, and Chapter 4 addresses this crucial aspect of skin health. The authors examine the role of natural products in managing these conditions, providing valuable insights for both practitioners and those seeking effective solutions.

In Chapter 5, we encounter the age-old challenge of scabies, and the authors explore how herbal medicines have historically been employed to alleviate this distressing skin condition.

The pursuit of beauty and self-care is a timeless endeavor, and Chapter 6 takes us into the world of natural cosmetics. With a focus on future applications, this chapter highlights the potential of botanicals in transforming the skincare industry.

Chapters 7 and 8 push the boundaries of innovation, exploring the realm of nanoparticle skin delivery and smart drug delivery systems for natural products. As technology continues to advance, these chapters present a glimpse into the promising possibilities that lie ahead.

As we journey through these chapters, it becomes evident that the study of plants in the context of skin health is both rich and dynamic. The contributors to this book have poured their knowledge and passion into their respective fields, resulting in a collective work that is both enlightening and inspiring.

It is with great pleasure that we present this book, hoping that it will serve as a valuable resource for researchers, healthcare professionals, and all those seeking to harness the healing power of nature for the benefit of healthy skin.

Tsong-Long Hwang
Distinguished Professor and Vice President
Chang Gung University of Science and Technology
Taiwan

PREFACE

Mother Nature has always been the treasure trove for biologically active compounds that helped humanity to survive and thrive. Medicinal plants have played a major role in the development of human civilizations. Since antiquity, humans have been searching for natural sources to cure diseases, and found their target in medicinal plants. The Egyptian, Greek, Indian, Chinese, and Aztec civilizations relied heavily on the use of medicinal plants to cure human and animal ailments. Medicinal plants have been used to treat all types of disorders, including cardiovascular, digestive, skin and kidney disorders. Skin disorders differ from other disorders by being external, can be detected by the naked eye, medicinal plant extracts can be easily applied to the disorders, and the healing effect can be easily tracked. Skin is the largest organ in the human body and the first line of defense against traumas, infections and radiation. Skin is a dynamic organ with millions of cells dying and regenerating regularly. It is affected by a plethora of disorders and should be treated to avoid the spread of invasion to internal organs.

Medicinal plants have been used to treat skin disorders and to improve skin condition. They have also been used in cosmetic preparations to remove wrinkles, black spots and provide a radiant appearance. In the current book, we take the reader on an enjoyable journey of medicinal plants treating skin-related disorders. The first chapter reveals "How to protect skin from harmful solar radiation." Pathologically solar radiation having UVA (320–400 nm) and UVB (290–320 nm) wavelengths may lead to serious hazards, especially to the skin. On one side, sunlight is essential for Vit D creation but on the other side, continuous exposure to it may lead to risk from sunburn to skin cancer. UV radiation can produce harmful compounds called free radicals or reactive oxygen species or ROS, which leads to skin cancer and premature aging. Traditionally herbal formulations and herbal extracts have been used as a sunscreen for photoprotection for a long time and are considered more vigorous compared to allopathic topical preparations due to their complex composition and high sun protection factor or SPF value. Vitamins C and E and flavonoids herbs not only show antioxidant properties but also indicate a strong potential against adverse skin reactions ensuing UV exposure. The second chapter clarifies "Natural products and burns: A tough case to crack". Burns are a type of skin injury that occurs due to close contact with a heat source or corrosive chemicals. The use of natural products to treat burns dates back to ancient civilizations. In this chapter, naturally derived products from plants, animals and fungal sources are discussed. The extraction and preparation methods, burn healing mechanisms, clinical studies, and pharmaceutical formulation are covered. The third chapter discusses "Wound healing". Wound healing is quite a complicated process in the human body, consisting of the action of constricting injured blood vessels, activating the immune system, angiogenesis, remodeling, *etc*. Under intensive mechanical stress, a fibrotic scar, which is unfavorable with respect to the beauty of the skin, can be formed to patch the wound. Moreover, chronic wounds due to the disruption in wound healing is another clinical problem for patients with diabetes or vascular diseases. Of note is that natural remedies, especially natural products, are demonstrated to be able to elicit certain positive effects on many aspects of wound healing. The fourth chapter discusses "The role of natural products in the management of pigmentary anomalies". The skin is one of the most important organs of the human body. Dermatological ailments and pathologies are of importance for public health because, since to represent physical damages, they manifest emotional and psychological repercussions, which sometimes present higher costs than the former. Some of the most important pathologies are eczema, psoriasis, acne, rosacea, vitiligo, pyoderma, scabies, tinea capitis, dermatitis, reactions of poisonous insect or reptile bites hives, pigmentary anomalies, and injuries such as burns and scars. These skin and subcutaneous disorders were the 4th leading cause of nonfatal disease burden worldwide in 2010 and 2013, emphasizing the role of dermatology in the ever-expanding field of global health. The fifth chapter deals with "Treatment of scabies with herbal medicines". Scabies has been acknowledged as a neglected tropical disease by the world health organization. Scabies is the most stereotypically occurring skin disease in developing countries, greatly contributing to mortality and morbidity worldwide. More than 0.3 billion of the global population is getting affected with a high prevalence rate in tropical countries that have poor resources. Skin is the largest organ of the body which acts as the instinctive fencing between external and internal conditions playing a significant role in some crucial biological processes like protecting from chemical and mechanical injuries. Scabies also cause a wide range of skin ailments such as abscesses, impetigo, and cellulitis, consequently leading to critical abnormal conditions like rheumatic heart disease, septicemia, and kidney disease. The sixth chapter summarizes "Back to the Roots: Natural cosmetics and their future applications". Numerous concerns have been raised on the side effects of the prolonged usage of synthetic compounds in cosmetics production, including skin damage due to inflammations, rashes, and itching, just to mention a few. These skin side effects have been reported to be linked to the breakdown of homeostasis of the repair system against deoxyribonucleic acid (DNA) and tissue destruction and these can lead to accelerated aging, melanogenesis, cell senescence or even cancer of the skin. Efforts to overcome these problems associated with synthetic cosmetics have led to the use of natural cosmetics of plant and animal origin. The seventh chapter discusses "Natural products and nanoparticle skin delivery". The use of synthetic products is usually associated with side effects, while natural products are also not completely without demerits, including poor solubility and/or stability. The application of nanoparticles is cutting across all human endeavors, with product development not being an exception. Skin disease treatment is one aspect of medicine that is as distinct as it usually involves topical application, and eventual absorption onto the skin surface. The use of nanoparticles has proven to be an effective way to solve the problems associated with the use of natural products in skin care and treatment. The eighth chapter deals with "Smart drug delivery systems for the topical administration of natural products". The effectiveness of natural products in the treatment and prevention of human diseases has been widely demonstrated by the world scientific community. The skin is often subject to the onset of pathologies induced by chemical or physical insults, such as the collateral effects of certain drugs, tumors, or photo-induced damage. The current treatments of skin diseases are focused, in most cases, on the systemic or oral administration of the drugs, since the classic topical administration does not allow it to reach the pharmacological objectives.

We covered in this book a wide array of skin disorders and how to treat them using medicinal plants. We included researchers from different countries to discuss their experience in using medicinal plants for the treatment of skin disorders. This book will guide researchers all over the world to understand the value of medicinal plants in treating skin disorders and how to move forward in their research.

ACKNOWLEDGEMENTS

The authors would like to express their deep appreciation for the professional assistance of the assistant editors and the publishing house. We are also grateful to our families for their continuous support and help. We are thankful to our colleagues for their insightful comments on how to improve the content of the book.

Heba Abd El-Sattar El-Nashar
Department of Pharmacognosy
Faculty of Pharmacy
Ain Shams University
Cairo
Egypt

Mohamed El-Shazly
Department of Pharmacognosy
Faculty of Pharmacy
Ain Shams University
Cairo
Egypt

&

Nouran Mohammed Fahmy
Department of Pharmacognosy
Faculty of Pharmacy
Ain Shams University
Cairo
Egypt

Dedication

To

THE SOUL OF MY FATHER,

Who taught me to trust in ALLAH,

encouraged me to believe in myself

MY MOTHER,

A strong woman whose loving spirit always sustains me.

&

MY HUSBAND AND MY LITTLE ANGLE LAYLA

A constant source of love, concern, support, strength, never-ending motivation, and patience.

List of Contributors

Abimbola Koforowola Onasanya	Forestry Research Institute of Nigeria (FRIN), Jericho, PMB 5054, Ibadan, Nigeria
Adegboyega Ayo Ogunbela	Forestry Research Institute of Nigeria (FRIN), Jericho, PMB 5054, Ibadan, Nigeria
Adeola Ahmed Ibikunle	Department of Chemical Sciences, Olabisi Onabanjo University, Ago-Iwoye, Nigeria
Ali Raza Ishaq	State Key Laboratory of Biocatalysis and Enzyme Engineering, Environmental Microbial Technology Centre of Hubei Province, College of Life Sciences, Hubei University, Wuhan, China
Amita Pandey	Herbal Bioactive Research Lab Faculty of Pharmacy, Integral University, Dasauli, Kursi Road, Lucknow, Uttar Pradesh, 226 026, India
Dongbo Cai	State Key Laboratory of Biocatalysis and, Enzyme Engineering, Environmental Microbial Technology Centre of Hubei Province, College of Life Sciences, Hubei University, Wuhan, China
Erick Paul Gutiérrez Grijalva	Catedras Conacyt-Centro de Investigación en Alimentación y Desarrollo, A.C., Culiacán, Sinaloa, México
Gang Chen	School of Traditional Chinese Materia Medica, Shenyang Pharmaceutical University, Shenyang, China
Jingsong Yan	School of Traditional Chinese Materia Medica, Shenyang Pharmaceutical University, Shenyang, China
José Basilio Heredia	Catedras Conacyt-Centro de Investigación en Alimentación y Desarrollo, A.C., Culiacán, Sinaloa, México
Kingsley Igenepo John	Lab of Department of Pure and Applied Chemistry, College of Natural Sciences, Veritas University, Abuja, PMB 5171, Abuja, Nigeria
Luis Alfonso Jiménez Ortega	Centro de Investigación en Alimentación y Desarrollo, A.C., Culiacán, Sinaloa, México
Maliha Fatima	Department of Botany, College of Life Sciences, Hubei University, Wuhan, China
Manuel Adrián Picos Salas	Centro de Investigación en Alimentación y Desarrollo, A.C., Culiacán, Sinaloa, México
May Abu Taha	Faculty of Pharmacy, Applied Science Private University, Amman, Jordan
Muhammad Asad Mangat	Department of Zoology, Government College University, Faisalabad, Pakistan
Muna Barakat	Faculty of Pharmacy, Applied Science Private University, Amman, Jordan
Muyideen Olaitan Bamidele	Department of Chemistry, Faculty of Natural and Applied Sciences, Lead City University, Ibadan, Nigeria
Nadeem Rais	Department of Pharmacy, Bhagwant University, Ajmer, Rajasthan, 305 004, India
Ning Li	School of Traditional Chinese Materia Medica, Shenyang Pharmaceutical University, Shenyang, China

Nurudeen Olanrewaju Sanyaolu	Department of Chemical Sciences, Olabisi Onabanjo University, Ago-Iwoye, Nigeria
Olayinka Oderinde	Department of Chemistry, Faculty of Natural and Applied Sciences, Lead City University, Ibadan, Nigeria
Om Prakash	Goel Institute of Pharmacy and Sciences, Ayodhya (Faizabad) Road, Lucknow, Uttar Pradesh, 226 028, India
Onome Ejeromedoghene	School of Chemistry and Chemical Engineering, Southeast University, Jiulonghu Campus, Nanjing 211189, PR China
Priyanka Bajpai	Goel Institute of Pharmacy and Sciences, Ayodhya (Faizabad) Road, Lucknow, Uttar Pradesh, 226 028, India
Rajesh Kumar	Narayan Institute of Pharmacy, Gopal Narayan Singh University, Jamuhar,Sasaram, Bihar, 821 305, India
Rana Abutaima	Faculty of Pharmacy, Zarqa University, Jordan
Ruchi Singh	Goel Institute of Pharmaceutical and Sciences, Ayodhya (Faizabad) Road, Lucknow, Uttar Pradesh, 226 028, India
Safa Daoud	Faculty of Pharmacy, Applied Science Private University, Amman, Jordan
Samar Thiab	Faculty of Pharmacy, Applied Science Private University, Amman, Jordan
Shazia Usmani	Herbal Bioactive Research Lab Faculty of Pharmacy, Integral University, Dasauli, Kursi Road, Lucknow, Uttar Pradesh, 226 026, India
Tahira Akbar	Department of Zoology, Government College University, Faisalabad, Pakistan
Tahira Younis	Department of Zoology, Government College University, Faisalabad, Pakistan
Xue Li	School of Traditional Chinese Materia Medica, Shenyang Pharmaceutical University, Shenyang, China

CHAPTER 1

How to Protect Your Skin from Harmful Radiation

Ali Raza Ishaq[1,*], Tahira Younis[2], Tahira Akbar[2], Muhammad Asad Mangat[2], Maliha Fatima[3] and Dongbo Cai[1]

[1] *State Key Laboratory of Biocatalysis and Enzyme Engineering, Environmental Microbial Technology Center of Hubei Province, College of Life Sciences, Hubei University, 368 Youyi Avenue, Wuhan 430062, Hubei, People's Republic of China*

[2] *Department of Zoology, Government College University Faisalabad, Pakistan*

[3] *Department of Botany, College of Life Sciences, Hubei University, Wuhan, China*

Abstract: Our interaction with the sun is still equivocal, to say the least. We like its soothing influence on the body and soul, but we are afraid of its highly hazardous heating ability and the long-term skin damage that can emerge from chronic sun exposure. Scientists are consistently seeking to enhance sunblock products in accordance with a need for better skin protection from the sun. Once human skin is exposed to solar ultraviolet radiation (UVR), the synthesis of reactive oxygen species (ROS) skyrockets. The influx of ROS leads to oxidative stress by mutating the natural equilibrium toward a pro-oxidative state. Alteration in proteins and lipids, stimulation of inflammation, immunodeficiency, DNA damage, and activation of signaling pathways that influence gene transcription, cell cycle, proliferation, and apoptosis are all illustrations of the detrimental effects of oxidative stress. This chapter provides new insight into several Phyto-products having an antioxidant activity to suppress the UV rays impact, the relationship between UVR-aging, current understanding of the regulation of constitutive human skin pigmentation and responses to UV radiation, with emphasis on physiological factors that influence those processes.

Keywords: UV rays, Skin, pigmentation, Microbial Products, Plant Extracts, Aging.

INTRODUCTION

The skin is the body's largest organ and works as the body primary line of protection against external problems, such as UV rays, toxic compounds, traumas, oxidative stress, and pathogens [1]. Keratinocytes are the epidermis main cellular component, but it also comprises melanocytes, Merkel cells, gamma delta T-lym-

---

* **Corresponding author Ali Raza Ishaq:** State Key Laboratory of Biocatalysis and Enzyme Engineering, Environmental Microbial Technology Center of Hubei Province, College of Life Sciences, Hubei University, 368 Youyi Avenue, Wuhan 430062, Hubei, People's Republic of China; E-mail: 202123107010001@stu.hubu.edu.cn

Heba Abd El-Sattar El-Nashar, Mohamed El-Shazly & Nouran Mohammed Fahmy (Eds.)

phocytes, and Langerhans cells. Keratinocytes in the epidermis's basal layer retain their potential to proliferate, establishing the spinous and granular layers. Keratinocytes terminally differentiate into corneocytes, leaving the granular layer. Corneocytes (compact keratinocytes without nuclei) and the intercellular lamellar compartment (lipids) contribute to the construction and function of the stratum corneum in the epidermis's outer layer (SC) [2]. Ultraviolet (UV) radiation is regarded as a complete carcinogen and one of the most prevalent oncogenic exposures for humans. Several physiological changes occur after exposure of skin to UV rays, like skin pigmentation, upregulation of free radicals, skin cancer, and skin aging [3]. Natural ingredients are endless sources of antioxidants that have been used as alternative remedies by people since the beginning of humanity [4].

The international cosmetics market is expected to reach $429.8 billion in profits by 2022, with a compound annual rate of 4.3% to 2022. (Research and Markets). America, Europe, and Asia–Pacific are the three largest worldwide cosmetics sectors. India is an emerging marketplace for a diversity of cosmetic products in Asia–Pacific, and it has developed swiftly in recent years. Due to globalization and industrialization, solar radiations affect skin tones, that's why the main target of the population is to preserve the skin nature from damage *via* the application of cosmetics. Cosmetics are the chemical derived from natural sources (microbial as well as Phyto-products) that can regain the nature of skin by targeting various metabolic pathways like inhibiting ROS formation, modulating the expression of oxidative stress-responsive enzymes such as heme oxygenase-1 (HO-1), activating the Nrf2/HO-1 antioxidant pathway, upregulating antioxidative enzymes superoxide dismutase 2 (SOD2), catalase (CAT) and glutathione peroxidase 1 (GPX1), boosting of xanthine oxidase (XO), reducing nicotinamide adenine dinucleotide phosphate (NADPH) oxidase (Nox), inhibiting interleukin-1β (IL-1β), interleukin-6 (IL-6) and tumor necrosis factor-α (TNF-α), nuclear factor-kappa B (NF-κB), stimulating the DNA Repair process and promoting immune response [5].

This chapter provides new insights into the molecular defense mechanism of skin against UV rays, types of UV rays, UV rays as a biological evolution in the skin, types of natural products used in skin photoprotection, and the relationship between skin pigmentation *vs.* UV rays.

DETRIMENTAL EFFECT OF UV RAYS ON HUMAN SKIN

Ultraviolet rays, a type of electromagnetic radiation, contain high-energy packet photons, coming from different sources, including sunlight, sunlamps, and sunbeds, into an atmosphere that a living community utilizes for survival. When ultraviolet (UV) radiation engages with the human body, it has multiple health benefits, including the synthesis of vitamin D3 and the potential for UV photons to be employed in treatments for skin ailments [6]. The electromagnetic spectrum of UV light coming from the sun has three characteristic regions, each specifies by a distinct wavelength range, as shown in Table **1**. UVC radiation is the shorter wavelength area of the UV spectrum, UVB is the medium wavelength zone, and UVA is further divided into UVA1 and UV2, having lower frequency waves. The ozone layer in the stratosphere serves as a buffer against destructive radiation. Due to the ozone layer's high transparency, only a small quantity of UVB radiation affects the earth's biosphere. Human activities on either side have eroded the ozone layer, enabling a considerable portion of UVB radiation to reach the stratosphere [7].

Table 1. Classification and spectrum of Ultraviolet radiation.

Categories	Wavelength (nm)	Nature of Wavelength	Absorption by the Ozone Layer	References
UVA1	315-340nm	Longer wavelength	0%	[8]
UVA2	340-400nm	-	0%	[7]
UVB	280-315nm	Medium wavelength	95%	[9]
UVC	200-280nm	Shorter wavelength	100%	

UV radiation can cause disorders such as skin cancer, eye cancer, immunosuppression, immunotoxicity and genotoxicity [10]. There is a positive correlation between the penetration depth and the damage intensity. UV radiation mainly causes damage to human skin because, in skin layers, many biomolecules are absorbed in the UV range, and UV rays have a limit on transmission. It is shown in Table **2** that muscles, bones and internal organs are least to be affected by UV radiation, as these are lying at a distance greater than the penetration range of UVR. Human skin is a remarkable physical barrier and plays an important role in protection, providing a large absorbing surface area for UV exposure. Due to the shorter wavelength and high frequency, UVA gets penetrated deep into the dermis and epidermis, which induces tanning effects by darkening the melanin functional components of human skin [9]. UVA also significantly participates in the premature photoaging of the skin cells by destroying the biological structure in the corium.

UV-Induced Damaging Mechanisms

During transmission of light rays through skin layers, two specific types of cellular molecules, namely photosensitizers and, chromophores, absorb UV electromagnetic radiation, which exerts numerous biological effects like unstable the concentration of reactive oxygen species. The absorption of UV light by these molecular species sows the seeds of many chemical reactions, which result in divergent upshots of redox reactants. These chemical reactions of different natures are kept to two types of fundamental mechanisms. One mechanism follows the direct absorption of UV energy by cellular chromophores that brings about UV photo-induced reactions. Human skin has many chromophoric biomolecules that absorb within the UVB wavelength range and passes through various de-excitation processes. Some of them are aromatic amino acids, quinones, NADH, NADPH, porphyrins, 7-dehydrocholesterol, nucleic acids, flavins, carotenoids, urocanic acid (UCA), and eumelanin [11 - 13]. Except for *trans*-UCA and melanin, other UVA-absorbing cellular chromophores are not reported in the literature yet [11].

Table 2. Penetration power of ultraviolet radiation into human organs.

Organs	Penetration Capability of UV	UV-Radiation Effects	Reference
Skin	Highly permeable	Highly affected	[10]
Eyes	Considerably permeable	Moderately affected	
Muscles	Less permeable	Less affected	
Bones	Lightly permeable	Least affected	
Internal organs	Impermeable	Not affected	

Proteins are structurally built-up of histidine, tyrosine, phenylalanine, cysteine, and tryptophan chromophoric amino acids that absorb UV light. By transit across a photo-oxidation reaction, the excited amino acids produce a cluster of radicals [14]. Urocanic acid (UCA) is a histidine derivative UV absorbing chromophore, and its commonly known whereabouts are the stratum corneum of human skin. On exposure to UV-B rays, UCA undergoes the isomerization process, because of which *trans*-urocanic acid isomeric form is configured into *cis* isomer. The conversion reaction stops when the aqueous solution attains an equilibrium ratio of 1:1 [15]. Urocanic acid in *trans*-configuration is a weak endogenic UV protector, while its *cis* isomer causes immunosuppression, like decreased level of pro-inflammatory response [16]. In direct mechanism, all chromophoric structures directly absorb UV rays and obey the basic excitation or de-excitation principle. According to this, chromophores absorb energy packets in the form of UV photons and show subsequent changes in electronic configuration.

By absorbing the wavelength of required energy, electrons from the ground state jump to the single high-energy state, and thus, electronic configuration gets disturbed, which ultimately destabilizes the molecules. The excited molecular system needs to stabilize, and to do so, the electrons in the single excited state need to come back to their initial state of low energy. To attain the original configuration, photo-excited molecules undergo vibrational relaxations and internal conversion (non-radiative transitions) and release energy in the form of heat which is transferred to the neighboring molecules. On the other hand, relaxation of some photoexcitation is accomplished by intersystem crossing and by exhibiting fluorescence. Similarly, a long-lived state is also generated, called the triplet excited state, which may elicit photochemical reactions, photo products, and phosphorescence by the molecules while returning to their ground state [17].

The indirect mechanism is related to the activation of endogenous and exogenous sensitizers of the skin, which leads to a group of photosensitization reactions [6]. Based on the chemical characteristics of photosensitizers, the indirect photo-damaging mechanism is subdivided into two major pathways, Type I and Type II. In the Type I mechanism, excited photosensitizers make direct interaction with the other biomolecules *via* the transfer of one electron, as shown in Fig. (**1**). As a result of direct interaction, many free radicals are formed. The specificity of this reaction lies in the fact that this pathway damages the cellular components with no involvement of oxygen elements. Conversely, molecular oxygen is the primary agent in the Type II pathway. The molecular oxygen gets energy from the excited sensitizers and becomes active. The activated oxygen molecules then initiate a massive production of reactive oxygen species (ROS). Usually, after getting energy from the photosensitizers, molecular oxygen transforms into a singlet excited state, which is a long-lived species; due to its long lifetime, oxygen in this high-energy state acts as a powerful oxidant.

Seldom, in some of the reactions, superoxide anions are formed, which leads to the formation of Hydrogen peroxide. Although, hydrogen peroxide itself has no potential to cause any damage, in the presence of transition metal cations (Fe, Cu), hydrogen peroxide undergoes the Fenton reaction. The simple description of the Fenton reaction is that it is a reaction between two species, one is ferrous ions, and the other is hydrogen peroxide. The resultant products of this reaction include hydroxyl radical, hydroxyl ion, and ferric ion [19].

Fenton reaction is one of the advanced oxidation processes (AOPs), which involves mainly the generation of. OH, radicals. Fenton's reagent is called a good oxidation agent and has a high oxidation potential (E^0=2.8V). The reason behind its superiority is the capacity of this radical to oxidize a wide range of organic compounds. The basic principle behind the catalytic process of the Fenton reaction is the transformation of electrons between the peroxides and metals. The success of this system lies in the fact that there is a continuous supply of Fe^{+2} in the acidic aqueous medium [20].

1. $Fe^+ + H_2O_2 + H^+ \rightarrow Fe^{3+} + \;^\cdot OH + H_2O$ $(k_1 = 58\; mol^{-1}dm^3s^{-1})$

2. $Fe^{+3} + H_2O_2 \rightarrow Fe^{2+} + \;^\cdot OOH + H^+$ $(k_2 = 0.02\; mol^{-1}dm^3s^{-1})$

whereas, the hydroxyl radical is called superoxide radical. The capacity of the hydroxyl radical to degrade organic matter heavily depends on its concentration [21]. There are some factors on which these reactions depend, namely the distributive pattern of the chromophores, photo susceptivity of the skin cells and tissue, and thickness of epidermal skin layers.

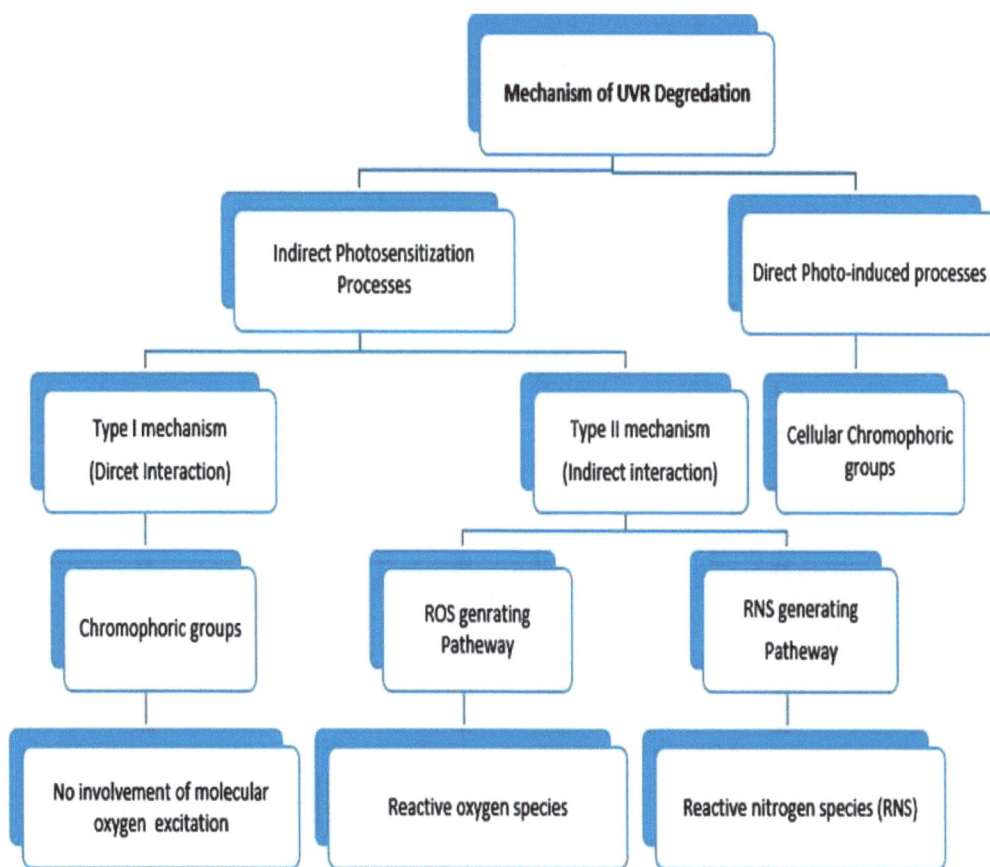

Fig. (1). Classification of UVR-induced degradation mechanism [17, 18].

Different Effects of UV-Irradiation on Human Skin

On exposure to UV radiation, a set of complex biochemical reactions come into existence. Apart from inflammation, photodamage also involves in the production of ROS. In general, these two said processes consolidate to produce destructive effects [22]. The possible damage that ensues from ROS and the inflammation process is oxidative cleavage of cellular biopolymers, such as carbohydrates and proteins. Similarly, lipids and other cellular components are also getting the baneful influence from these residual processes. The damaged cellular components tend to accumulate in dermal and epidermal parts and participate in photoaging. Further, intermittent exposure to UV radiation puts a stop to antioxidant enzyme systems by exhausting the cellular antioxidants, hence damaging DNA. On accumulation, thymidine dimers institute a large number of proinflammatory mediators by activating the neuroendocrine system [23]. The following paragraphs thoroughly describe all the possible damages caused by UV rays on human skin.

UV-Induced Damage to Macromolecules of the Skin

Many macromolecules of skin get damaged by UV light. The damaging pathways, either direct Photo-induced or Indirect Photosensitization, depend on the nature of the macromolecules. For example, DNA molecules can be mutilated by both the damaging mechanisms, while lipids and polysaccharides cannot be affected by direct Photo-induced pathways because these macromolecules do not absorb in the UV region. Therefore, oxidative processes are the only cause of their destruction. Among all the other environmental agents, UV radiation plays a prominent role in damaging the DNA of the skin. Consequently, many reactions of various natures get initiated in the skin having long-term consequences; modified nucleic acids cause several biological reactions of critical nature in the skin. In the most peripheral proteinaceous layer of skin, called stratum corneum, UVB-absorbing aromatic amino acids are present due to which the maximum intensity of UVB rays is absorbed by this layer, and a very small fraction of radiation leaves behind for the nucleic acid of the viable cells, which also absorb in the UVB rang [8]. Ultraviolet radiation causes damage to DNA in many ways. The resultant effect depends on the nature of the UV light exposure and follows the mechanism. UVB and UVA show a different damaging effects on DNA even by following the same damaging mechanism.

DNA Damage Induced by Direct Mechanism

It was experimentally ascertained that acute UVB radiation damages DNA in a direct degradation mechanism and produces several dimeric photoproducts which are formed between the pyrimidine bases adjoining the same strand. These dimeric photoproducts exist in two basic forms: [6, 4] pyrimidine pyrimidone dimer and cyclobutyl pyrimidine dimer (CPD). One basic [6, 4] Pyrimidine pyrimidone dimer is a covalently bonded photoproduct where the covalent bond locates between carbon atoms at positions C6 and C4 of two pyrimidines next to each other. Furthermore, isomerization of [6, 4]-PP into Dewar valence isomer occurs on the absorption of UVA/B radiation (Fig. **2**). The reverse conversion of the Dewar valence isomer to [6, 4]-PP is possible by the absorption of the photons of a shorter wavelength. While the covalent bonding between the carbon atoms at C5 and C6 results in the formation of CPDs photoproduct [24, 25]. Cytosine-cytosine (CC) and thymine-cytosine (TC), CPD dimers, have a high potential for mutagenicity. UV-induced cancerous cells usually have a mutated p53 gene, which is mainly caused by a mutation in thymine-cytosine and cytosine-cytosine thymidine dimers [26].

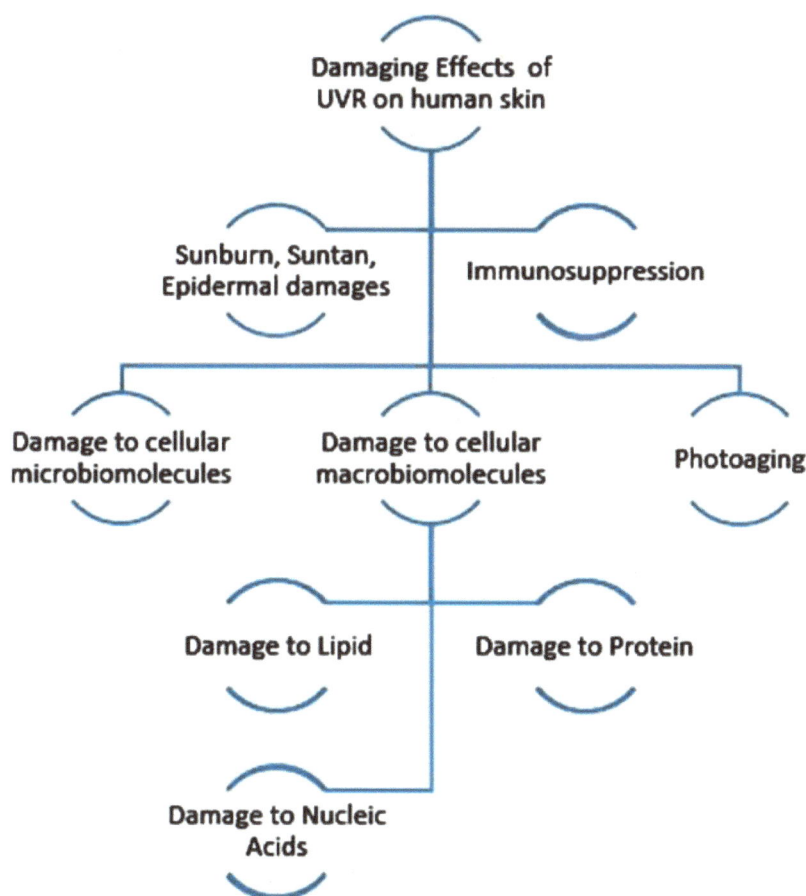

Fig. (2). Different deleterious effects of ultraviolet exposure on human skin.

Acute UVA radiation also supports the formation of pyrimidine dimers, as does UVB, but it requires more energetic waves at 365nm. It was experimentally investigated by Mouret *et al.*, that UVA triggers the formation of thymine dimers in the cells of humane skin [27]. It was also mentioned in those studies that thymine dimers are more highly yielded than that 8-OXO-deoxyguanosine (8 OXO-Dg), which causes oxidative damage. Acute UVA commences an indirect photoactivation mechanism that activates the endogenous photosensitizers, *e.g.*, riboflavin. Porphyrins are quinones, which act as reactive oxygen species (ROS). Many studies also authenticated the damaging of cultured cells and skin biopsy specimens, and the breakage of DNA on the exposure to acute UVA irradiation [28, 29]. Reactive oxygen species (ROS) are pyrimidines and purine modifiers, for example, 8 OXO-Dg, which is an oxidative product of guanine moiety [30, 31].

The long-term damaging effects due to chronic UV exposure, are associated with those photoproducts which are not efficiently repairable. For example, in mammals, photoproducts of CPDs nature are irreparable, as compared to [6, 4] pyrimidinone, and thus make a major contribution to mutations. Any failure in repairing these DNA lesions can root the mutagenic changes in the epidermal cells, and, as a result, permit the formation of cancerous cells. The mutated gene replicates, and the mutation gets transferred further. Pyrimidine's dimerization engenders structural deformations in DNA, which directly or indirectly induces cell signaling pathways, in addition, results in mutagenicity and cytotoxicity. Moreover, pyrimidine dimers question cell survival by shutting off DNA replication and cell division. It also interferes with the synthesis of messenger RNA, which is obligatory to produce cellular proteins.

It was mechanistically determined in one of the recent studies that mutation induced by both UVB and UVA radiation is the same. Differences are due to the degree of cellular responses to both types of UV rays. For instance, p53 is weakly activated by UVA irradiation and strongly activated by UVB exposure, which leads to the formation of different dimers. The author also mentioned that in comparison to strong activation by UVB, the weakly activated p53 has more probability of causing mutation. The grounds behind such inclusive mutation are weaker cell cycle arrest, less p53-mediated induction of the DNA repair system, and apoptosis. In consequence, the impaired template passes through the replication process, the damaged DNA molecule, and the sustainability of mutation stimulates the formation of skin cancer. According to this hypothesis, due to the absence of considerably protective DNA responses against dimers that are formed on UVA exposure are more mutagenic in order.

DNA Damage Induced by Indirect Mechanism

UV radiation, when it falls on tissues of the skin, vitalizes two types of radicals and unstable species-producing mechanisms. One is the reactive oxygen species (ROS) generating system, this system consists of active precursors like $^1O_2$, hydrogen peroxide and ozone. These precursors generate active metabolites, such as hydroxide radicals, superoxide and peroxide radicals. Another one is a reactive nitrogen species (RNS) generating system that involve the generation of nitric dioxide and nitric oxide (NO). ROS are highly unstable productive species that form naturally in cellular metabolism. Fibroblasts and keratinocytes in the skin are the ROS-yielding sites; these sites have antioxidants such as nonenzymic (glutathione (GSH)), tocopherol, ubiquinol, ascorbic acid and enzymic (superoxide dismutase (SOD), glutathione peroxidase (GPx), catalase (CAT), glutathione reductase) and thioredoxin reductase. These antioxidants operate to swab away the harmful species and give rise to a balance between the pro-oxidant and antioxidant concentrations and bring forth stability to cells and tissues [32, 33].

The overflow of ROS develops from UV exposures and produces oxidative stress in the skin. Oxidative stress is a condition in which disequilibrium occurs in pro-oxidant/AOx concentration due to the overwhelming performance of the antioxidant (AOX) defense mechanisms [34]. Oxidative stress is greatly impacted by UVA exposure than UVB. UVA light induces ROS/ RNS, which crosses the threshold that is necessary for maintaining equilibrium and damaging DNA, lipids, and protein. Skin cells facing oxidative stress become energy depleted as NADH is also under the influence of a damaging process [35].

Alteration of Mitochondrial DNA

UV-induced oxidative stress alters both nuclear and mitochondrial DNA content but at different rates. The possible alteration is negatively correlated with the efficiency of the DNA repair system. An efficient DNA repairing process would suppress the degree of alteration. In mitochondria, the DNA repairing process is not that much efficient as in nuclei. As a result of this, mutation accumulates at a rapid rate; therefore, the cell capacity of oxidative phosphorylation is altered [36].

ROS/RNS systems cause oxidation of the DNA lesions and fuel the initiation of carcinogenesis [37]. DNA lesions are more susceptible to UVB radiation, as it stimulates tumorigenic, lethal, and mutagenic responses. These highly unstable and reactive species not only break the DNA into single strands, but also activate the cross-linking of DNA proteins, and make structural changes in the DNA bases. Type I and Type II mechanisms strongly affect guanine bases because these bases have low ionization energy and become unionized easily. Radical cations are the primary intermediates of Type I reaction; these cations get solvated by the water molecules due to electrostatic interactions or undergo deprotonation. A radical intermediate that acts as a reducing agent is formed because of the hydration of the guanine radical cation. This radical acts differently under different conditions of the reaction. In the presence of molecular oxygen, the guanine radical cation converts to 8-oxo7,8-dihydro-2-deoxyguanine (8-oxo-dG). The same radical produces 2,6-diamino-4-hydroxy-5-formamidoguanine under reducing conditions.

Imidazole ring and singlet oxygen undergo cycloaddition reaction and the products of these reactions are endoperoxides. The 8-oxo-dG is a mutagenic lesion and is a decomposition product of endoperoxides [1] UVA rays, more specifically, produce 8-oxo-dG lesions and play a minor role in the DNA breakage and crosslinking of DNA-protein. 8-oxo-dG pairs up with adenine and generates GC → TA transversion during replication, while it does not pair up with cytosine [37].

RNA is important to produce functional proteins. RNA is also damaged by UV radiation in direct or indirect ways. The direct damaging results in the structural changes of the genes, which cause the failure of the production of functional proteins Indirect damaging roots from the formation of the DNA photoproducts initiates apoptosis of cancerous keratinocytes [11].

ROS-Induced Damage to Proteins

UV radiation marks its deleterious effect on human skin in many ways; one is extensively elaborated on in the previous paragraphs. The following paraphrase will illustrate the possible damage to the proteins and expression of enzymes. In skin tissues, carbonyl derivatives are formed by the modification of proteins by ROS. Here, is the explanation of the influence that UV irradiation cause on the expression of different enzymes, which play important structural and catalytic functions in a cell.

Many signaling molecules, including mitogen-activated protein kinases (MAPKs), NF-Kb, activator protein-1 (AP-1), and interrelated inflammatory cytokines, encounter changes in gene expression under the influence of URA/UVB irradiation. These signaling molecules engage in the induction of matrix metalloproteinases (MMPs) and heme oxygenase-1 (HO-1) in the skin. Iron will be available in high concentration in a cell by increasing the concentration of heme oxygenase-1 (HO-1), because of which the Fenton reaction will start. The following mechanism of complex aromatic degradation supports the fact that more ROS will be generated in the presence of free iron in the cellular matrix, resulting in more damage. Degradation mechanism of the aromatic compounds:

The Fenton degradation process has been under consideration for the last decades. This process was equally applied to the degradation of the aromatic and heterocyclic rings as well. The following mechanism is generally proposed for degradation. The radical adds to the aromatic ring or heterocyclic rings. This radical can initiate radical chain oxidation by abstracting a hydrogen atom from the compound [38]. The following reaction mechanism shows that produced organic radical in the first step will be oxidized by the ferric ions and then reduced by the ferrous ion, as shown.

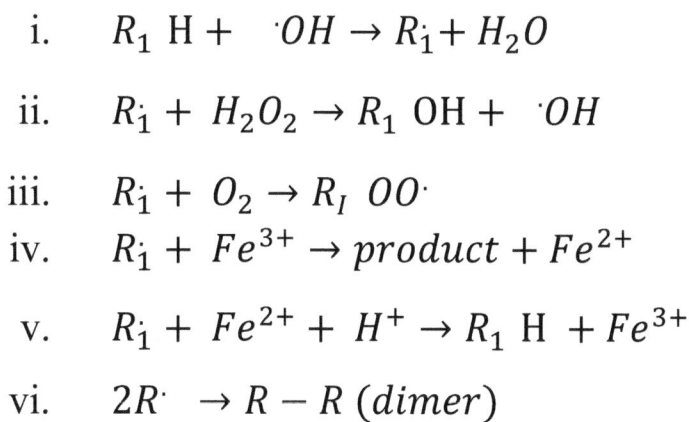

i. $\quad R_1 H + \ \cdot OH \rightarrow R_1^{\cdot} + H_2O$

ii. $\quad R_1^{\cdot} + H_2O_2 \rightarrow R_1\ OH + \ \cdot OH$

iii. $\quad R_1^{\cdot} + O_2 \rightarrow R_I\ OO\cdot$

iv. $\quad R_1^{\cdot} + Fe^{3+} \rightarrow product + Fe^{2+}$

v. $\quad R_1^{\cdot} + Fe^{2+} + H^+ \rightarrow R_1\ H + Fe^{3+}$

vi. $\quad 2R\cdot \ \rightarrow R - R\ (dimer)$

The turning production of endopeptidases from their normal production pathways will be initiated by UV irradiation. This unusual production will become the reason for wrinkle formation because endopeptidases start degrading the extracellular matrix proteins. Cyclooxygenases (COX) enzymes are important for many functions in cells. The major function is the catalytic formation of lipid signaling mediators PGs from AA. These mediators are important in many inflammatory and normal processes [39]. Among all the other COX enzymes, COX-1 is expressed in all the cells, while its inducible form is COX-2. Both UVA and UVB irradiation stimulates the formation of an inducible form of COX-1 enzyme [40]. Phospholipases' continuous release of AA, and high concentration of COX-2 meld together to increase the level of PGs in skin cells. COX-2 unusual expression generates PGE_2, which is a distinguishable agent, assists the proliferation of damaged skin cells and eventually forms tumors in the human skin, skin cancers, pre-malignant skin lesions formation, force out skin cancer cell lines, and cause immunosuppression by interacting with IL-4 and IL-10 (cytokine).

Heme Oxygenase (HO): These enzymes catalyzed the redox reaction, which degraded the heme. These enzymes exist in two isoforms one is constructive HO-2, and the other is inducible HO-1 form. The expression of these enzymes can be mediated by UVA and other factors like the presence of hydrogen peroxide molecules [41]. On mediation, HO-1 causes a reduction in the intracellular GSH levels and integration of the cytoplasmatic membrane [42]. Cells under UVA irradiations generate microsomal heme-containing proteins which produce free heme. The free heme directs transcriptional activation and repression of the HO-1 gene [43].

Ornithine decarboxylase (ODC) is an enzyme that regulates the cellular proliferation mechanism and promotes the formation of tumors. Chronic and acute UVB irradiation initiates several epidermal activities and protein expression of the Ornithine decarboxylase enzyme [44].

Cytochromes P45 (CYP) represents a sub-class of microsomal membrane-bound monooxygenases. These enzymes metabolically activate the endobiotic and xenobiotics. They also participate in those processes which run for the protection of the skin. Extrahepatic tissues show the high strength of CYP1A1 under exposure to UV rays. More specifically, UVB irradiation induces the gene expression of both CYP1A1 and CYP1B1 in human skin. The abnormal expression will enhance the activation tendency of organic pollutants, *i.e.,* polycyclic aromatic hydrocarbons. This will make the human skin susceptible to allergic reactions and UVB-induced skin cancers [45, 46].

UV-Induced Damage to Lipids

The cell membrane has a phospholipid structure which gets damaged by the peroxidation reaction of fatty acids with ROS. This reaction produces various products, many of which are oxidative, including lipid hydroperoxides, lipid peroxide radicals, and fragmented products [32]. Among all the other oxidizing products, lipid peroxides have a long life and cause oxidative damage on a large scale due to the initiation of oxidative damage [18]. UVA rays also induce active unstable species by launching the ROS system, which empowers the arachidonic acid (AA) formation. The acidic molecules make a worthwhile contribution in changing the membrane's characteristic features like altering the fluidity of the membrane. Further, UV-response genes are activated by turning on the functionality of nuclear messengers and secondary cytosolic [47].

Other Damaging Caused by UV Irradiation

It was observed that human skin, after exposure to sub-erythematic UVA dose for one month, showed many histological changes, including epidermal hyperplasia, dermal inflammatory infiltrates, deposition of high concentration of lysozymes on the elastic fibers, Langerhans cell depletion, and stratum corneum thickening [48]. It can be concluded from the above description that dermal collagen and elastin both get change even for casual radiation exposure, hence the use of UVB-absorbing sunscreen is not well appreciated in terms of protection from photoaging [49]. Moreover, Chronic exposure to UV radiation hurdles the going of apoptosis process or complete closure of p53 and the Fas-Fas ligand pathway. As a result of all these phenomenon breakthroughs, many changes will occur including DNA damage by abnormal proliferation of keratinocytes, reduction in the Fas-Fas ligand interactions, and accumulation of p53 mutations. The cell passing through all these damaging phases will face carcinogenesis. The following passages illustrates the other detrimental effect of UVR.

Skin inflammation is another harmful effect of UV radiation. In contrast to UVB rays, the wavelength of the UVA spectrum plays a key role in causing skin inflammation. However, cutaneous inflammatory response is developed by UVB substantial participation [47]. The inflammation process is a dangerous process in terms of the other events that it stirs up. These events cause damage to the unrecoverable nature. These include the inflammation of blood leukocytes, infiltration of macrophages and neutrophils, increase in the production of lipid peroxidation (LPx) by forming the prostaglandins (PGs) in large concentration, stimulate the generation of tumor necrosis factor-alpha (TNF-α), nuclear factor-κB (NFκB), and an increase oxidative stress by initiating the formation of ROS due to influential release of inflammatory cytokines (interleukins; IL-1α, IL-1β, IL6). Skin cancer is also developed by inflammation; inflammatory cells are power sources to produce ROS, which malignantly convert benign human solar keratosis into SCC. In this way, skin inflammation oxidative damages DNA.

The human immunity system gets suppressed on exposure to both UVA and UVB rays. The suppression of the immune system by UVA is more complicated, and its impact varies according to genetic makeup. According to recent studies, in low doses (below 840 mJ/cm^2), UVA boosts the memory of cell development; in medium doses, UVA causes the modulation of the immune system. UVA also does interference with the suppression effect induced by UVB; for example, in high dose, UVA shows protective capability for the immune system and prevent its suppression by the UVB.

PHYSIOLOGICAL RELATION BETWEEN UVR-AGING

Photoaging is a complicated biological process that damages skin layers, more specifically, the cognitive tissue of the dermis. It is caused by chronic exposure to sun radiation. The clinical symptoms that ensure the photoaging include anomalous pigmentation, wilting, patchy pigmentation, sagging, laxity, wrinkling, telangiectasia, dryness, and elastosis. Additionally, a massive accumulation of deranged elastic fibers occurs in the skin dermis, disorganization of collagen fibers, dilation of a blood vessel with sinuous structure, increased number of inflammatory cells in the skin dermal, reduce in the polarity of Keratinocytes, irregularity of Keratinocytes, fewer melanocytes, and a high number of abnormal Melanocytes are all symptom of post-sag. UVB photons are high-energy packets that, on absorption by the epidermis, cause photo carcinogenesis, sunburn, and suntanning [36]. The molecular changes in epithelial cells of the skin are shown in Fig. (**3**).

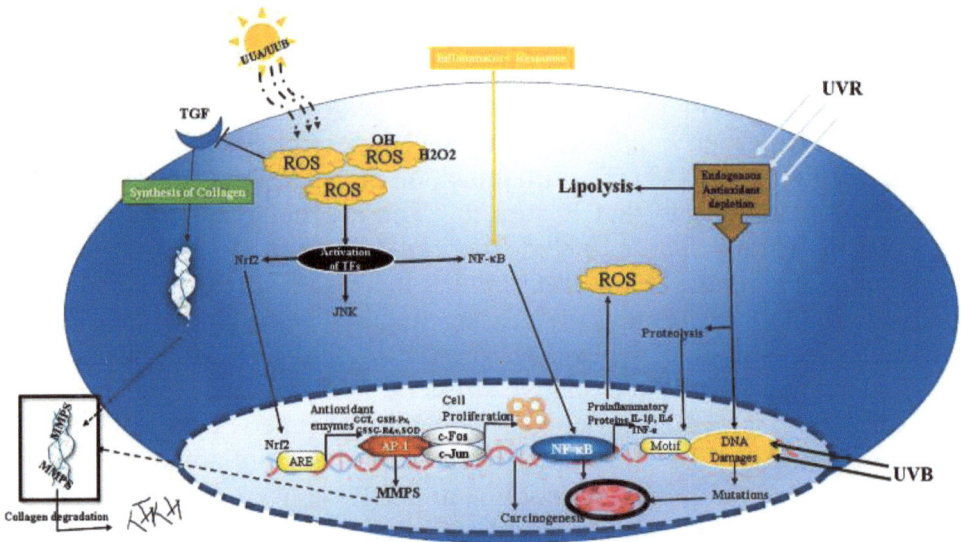

Fig. (3). Effect of UV rays on keratinocytes-a molecular mechanism.

UVA-induced matrix metalloproteinases (MMPs) are a class of zinc-dependent endopeptidases produced largely by some skin cells such as macrophages, fibroblasts, eosinophils, endothelial cells, mast cells, and keratinocytes. On the inhibition of the synthesis of procollagen, MMPs have great potential to degrade the framework of collagen in the skin. Collagen of type I gets cleave by MMP-1, and collagen type IV and VII, which are compounds of the basement membrane, are degraded by MMP-2, which also causes elastin degradation. MMP-3 is a substrate-specific endopeptidase and participates in the degradation of proteoglycans, laminin, fibronectin, and collagen type IV. UVR decreases the level of procollagen I proteins, activates NFκB, and activates matrix degradation by initiating neutrophil attraction which accumulates the neutrophil collagenase

(MMP-8) on the irradiation sites. Oxidative stress can influence the functioning of dermal fibroblasts by accumulating the elastin mRNA. This accumulation triggers a mechanism that results in the elastolysis changes in the dermis layer.

SKIN PIGMENTATION

For the maintenance of body's internal environment, the skin acts as a barrier that serves diverse functions by maintaining homeostasis and immunological protection from the harms of the external environment. The two major factors responsible for skin-related issues are modifiable factors, such as UV radiation and others are non-modifiable factors, like genetic. Though melanogenesis protects skin against damage induced by UV but excessive melanin production can cause hyperpigmentation as well as many other pigmentation disorders [50]. Melanin pigmentation is a critical phenomenon for the protection of skin from the damage of sunlight, *i.e.*, UV radiation [51]. Pigmentation leads to human skin aging. Melanin formation in melanocytes, transfer of melanosomes to keratinocytes and degradation of melanosomes mainly determines skin pigmentation. Melanosomes are restricted to melanin production because they contain tyrosinase which is a major regulatory enzyme for melanogenesis & TRPs (tyrosine-related proteins). TRPs are involved in the early steps of dopaquinone synthesis, which causes two types of melanin's. These are eumelanin (brown, black) and pheomelanin (yellow, red). Amongst them, pheomelanin is phototoxic and promotes UV damage and photoaging [52].

Oxidative stress could also be a reason for skin pigmentation abnormality. Melanin production is induced by sunlight which in turn protects skin from damaging UV radiation, as shown in Fig. (**4**). Substantially oxidative stress play's role in the production of melanogenesis (UV induced) and directs the association between UV-induced skin pigmentation and oxidative stress by antioxidant therapy [53, 54]. Sunlight has the capacity to produce free radicals and energy, which causes these stresses [55].

Solar radiation found on our planet consist of an ample amount and range of ER (electromagnetic radiation), which include UV (wavelength range from 180nm to 380nm), Vis (visible, nearly 380-800nm) & infrared light (1nm to 3nm). All radiation reaching planet earth ultraviolet radiation has the greatest energy and carries potential harm. Subdivision of this radiation includes UVA, UVB & UVC. Among these three regions, UVA has the highest wavelengths (320 to 380nm). UVB is in the middle of these radiations comprising (280 to 320 nanometers), and rays with the shortest wavelength 180 to 280 nanometers but has the highest energy [55]. In the case of human skin, UVB, which is highly energetic, does not show penetrance due to epidermal cellular biochromes; these are mainly kept to the epidermis. UVA & visible light display major penetrance & they affect cellular structures inside the epidermis. Ultraviolet light affects the skin in two ways first way is by increasing lesions by DNA absorption of mutagenic radiations called UV signatures. The second way is indirect interaction with many biochromes, which generate ROS that retain their harmful effects on cells, causing oxidative modifications & strand breaks [56]. Physiological responses of the skin to solar radiation exposure are determined by the distribution, production, types and quantity of melanin produced by melanocytes & their transfer to keratinocytes [55]. Every component of UV affects diverse cells, tissues & molecules. Geographic variations also affect the intensity and exposure of UV rays. UV dosing per person depends on the strength of UV radiation, time spent outdoors, use of UV radiation protective clothes, shady areas, and sunblock. There is no surprise that skin tone people have higher tendencies to get skin cancer and higher pigmentations because they have sensitivity to UV rays [57, 58].

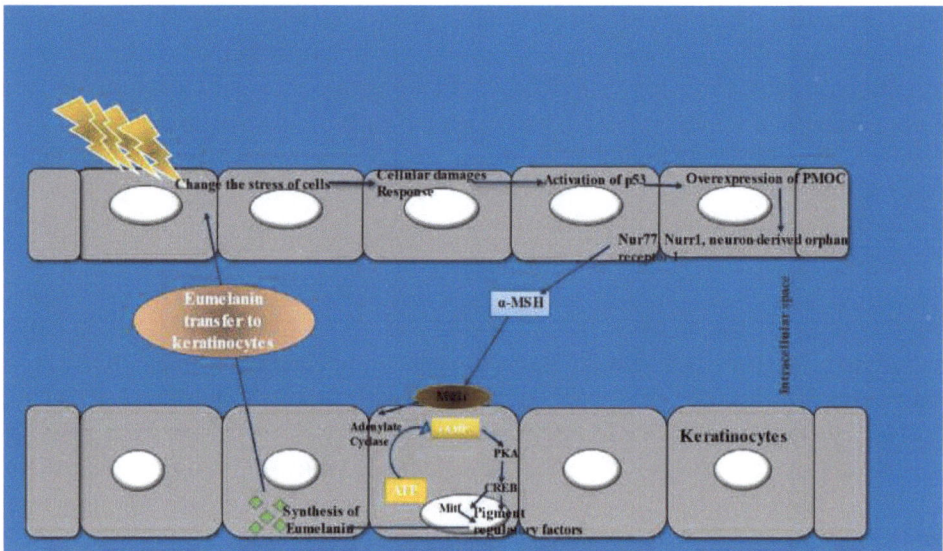

Fig. (4). UV rays induced the hormonal changes inside the keratinocytes to provoke skin pigmentation.

The spectrum of UV radiation reaching the earth, and its biochemical effects on the skin. Penetration of UV depends upon wavelength; the longer the wavelength, the deeper the penetration into the dermis and reaches soundly into the dermis. UVC is predominantly absorbed by the ozone in the atmosphere, so sunlight that reaches human skin is usually UVA & UVB. Contrary to UVC, UVB completely penetrates the epidermis very little amount of it reaches the dermis, but UVA is the one that gets absorbed into the dermis completely due to its higher ROS production capacity.

Melanogenesis is a biochemical process that leads to the formation of melanin. The mechanism behind the production of melanin is initiated and catalyzed by the enzyme tyrosinase. This enzyme catalyzes 2 consecutive processes, *i.e.*, L-tyrosine hydroxylation to L-dopa & oxidation of o-diphenol into dopaquinone. Production of leukodopachrome (known as cyclo-dopa) is done spontaneously by dopaquinone. These intermediates quickly undergo redox disproportionation into dopa & dopachrome. Tyrosinase action leads to the recruitment of dopa in this pathway, dopachrome then continues to the production of eumelanin. O-quinones are produced by the action of enzymes tyrosinase or its relevant proteins on DHI & DHICA. Finally, these species produce eumelanin. TRP1 acts as a stabilizing protein for the enzyme tyrosinase [59, 60]. Dopaquinone are being conjugated with compounds containing thiol (L-cysteine, glutathione) for the branching of the pathway to get products containing sulfur products, leading to pheomelanin. Human skin contains these two forms of melanin (eumelanin & pheomelanin). From dark to black coloration of Eumelanin depends upon the ratio of DHI/DHICA [61]. While pheomelanin is a yellow or red pigment, it is common in light phenotypes like blond hairs or red hairs. Photoreception of Eumelanin is higher than the pheomelanin. After exposure to UV, pheomelanin quickly becomes a photosensitized agent by the stimulation of lipid peroxidation & reactions which lead to higher levels of ROS and then consequent undesirable reactions [62]. As photoprotection from solar radiation is because of the darker skin pigmentation, which is linked to eumelanin. Despite melanin inside human skin, it is not enough as compared with light photo types as they preferentially have pheomelanin [63]. Consequently, complementary sunscreens are vital for photoprotection. Without skin protection, sun exposure can be very damaging for the skin anytime, predominantly during the summer season.

Sunscreens are the most fundamental part of the photoprotection strategy world widely [64]. It is an assumption that sunscreens can be very effective against all kinds of UV, as already assumed protection from sunburning may not be linked with cancer (skin) protection. The efficacy of sunscreens can be determined by two parameters: SPF (sun protection factor) & PA (protection grade of UVA). According to FDA (food & drug authority), USA products are essentially labeled with values of SPF to designate how long they protect against UVB. SPF ranges are from 10 to 25 & from 50 to 100, which are related to low, high, and very high levels of protection from UV rays. Sunscreen usually focuses on UVB protection, but it should protect against other UVA, infrared and blue light. As UVA displays deeper penetrance in the dermis & at the junction of the dermis and epidermis, where most of the melanocytes are located. Induction of pigmentation is also possible due to the effects of UVA [55].

NATURAL PRODUCTS ACT AS PHOTO-PROTECTIVE AGENTS

Microbial Substances as Photoprotective Agents

Aside from the pharmaceutical, medical and food industries, biological chemicals have a sporadic application in the cosmetics industry. Numerous biological molecules have played a significant role in the development of different compounds, such as various fragrance compounds, active substances and esters, that are widely employed in the cosmetics industry, either directly or indirectly. The main benefit of employing microbial components is their biocompatibility; however, they also have other advantages, such as a simplified procedure, enhanced product quality and a lower environmental imprint. Bacteria are one type of microorganism that secretes biologically active chemicals with significant commercial value, to name a few biosurfactants, other exopolysaccharides (EPS), oligosaccharides, as well as enzymes, peptides and vitamins; these chemical compounds have been found in a wide variety of cosmetic items that are used for either beauty appearances or maintain the health of the subject, as shown in Table **3**.

Bacteria and their Associated Products Use in Photoprotection

Biosurfactants

Biosurfactants, in addition to cyclodextrin, are employed in the manufacture of several cosmetic products due to their multi-functional properties as an emulsifying agent, skin moisturizing agent, foaming agent as well as detergent and are non-biodegradable. Biosurfactants are frequently made by bacteria, fungi, and other microorganisms. Additionally, biosurfactants such as rhamnolipids have been authorized for use in cosmetics, food and pharmaceuticals by the US EPA s [78]. Mannosylerythritol lipid is one of the most widely used biosurfactants (MEL) and is frequently used in the manufacturing of a variety of cosmetic products, including eyeshadows, Lipsticks, nail polish, body massage oils, various soaps, sprays, powders and accessories are all available [79, 80].

Anti-wrinkle cosmetics and hygiene products are other prominent applications for biosurfactants. The Japanese cosmetic industry has benefited tremendously from the use of surfactant derivative lipopeptides [81]. Surfactants are widely used in dermatological items that are administered directly, as well as in cosmetic formulations of water and oil emulsions [82]. Bacillus species are the most common source of surfactants [83, 84].

Table 3. Microbial products as photoprotective agents.

Source	Compound	Biological Activity	Skin Protect Mechanism	References
Microbial				
Pseudonocardia sp. *Actinosynnema mirum* *Streptomyces avermitilis* *Streptomyces lividans* *Corynebacterium glutamicum*	Mycosporine-like amino acids (MAAs)	Antioxidative, anti-inflammatory, anti-aging	UV-B absorbing/screening compound scavenging potential for hydro soluble radicals, antioxidant activity in a lipid medium, and the scavenging capacity for superoxide radicals shikimate or pentose-phosphate pathway	[65]
Paracoccus, Agrobacterium aurantiacum Thraustochytrid, Rhodotorula, Phafa rhodozym	Astaxanthin	Anti-oxidation Anti-inflammatory Anti-cardio-cerebrovascular diseases	Inhibits ROS formation Modulates the expression of oxidative stress-responsive enzymes such as heme oxygenase-1 (HO-1) Activates the Nrf2/HO-1 antioxidant pathway Upregulation of antioxidative enzymes superoxide dismutase 2 (SOD2), catalase (CAT), and glutathione peroxidase 1 (GPX1) Upregulation of xanthine oxidase (XO) Reduced nicotinamide adenine dinucleotide phosphate (NADPH) oxidase (Nox) Inhibit interleukin-1β (IL-1β), interleukin-6 (IL-6), and tumor necrosis factor-α (TNF-α), nuclear factor-kappa B (NF-κB)	[5, 66]

(Table 3) cont.....

Source	Compound	Biological Activity	Skin Protect Mechanism	References
Microbial				
			Induced the DNA Repair process Promote immune response	
Corynebacterium autotrophicum	Zeaxanthin	Antioxidation Anti-inflammation Structural actions	Protected against UV rays Reduce inflammation Reduce sunburn Skin lightening and improve skin health conditions Provide protection against skin swelling (edema) and hyperplasia Inhibit lipid peroxidation, Quench the triplet state of photosensitizers Quench the singlet state of molecular oxygen, and intercept the propagation step of lipid peroxidation	[67, 68]
L. mesenteriodes Streptococcus mutans	Dextran	Inhibitory effect on thrombocyte aggregation and Coagulation factors Plasma volume expander	To decrease vascular thrombosis to reduce inflammatory response to prevent ischemia–reperfusion injury skin appendage regeneration	[69, 70]
P. aeruginosa A. vinelandii	Alginate	Anti-tumor, anti-oxidative, immunoregulatory, anti-inflammatory, neuroprotective, antibacterial, hypolipidemic, antihypertensive, and hypoglycemic properties	Lower cytotoxic effects on human dermal fibroblasts expression profiles of inflammatory cytokines	[71, 72]
Xanthomonas spp.	Xanthan	Antioxidant, anti-inflammatory and antibacterial	Stimulates keratinocyte growth Photoprotective agent	[73]

(Table 3) cont.....

Source	Compound	Biological Activity	Skin Protect Mechanism	References
Microbial				
Sinorhizobium meliloti M5N1CS and Gluconacetobacter hanseni	Glucuronan	Anticancer, antioxidant, antihyperlipidemic, and anticoagulant	Photo-protective Mechanism not clear	[74]
Streptococcus thermophilus	Hyaluronic acid	Anti-inflammatory, anti-oedematous, and anti-bacteria	Expression of HAS-1 and HAS-2 in the dermis upregulated by TGF-β1	[75]
Pseudomonas sp.	Viscosin, Rhamnolipids	Antiviral Antibiofilm Immunomodulatory Cholesterol-lowering activity Antioxidant Antimicrobial Anticancer	Wound healing with reduced fibrosis, cure of burn shock and treatment of wrinkles	[76]
Pseudozyma sp., Ustilago sp., Candida antartica	Mannosylerythritol lipid		Moisturization of dry skin, activation of fibroblast and papilla cells and antioxidant and protective effects in skin cells	[77]
Bacillus subtilis, Bacillus pumilus A, B. licheniformis B. amyloliquefacien	Surfactin			

Exopolysaccharides

The utilization of microbial exopolysaccharides (EPS) has greatly facilitated its use in the cosmetic market. Dextran is one of the most well-known EPSs derived from glucose polymer. Dextran is produced from bacteria belonging to the *Leuconostocaceae* family, such as *Leuconostoc mesenteriodes* and *Streptococcus mutans*. Dextran is utilized as a skin smoothing and whitening agent in cosmetic products because it increases skin cleanliness, brightness, and plays an important role in wrinkle reduction [81]. The bacterial genus *Xanthomonas* has been reported to produce Xanthan, a complex heteropolymer EPS [85]. Xanthan possesses thickening and gelling qualities, thus it's employed in skin formulations to assist skin smoothness and conditioning [86]. In keratinocyte cells, it also lowers *trans*-epidermal moisture loss. Secondly, Xanthan is exploited as an agitator and foaming agent in a variety of products for the skin [87].

Hyaluronic Acid

The glycosaminoglycan (GAG), hyaluronic acid (HA) is usually employed as a dermal filler in cosmetic surgery [88]. Moreover, sodium hyaluronate is an active ingredient in many skin moisturizers and serums because it increases hydration, reduces wrinkles, and enhances skin flexibility [89]. For the synthesis of HA, genetically modified bacillus species have recently been employed [90].

Oligosaccharides

Cyclodextrins are used to decrease the volatility of esters in beauty products and room freshener gels, and they play an important role in creams and lotions [91]. They are also often utilized in detergents for a consistent and long-lasting infusion of fragrance, leading in a long-lasting impact. Smaller cyclodextrin powders are being used to decrease the smell in pads, napkins, nappies, menstruation discs, and other commodities [92]. Enzymatic transformation instead of chemical synthesis is the primary way for commercial cyclodextrin synthesis [93]. As a result, bacteria strains have been used significantly in the production of cyclodextrinase enzyme [94] and some of the most common strains utilized to make cyclodextrin are bacillus strains [95]. The alkalophilic *Bacillus agaradhaerensis* enzyme cyclodextrin glucano-transferase is extensively used in possible cosmetic formulations [96].

Proteins, Enzymes and Peptides

Proteins and peptides, in addition to biosurfactants, have made significant contributions to the cosmetic industry. Proteins and peptides have been utilized to increase the effectiveness of hair, nails, and skin. As an exfoliant, superoxide dismutase (SOD) and peroxidase (lactoperoxidases, catalase and glutathione peroxidases) operate together. When administered to the skin surface, these enzymes act as a natural antioxidant and protect the skin from UV rays [97]. Proteases are well-known enzymes that hydrolyze the peptide bonds in the skin's collagen, keratin, and elastin. Numerous alkaliphilic bacterial sources of alkaline aspartic proteases have been primarily used to treat skin issues such as psoriasis, xerosis and ichthyoses [98].

Stretch marks, scar tissues, and epithelial cell regeneration are all known to be treated with keratinases. Keratin hydrolysates are commonly used in skin ointments and lotions for knees, elbows, and heels by providing smoothness and reducing skin damage. Keratinase is also employed in hair removal and enzymatic peeling. Commercially utilised bacterium for keratinase synthesis is *Bacillus licheniformis. Chrysosporiu, Microsporum, Trichohyton* and *Epidermophyton* fungi are well-known keratinophilic fungi possessing the ability to break the keratin strands [99]. Specific peptides, in addition to enzymes, have been frequently employed in cosmetic formulations. Non-soluble peptides are utilized in face masks, while soluble peptides are employed in emulsions, gels, lotions and powders [100]. For economic uses, these peptides are manufactured by the guided action of proteases [101] which are primarily produced by numerous *Bacillus* species [102]. Pentapeptides are also known to decrease wrinkles and dullness on the face [103].

Algae and its Associated Products in Photoprotection

Algae are a diverse group of organisms, consisting of more than 72500 evolutionary classifications [104]. Changing and controlling the physiological culture conditions can easily manipulate the production of bioactive chemicals from algae [105]. Phycobilin's, polysaccharides, lipids, proteins, carotenoids, fatty acids, vitamins, sterols and polyphenols are extracted from algae that have shown photo-protective, antioxidant, anti-inflammatory and anti-aging properties [106].

Recent research has shown that different types of multicellular algae exhibit photoprotective properties, as shown in Fig. (**5**). Mycosporine-like-like amino acids (MMAs) are powerful UV-absorbing chemicals generated in large quantities by a variety of algae species and have long been used in commercial sunscreens [107]. Algae extract has UV absorption qualities as well as the ability to protect against UVR-induced ROS. *Corallina pilulifera* (a red algae) was extracted in methanol and shown to have high antioxidant activity, protecting against UVA-induced oxidative damage. The extract was found to reduce the expression of the matrix metalloproteinases MMP-2 and MMP-9 at the molecular level [108]. Brown algae have been shown to offer photoprotective properties in a variety of species. *Ecklonia* cava is high in polyphenols, which can help protect you from photo-oxidative stress [109]. In keratinocytes, extract from *Unidaria crenata* was found to have strong free radical scavenging properties and to reduce UVB-induced apoptosis as well as lipid and protein oxidation [110]. Fucoxanthin, a carotenoid extracted from the brown algae *Sargassum siliquastrum*, has been demonstrated to inhibit fibroblast apoptosis caused by UVB radiation. Many additional brown algae species, such as *Undaria, Sargassum*, and *Hijikia* contain fucoxanthin, which has been demonstrated to reduce UVB-induced photoaging in mice by lowering VEGF and MMP-13 expression. Other components of the brown algae Sargassum sagamianum, such as plastoquinones, sargachromenol, and sargaquinoic acid have been proven to provide UVB protection, confirming the abundance of photoprotective chemicals found in the algal extract [111].

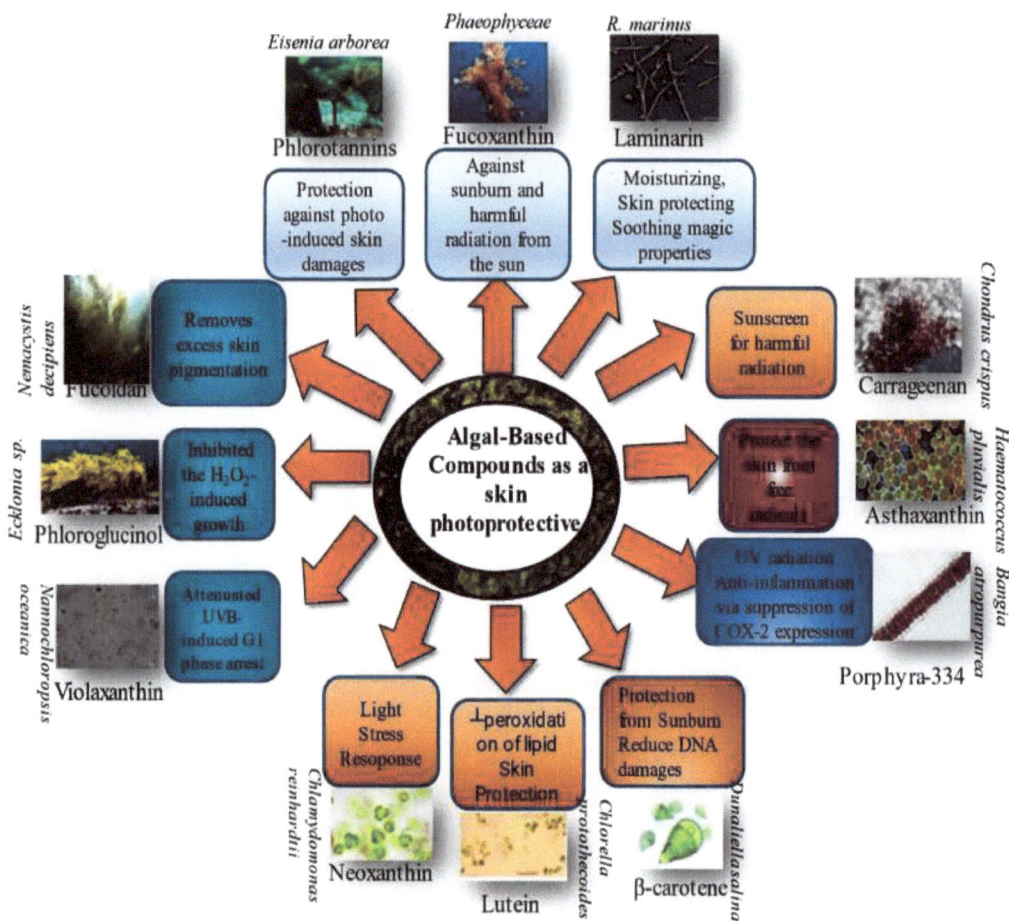

Fig. (5). Diagrammatic representation of algal-based compounds; source and their photo-protective compounds.

Anti-Photoaging Compounds and UV Photoprotection

Algae have been found to create a variety of UV-protective compounds, including mycosporine-like amino acids (MAAs), phycobiliproteins, flavonoids [112], carotenoids [113] and scytonemin [114]. Most algae and cyanobacterial species contain MAAs are used as UV photoprotective compounds [115]. They have characteristics that let them absorb UV light more effectively and disperse it without producing free radicals. Additionally, when members of the Rhodophyceae, *Ochrophyta, Phaeophyceae*, and *Chlorophyceae* were subjected to high levels of intense solar radiation, they developed a high level of MAAs act as a defensive shield and inhibited cell desiccation. Helioguard 365™ and Helionori™ are examples of sunscreen lotions and creams which contain these MAAs. Anthocyanins, which are derived from algae, have been shown to be effective in treating radiation dermatitis during radiotherapy [116].

Agents for Skin Lightening and De Pigmentation

Melanin pigment gives the skin its hue and shields it from harmful UV rays. It also helps to prevent carcinogenesis. Overproduction of melanocytes, on the other hand, causes hyperpigmentation, or skin darkening. Moreover, as people age, their melanocyte regulation, control, and dispersion become unpredictable, resulting in dark and discolored areas on the skin. Tyrosinase is a key enzyme in the production of melanin, and blocking it is an effective way to minimize hyperpigmentation. *Ecklonia* cava has been shown to reduce melanogenesis and has the potential to be utilized as a skin-lightening agent [117]. Zeaxanthin, derived from the microalgae *Nannochloropsis oculata,* has been shown to have anti-tyrosinase properties and can be used for skin whitening [118]. In topological testing, the fucoidan present in *Undariapin natifdaand, Fucus vesiculosus* extract exhibited antioxidant potential and enhanced the efficacy in skin whitening, spot reduction, and skin protection [119].

Hair Care

Algal oil enriched in omega 3 fatty acids is known for its potential to treat dryness, thin hair, itchy, scratchy scalp, dandruff, and loss of hair. Docosahexaenoic Acid (DHA) and Eicosapentaenoic Acid (EPA) derived from microalgae are widely used in hair oils, serums, gels, and sprays to provide deep nourishment to the hair follicles and scalp, making the hair healthier and longer. Sericin protein, a commonly used component in hair conditioning and skin treatments, is produced primarily by *Bombixmori,* but it can also be obtained from microalgae such as *Chlorella vulgaris* and *Arthro spiraplatensis* [120]. In dermal papilla cells (DPCs) and outer root sheath cells (ORS), 7-phloroeckol has been shown to promote hair development [121].

Skin Ageing

Collagen has been shown to slow down skin wrinkling and improve skin elasticity [122]. Collagen alongside elastin fibers that are naturally found in skin assists in the maintenance of bright skin by keeping it elastic and resilient after stretch. *Eiseniabicyclis* and *Ecklonia* cava have been shown to improve the skin by greatly reducing the elastase action [81].

However, green microalgae, such as *Chlorella*, maintain skin firmness by preserving collagen and elastin fibers from the degrading enzymes collagenase and elastase, which are popularly exploited as anti-wrinkling agents in skin creams [123]. Hexadecatetraenoic acid is derived from the Antarctic Sea ice diatom, Stauroneisamphioxys, and Hexadecapentaenioic acid is derived from the marine green microalga *Anadyomene stellata*. It is utilized in cosmetic preparations to prevent creases, dragging, anti-aging, and collagen deposition. By stimulating the production of syndecan-4 in the extracellular matrix of dermal tissues, the brown algal extract of *Macrocys tispyrifera* is reported to boost hyaluronic acid synthesis [124].

Anti-Oxidants

The increase in lipid peroxidation, which is mediated by superoxide anion, OH radicals, and H_2O_2 enhances the ageing processes in dermal cells. Antioxidant compounds are essential to protect human dermal tissues from the scavenging effects of free radicals. *Rhodophyceae* are known for their anti-oxidant action due to the presence of colorful pigments such as phycocyanin, allophyco-cyanins, carotenoids, phycoerythrin and xanthophylls [125]. These algal pigments have been used in a variety of cosmetics, including the Pure Clay Red Algae Mask. Scytonemin, asterina-330, shinorine, and palythine, among other cyanobacterial MAAs, successfully neutralize the free radicals generated by photo-oxidation in skin cells [114]. Dunaliellasalina also produces β-carotene, which is changed into vitamin A that plays a vital role in the maintenance of healthy skin as well as in preserving the mucous membrane [113].

Fungi-Associated Product Use in Photoprotection

Fungi are a complex and varied group of creatures. Fungi is an amazing biodiverse kingdom with members spanning a wide range of living habitats, life forms, shapes, and size. According to current high-throughput estimates, our ecosystem has 5.1 million fungal species [126]. Fungi are being used to generate a variety of possible cosmetics items, including skin care, antioxidants, and hair products. Mushrooms are high in secondary metabolites, which have a variety of therapeutic benefits. Compounds produced from *Schizophyllum commune*, such as Schizophyllan, are known to protect the skin from UV radiation and aid in skin inflammation reduction [127].

Chitin-Glucans

Chitin-glucans are copolymers derived from fungi's cell walls that act effectively as moisturizers [128]. Chitosan is a well-known example of chitin-glucan. Chitosan is commonly used in toothpaste formulations as an antibacterial agent against dental plaque. In hair-setting lotions and gels, chitosan is combined with hyaluronic acid and collagen to create a coating that adds thickness, volume, strength, and protects hair from damage. Moreover, chitosan nanoparticles preloaded with minoxidil are employed to provide effective transdermal transfer and hair growth *via* continuous release of minoxidil.

Ceramides

Ceramides are utilized in cosmetics as skin moisturizing agents since they are abundant in the stratum corneum of the human epidermis. Ceramides are found solely in eukaryotic cells and are derived from animals (*e.g.*, cows). Concerns about infectious illnesses, on the other hand, have prompted researchers to look for other sources of ceramides. Furthermore, plant-derived ceramides differ structurally from animal ceramides, limiting their usage in cosmetics. Ceramides have been generated and utilized in cosmetics from a variety of fungal species [129]. Glycosly ceramides are made by *Candida albicans*, *Armillaria tabescens*, and *Agaricus bisporus* [130]. Attempts to generate ceramides using yeast (*Saccharomyces cerevisiae*) metabolic engineering have also been developed [131].

Lactic Acid

Lactic acid is found in high concentrations in cosmetics and skin creams to help skin maintain hydration, suppleness, and smoothness. Lactic acid in high concentrations (up to 12 percent) is used in skin peeling creams as an exfoliant, skin lightener, and acne reducer [132]. In addition, poly-l-lactic acid (PLLA) is employed as a bio-stimulatory filler and in the elimination of facial folds, reduction, wrinkles, and photodamage reduction [133]. Fungi of the Rhizopus genus are known to create lactic acid from aerobic glucose fermentation and have a lower substrate cost than bacteria such as *Lactobacillus* [134].

Antioxidants

The anti-oxidant l-ergothioneine is isolated in high amounts from mushrooms like *Criminis* and *Portabellas* species [135]. Ergothioneine is utilized in anti-aging skincare products because of its outstanding antioxidant qualities, which protect the skin from oxidative and DNA degradation. Gallic acid, on the other hand, is thought to have antimicrobial and free radical scavenging properties. Gallic acid is produced by *Aspergillus niger*, *Trichoderma viridae*, and *Fusarium solani* [136]. Trehalose is an antioxidant chemical found in *Lentinula edodes*, *Auricularia auricula-judae*, *Pholiotanameko*, and *Grifolafondosa* mushrooms. Terahalose has a high-water retention capacity and is a powerful antioxidant. This makes it suitable for use in cosmetics items such as moisturizing creams.

Application of Whole Plant Extract

Whole herbal extracts are made up of a variety of chemicals that work together to improve the skin's appearance. Antioxidant, anti-inflammatory, melanin-inhibiting, emollient antimutagenic, antiaging, and other characteristics may be found in a single plant extract. Plants extract are potent agents to stunt the UV rays fluctuation by absorbing the harmful radiations, as shown in Fig. (**6**).

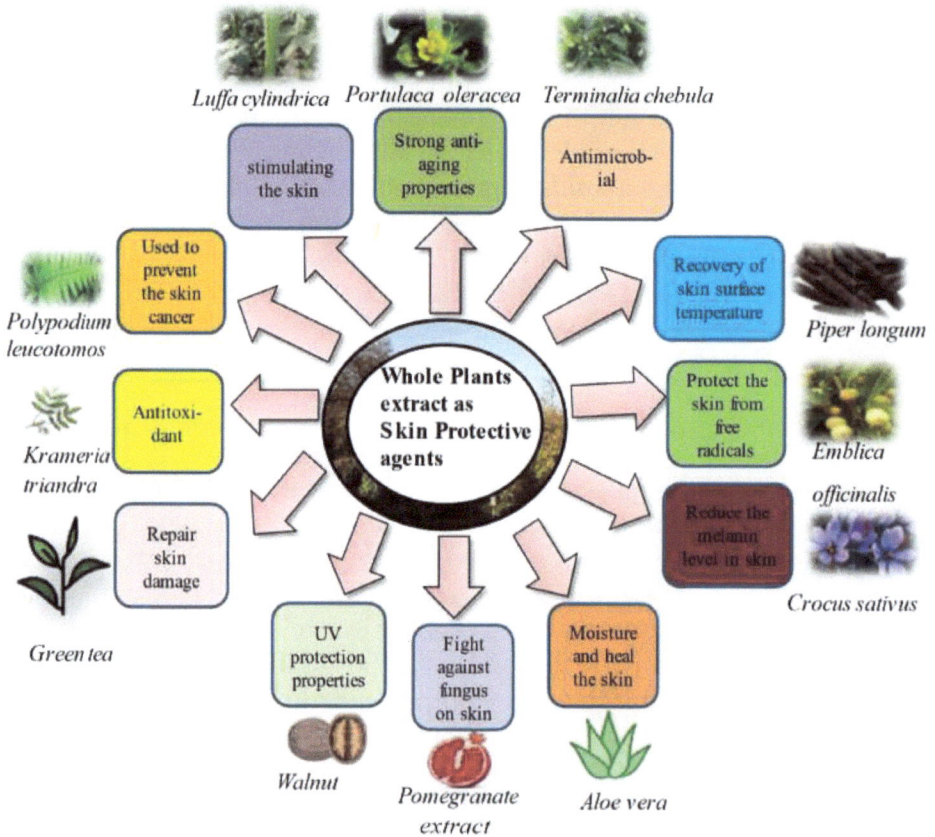

Fig. (6). Summary of various plants extract, source and skin protecting mechanism.

Aloe Vera

Aloe vera also known as *Aloe barbadense*, has been clinically demonstrated to help with all types of burns, including radiation, thermal, and sun. It has also been shown that using it before, during, and after these skin-damaging events has a preventive effect. The plant is clearly utilized for its relaxing and cooling effects; however, if used at less than 50%, the plant is worthless, and it is advised that it be used at 100% to ensure any good impact. Polysaccharides, mannose-6-

phosphate, and complex anthraquinones all work together to enhance the material's advantages [137]. *Aloe vera's* natural chemical contents may be divided into the following categories: vitamins, anthraquinones, Amino acids, enzymes, minerals, sterols, mono- and polysaccharides, lignin, salicylic acid, and saponins are among the many substances found in plants. *Aloe vera* not only enhanced the shape of fibroblast cells, but also increased the collagen manufacturing process. *Aloe vera* is a highly powerful moisturizer and healing agent for human and animal skin [138].

Pomegranate Extract

The juice, seed, and peel of the pomegranate fruit Punica granatum are used to make pomegranate extract. The phenolic components have strong antioxidant properties. The activity of catalase, superoxide dismutase, and peroxidase enzymes has been found to be restored *in vivo* after topical administration of the peel extract [139]. Pomegranate extract has been demonstrated to protect against UVB and UVA damage *in vitro* experiments [140]. Pomegranate has been found in animal experiments to play a preventive function in the development of skin cancer [141]. Human studies are scarce, even though pomegranate is frequently used in topical preparations for its antioxidant effects [142].

Walnut

The fresh green shells of the English walnut, Juglans regia, are used to make the walnut extract. The aqueous extract has been demonstrated to work well as a self-tanning sunscreen agent. Juglone (5-hydroxy-1,4- naphthoquinone), a naphthol related to lawsone, is the most essential component (2-hydroxy-1,4-naphthoquinone). Sclerojuglonic chemicals are formed when juglone reacts with keratin proteins in the skin. These are UV-protected and come in a variety of colors [143].

Green Tea Extract

Green tea is made from Camellia sinensis leaves and leaf buds. Green tea extract (GTE) is widely used for its anti-inflammatory properties in various parts of the world. The primary phenol component, epigallocatechin-3-gallate (EGCG), is capable of inhibiting metalloproteinase expression, oxidative stress, angiogenesis, and tumor carcinogenesis [144].

In human subjects, topical administration of ECCG reduced UV-induced penetration of the epidermis by hydrogen peroxide, lymphocytes, and nitric oxide. Participants were given a 250 mg GTE pill or a placebo in double-blind, placebo-controlled research. The GTE group demonstrated a decrease in photodamage after 6 months of clinical examination by a dermatologist ($P = 0.02$) [145]. At 6 and 12 months, the GTE group had much less erythema and telangiectasias than the control group. These differences did not persist at the 24-month mark, but the researchers speculated that the GTE group's photoprotective effect begins sooner. Brown spots and UV spots in the GTE group were reduced after one year using Visia Complexion Analysis, but no changes in other parameters (wrinkles, texture unevenness, pores) were seen at any period (wrinkles, texture unevenness, pores). There were no changes in histopathology between the GTE and placebo groups (total UV damage, perivascular inflammation solar, elastosis, epidermal melanin, dermal mucin, epidermal thickness, dermal elastin or dermal collagen [146]. In a separate double-blind trial, 30 women drank 1 litre of green tea every day while the other 30 women drank a neutral beverage; after the 12th week, several skin characteristics had improved [147].

Carotenes are natural antioxidants found in several fruits and vegetables that have long been known to have photoprotective properties. Supplementing with carotene was found to be useful in avoiding photo dermatoses, treating some photo-related illnesses, such as porphyria, and lowering MED in early clinical investigations [148, 149]. Carotenes may be found in abundance in tomatoes and tomato paste. In healthy participants, consuming 40 grams of tomato paste per day with 10 g of olive oil helped to reduce erythema and enhance MED. After UVR, there was a substantial rise in procollagen I and a decrease in metalloproteinase-1 (MMP-1) in the tomato paste group after 3 months of supplementation [150].

Krameria Triandra

The photoprotective ability of a standardized Krameria triandra root extract (15 percent neolignans) was tested in several cell models, including human keratinocytes cell lines and rat erythrocytes which were subjected to physical and chemical-free radical inducers. Krameria triandra root extract effectively and dose-dependently reduced cell viability loss and intracellular oxidative damage in cultured human keratinocytes exposed to UVB light. The extract's cytoprotective activity was validated in a more severe model of cell damage: keratinocytes were exposed to greater UVB levels, which resulted in 50% cell death. Cell viability was nearly entirely retained and more effectively than with (-)-EGCG and green tea in keratinocyte cultures supplemented with 10 g/ml. The findings suggest that Rhatany extracts standardized in neolignans might be used as topical antioxidants to protect skin from photodamage [151].

Polypodium Leucotomos Extract

Some plants have numerous photoprotective mechanisms and synergistic photoprotective effects. The most well-studied oral supplement with photoprotective properties is Polypodium leucotomos extract (PLE), which is taken from a fern that grows in tropical parts of the Americas. PLE has been established in several *in vitro* experiments to protect human keratinocytes from the harmful effects of UV exposure [152]. It has been shown that PLE treatment of keratinocytes reduces the synthesis of nitric oxide and tumor necrosis factor-alpha, as well as the activation of nuclear factor-kappa B (NFB), all of which have been linked to UVB-induced skin cancer. In an *in vitro* model of the human epidermis, PLE has been demonstrated to protect against UVB-induced damage, with a decrease in sunburned cells and the generation of cyclobutane pyrimidine dimers (CPD) [153].

Luffa Cylindrica

The climber *L. cylindrica* (Linn) M. Roem, has a thin, hairy stem with little furrowing [154]. The oil in the seeds of *L. cylindrica* contains linoleic acids and stearic, which are unsaturated fatty acids [155]. Free radical scavenging capabilities of naturally occurring unsaturated fatty acids and phenolic compounds have been reported. It was discovered in a study that the fixed oil extracted from the plant's seed kernels not only scavenges free radicals but also suppresses their formation [156].

Portulaca Oleracea

Portulaca oleracea (Common Purslane; also known as Verdolaga, Pusley, Little Hogweed, or Pigweed) is a small annual succulent in the Portulacaceae family that can grow up to 40 cm tall. It is native to India and the Middle East but has been naturalised worldwide and is considered an invasive weed in certain areas. Bactericide, Antiphlogistic, antidiabetic, calmative, diuretic, anaphrodisiac (opposite of aphrodisiac), emollient, and refreshing agent are all used to describe the complete plant [157, 158]. Sanja and colleagues used DPPH free radical scavenging, $FeCl_3$ reducing power estimate, nitric oxide free radical scavenging, and super oxide scavenging activity to demonstrate the antioxidant activity of the methanol extract [159]. The extract exhibits a proclivity for scavenging free radicals implicated in the ageing process and skin wrinkling, suggesting that it may have some photoprotective properties.

Terminalia Chebula

Terminalia chebula, popularly known as Harde, is a member of the Combretaceae family. It is extensively used as a laxative, cardiotonic, and diuretic in many Ayurvedic medicines, as well as in various health supplements [160]. Ascorbic acid, ellagic acid and gallic acid, are chemical components that have been shown to have free radical scavenging activities [161].

Piper Longum

Piper longum L., a member of the Piperaceae family, is widely distributed in Philippines Indonesia, and India. It is made up of a spike of fruits that is roughly 4 cm long and 6 mm in diameter. The fruit (pepper) includes a resin, 1 to 2.5 percent volatile oil, and 5 to 95 percent crystalline alkaloids piperettine and piperine. Because of its antioxidant efficacy *in vitro* and *in vivo* in mice, piperine isolated from this plant has been employed as a component in Ayurvedic formulations [162]. Piperine is used topically in a cream basis to treat sunburn conditions because of its antioxidant properties [163].

Emblica Officinalis

Amla, or *Emblica officinalis* Gaertn. is a good source of vitamin C, amino acids and minerals in the diet. It also includes phenolic chemicals in different forms. Amla extract has been shown to have powerful antioxidant effects and to protect human dermal fibroblasts from oxidative stress, hence it is thought to be effective for natural dermal care [164]. Amla extract has been shown to have an influence on human skin fibroblasts, namely on the formation of procollagen and matrix metalloproteinases (MMPs) [165]. 2 percent ascorbic acid and 29.4 percent polyphenols, including elaeocarpusin and gallic acid, are found in the aqueous extract from dry amla powder [166]. Amla extract stimulates the synthesis of procollagen in human skin fibroblasts *via* increasing mitochondrial activity. As a result of its putative anti-inflammatory, aesthetic, and medicinal properties, amla has been utilised for skin therapy since antiquity [167].

Crocus Sativus

Saffron, a spice and culinary colorant made from the dried stigma of the *Crocus sativus* L. plant, has been used in traditional medicine to cure a variety of ailments, including cancer. The colourful carotenoids crocetin and crocin, as well as the monoterpene aldehydes safranal and picrocrocin, are chemical components of saffron [168].

Saffron extract has been shown to have non-mutagenic and anti-promoting properties [169]. Crocins can protect against the harmful effects of hepatocarcinogenic substances and crocetin, the deglycosylated crocin derivative, can block intracellular nucleic acid production, according to Lin *et al.* [170]. Using a two-stage skin carcinogenesis model in mice, the anticarcinogenic impact of an aqueous infusion of saffron, provided orally, was investigated; the protective role of saffron against carcinogenic exposure was also investigated. Its influence on physiological detoxification processes was linked to it, and thus confirmed that

Saffron can help to reduce skin damage caused by chemicals. In Swiss albino mice, carcinogenesis occurs [171].

Peumusboldus Molina

Peumusboldus, a tree of the *Monimiaceae* family whose leaves have been used in folk medicine for centuries, is now extensively recognized as an herbal cure by several Pharmacopoeias. Its leaves are high in numerous aporphine-like alkaloids, the most abundant of which is boldine [172]. Boldine was shown to be one of the most effective natural antioxidants, according to research done in the early 1990s. It has anti-tumor promoting, cytoprotective, antiatherogenic actions, anti-diabetic, and anti-inflammatory, as well as some actions that do not appear to be associated with these activities, such as *vasorelaxing, cholagogic, anti-trypanocidal, choleretic actions*, and/or immuno- and neuromodulator, which are derived from its antioxidant properties. Most UV-induced skin lesions are thought to include free radicals in their progression or aetiology [173]. Experiments on boldine have shown that it possesses a UV light-filtering capability that is important as a photoprotective agent. Free radicals are thought to have a role in the aetiology and progression of most UV-induced skin lesions. Boldine has been proven to have a UV light-filtering property pertinent to a photoprotective activity by research done on it. Indeed, it has been demonstrated that Bodine is photo-unstable at wavelengths up to 300nm and that it has a photo-protector action against UV-B *in vitro* and *in vivo* in mice. The inhibition of UV-induced increases in the skin temperature of rats demonstrated photo-protection. The photo-filtering properties of boldine in humans were recently investigated, and it was discovered that applying boldine (25 mM) to a 12 cm^2 area of the back of volunteers protected their skin against erythema formation to a degree slightly lower than that of a commercial sun cream (Nivea sun spray LSF -5) with a UV-protection factor of 5.

UV Protection by Botanical Extracts

Several plant extracts or ingredients have previously been shown to reduce inflammatory reactions in animals, cells, and people owing to UV exposure.

In cultured human epidermal melanocytes exposed to UVB radiation, botanical extracts from *Sasa quelpaertensis*, Dryopteris crassi rhizome, and Althaea rosea, reduced melanin formation and cytotoxicity [173]. These plant extracts prevented an increase in ear thickness or dorsal skin redness when applied topically to the ears of C57BL/6 mice or the dorsal skin of the SKH-1 hairless mouse before and after exposure to UVB rays, suggesting that they have anti-inflammatory activity that reduces erythema and edoema. The most effective action was found in the Sasaquelpaertensis extract, which includes *p*-coumaric acid as one of its key ingredients [174].

Bambusae caulis in Taeniam has been utilised for the treatment of atherosclerosis, tiredness, hyperlipidemia, and hypertension, among other disorders [175]. Its bioactivity is thought to be linked, at least in part, to its strong antioxidant capabilities. Bambusae caulis in Taeniam extract, which also contains *p*-coumaric acid, increased the survival of UVB-exposed HaCaT human keratinocytes and inhibited apoptotic processes, such as procaspase 3 cleavage to its active form and an increase in the Bax to Bcl-2 ratio [176]. It also has antioxidant properties, as it reduces the production of reactive oxygen species (ROS) and lipid peroxidation in UVB-exposed cells. In addition, after UVB stimulation, it inhibited MMP1 expression and JNK phosphorylation [177].

As it contains different flavonoids, such as baicalin and bailcalein (baicalein-7-O-glucuronide), Scutellaria radix, the root of Scutellariabaicalensis Georgi, has been used in traditional medicine in Asia to treat inflammatory and allergic illnesses [111] In numerous experimental models, Scutellaria radix extract and its components have been proven to have anti-inflammatory and antioxidant properties [178]. Scutellaria radix extract was also found to have UV-protective properties [179].

The extract of Scutellaria radix has strong UV absorptivity and free radical scavenging activity, and it prevented UV-induced cell death in HaCaT keratinocytes, according to our findings. In human subjects, the use of Scutellaria radix extract in sunscreen lotion dramatically increased the sun protection factor (SPF) [180].

Propolis is a honeybee-produced combination of bee wax, resin, salivary gland secretions and pollen that contains phenolic chemicals [181]. Propolis and its components have been proven in previous research to have antioxidant properties by preventing oxidative changes in biomolecules [182].

Under various pathological situations, propolis extract has also been proven to have anti-inflammatory and immunomodulatory properties [183].]Propolis extract reduced total protein carbonyl content, a measure of protein oxidation, in HaCaT cells exposed to UVB radiation in recent research. In a model of reconstituted skin tissue, it also reduced oxidative photodamage caused by UVB exposure [184].

An extract of Portulaca oleracea, also known as Purslane [185], has been shown to reduce apoptotic cell death in human keratinocytes and fibroblasts after UVB irradiation, as mitochondrial membrane depolarization was detected using JC-1 staining, phosphatidylserine exposure was detected using annexin V-fluorescein isothiocyanate (FITC) staining [186]. Other extracts from broccoli sprouts, rosemary, blackberries, and citrus have been found to protect keratinocytes, humans and mice against UV damage [187].

Phyto-Compounds for Skin Protection

The growing prevalence of skin illnesses has created a strong need for researchers to investigate and develop better skin photo-protection options. Traditional sunscreens involve compounds that resist and scatter UVA and UVB rays, such as zinc oxide (ZnO) and titanium dioxide (TiO_2). These inert particles, on the other hand, frequently appear on the skin as an unsightly opaque film. Furthermore, there has been rising worry regarding the safety of these metal-based particles as well as their potential toxicity [188]. Recognizing UVA's harmful effects has prompted a substantial investigation into natural goods' active constituents. Antioxidants have the ability to boost the skin's endogenous antioxidant capacity and aid in the neutralization of ROS caused by external sources such as solar UV radiation [189].

Plant-derived compounds have been studied for their antioxidant activity in the hunt for efficient topical photoprotective agents, and the usage of natural antioxidants in commercial skin care products is on the rise. Today, we examine the chemical makeup of herbal treatments in order to figure out what, chemically and pharmacologically, is causing these results. Tocopherols, phenolic acids, flavonoids, nitrogen-containing compounds (monoterpenes, amines, amino acids, and alkaloids), and indoles are all effective plant antioxidant substances that are frequently utilised in traditional medicine. Botanical agents from a variety of chemical families, including polyphenols, indoles, monoterpenes, flavonoids, and organosulfides have been proven in mouse models to exhibit anti-mutagenic and anti-carcinogenic characteristics without producing considerable toxicity. These chemicals' mechanisms of action include immunological and anti-inflammatory response activation, gene expression manipulation, antioxidant regulation, and detoxification [190].

Phenolic acids, mycosporine-like amino acids, flavonoids, nonflavonoids, terpenoids, and lichen polyphenols are all essential secondary metabolites that function as UV blockers. These chemicals can prohibit radiation from penetrating the skin, resulting in reduced inflammation, oxidative stress, and DNA damage. In addition to their capacity to absorb UV radiation, several natural chemicals have been discovered to lower inflammation, influence numerous signaling pathways and oxidative stress, all of which help to protect the skin from UV-induced damage [191].

Many botanical compounds contain antioxidants, which are known to strengthen cell membranes and protect intracellular constituents from UV-induced cellular damage and consequent intracellular fluid loss. In addition, evidence is mounting that combining antioxidants with sunscreens improves photoprotection [192]. Some antioxidants are more powerful than others at neutralizing various free radicals in cells and specific areas of the body. Furthermore, some are more effective when taken in combination. Water-soluble vitamin C, for example, eliminates free radicals from cell structures made mostly of water and from places holding bodily fluids. Fat-soluble carotene and vitamin e are active in the lipid or fatty sections of the cell membrane as well as in fat tissue. Furthermore, certain antioxidants act as both free-radical scavengers and anti-aging catalysts.

Anthocyanins

Anthocyanidins and their derivatives, many of which may be found in everyday foods, protect against oxidants in various ways. In recent Japanese animal research, cyanidins, which are found in most fruit sources of anthocyanins, were discovered to "act as a strong antioxidant *in vivo* [193]. Cyanidins protected cell membrane lipids from oxidation by a range of hazardous chemicals in other animal tests [194]. Animal studies show that cyanidin is four times as potent than vitamin E as an antioxidant. Pelargonidin, an anthocyanin, shields tyrosine against the highly reactive oxidant peroxynitrite. Eggplant includes nasunin, a derivate of the anthocyanidin delphinidin that inhibits the hydroxyl radical-generating mechanism, which is a primary source of oxidants in the body [195].

Quercetin

Quercetin is the most frequent flavanol in the diet. Quercetin contains anti-inflammatory, immunomodulatory, and antioxidant properties. Quercetin is found in food as an aglycone (a sugar molecule connected to it). Only a small fraction of quercetin consumed is absorbed into the bloodstream. Many common foods contain quercetin, including apples, cabbage, onion, tea, almonds, cauliflower, and berries. When applied topically, a diet rich in quercetin has been shown to suppress the establishment of carcinogen-induced rat breast cancer, skin tumor growth, oral carcinogenesis, and colonic neoplasia in three models of skin carcinogenesis in mice [196]. Quercetin may be responsible for the anti-mutagenic and anti-carcinogenic actions of dietary fruits and vegetables on carcinogens and mutagens, such as metals. It may be found in a variety of vegetables and fruits, as well as drinks and plants. Onions have the greatest amounts. In humans, rutin and quercetin were investigated as possible topical sunscreen ingredients and shown to give UVA and UVB protection [197].

Genistein

The aglycone (non-sugar component) of the glycoside genistin is genistein. Genistein must be freed from genistin before it may function. Peapods, Soya beans and other legumes are the principal sources of genistein. Small levels of genistein can be found in other legumes, such as chickpeas. Genistein is a flavonoid that belongs to the isoflavone family. Genistein is classified as a phytoestrogen since its structure is like that of oestrogen. It has antioxidant and phytoestrogen properties. Topical administration of genistein and its gastrointestinal metabolites, such as equol, dehydroequol, and isoequol, to the skin of hairless mice, decreased UV-B-induced hydrogen peroxide (H_2O_2) generation, inflammatory edoema, and contact hypersensitivity [198].

Apigenin

Apigenin is a flavonoid found in plants that may be found in herbs, drinks, fruits, and vegetables. In SKH-1 mice, apigenin was found to be helpful in preventing UVA/UVB-induced skin cancer. Apigenin did not prevent NF-B from translocating to the nucleus, but it did stop NF-B from driving reporter gene expression [199]. Apigenin is also present in marigolds (*Calendula officinalis*), where the flavonoids were discovered to be responsible for the activity in the mouse ear test, with apigenin being more active than indomethacin. Plants like coneflower, arnica, purple eyebright, carrot, and agrimony all contain luteolin, apigenin and their derivatives [200].

Curcumin

Curcumin is an odourless yellow pigment extracted from the rhizome of turmeric (*Curcuma longa*). Curcumin has antitumoral, anti-inflammatory, and antioxidant effects [196]. UVA-induced ornithine decarboxylase (ODC) activity was shown to be considerably reduced by topical administration of curcumin in the epidermis of CD-1 mice. Curcumin's inhibitory effects have been related to its capacity to scavenge reactive oxygen species (ROS). Curcumin can protect human epidermoid carcinoma A431 cells from apoptosis caused by UV exposure.

Silymarin

Milk thistle (Silybum marianum) seeds contain silymarin, a flavonoid component. The main phytochemicals that makeup silymarin are silybin, silicristin, and silidianin. The most potent phytochemical is silybin [201]. The anticancer effect of topical silymarin has been demonstrated. UVB radiation decreased the number of tumours produced in the skin of hairless mice by 92 percent. Silymarin inhibited the development and death of UV-induced sunburn cells. The finding was unrelated to a sunscreen effect, and it's possible that an antioxidant mechanism is to blame. *in vivo*, silymarin therapy reduces immunological suppression and oxidative damage caused by UVB.

Proanthocyanidin

OPC (or proanthocyanidin) is a DNA mutation inhibitor. Furthermore, OPC inhibits elastase, preserving the integrity of elastin in the skin, and works in tandem with vitamin C and E to preserve and restore it. OPC has been studied and shown to be useful against the harmful rays of the sun in the form of a cream (UV rays). When OPC cream is massaged prior to exposure to the sun, the skin burns less. Grape seed OPCs demonstrated a solo antioxidant activity comparable to vitamin E in one investigation, protecting various polyunsaturated fatty acids against UV light-induced lipid peroxidation. Grape OPCs worked synergistically with vitamin E in this study, recycling the inactive form of the substance into the active ingredient and serving as a virtual vitamin E extender [202].

Grape seed proanthocyanidins (GSP) are powerful antioxidants and scavengers of free radicals. In bald mice exposed to carcinogenic UV radiation, GSP prevented skin tumor growth and reduced the size of skin tumors. The immune system can be suppressed by UV light, however, GSP reduced this inhibition in mice fed a GSP-rich diet. In a model designed to evaluate tumor development in skin cells, GSP treatment promoted tumor cell death.

Ascorbic Acid (Vitamin C)

The body's most essential intracellular and extracellular aqueous-phase antioxidant is vitamin C (L-ascorbic acid). Vitamin C has several skin advantages, the most notable of which are improved collagen production and photoprotection. Vitamin C's anti-inflammatory effects help to boost photoprotection. Photoprotection for several months helps the skin to repair prior photodamage; collagen production and MMP-1 suppression have been shown to reduce wrinkles; and tyrosinase inhibition and anti-inflammatory activities have been shown to depigment solar lentigines [203].

Carotenoids

Dietary carotenoids build in the skin because of a healthy, untreated diet, and their amount is linked to sun protection. Eating a lot of fish oil tends to give sun protection, up to SPF 5 in certain situations, and may lessen the UV-induced inflammatory response by lowering prostaglandin E2 levels. Lutein, and lycopene-carotene, were all shown to dramatically reduce lipid peroxidation caused by UVB in human fibroblasts. After a 12-week oral supplementation with lycopene, selenium, lutein, tocopherol, and carotene, one clinical research found substantial improvements in skin thickness, density, roughness, and scaling. Another human experiment found that oral lycopene-carotene, selenium, and tocopherol treatment reduced UV-induced erythema, the development of sunburn cells, and lipid peroxidation [204].

Vitamin E

Both animal and plant cell membranes may be protected from light-induced harm by the antioxidant vitamin E (tocopherol). These antioxidants have been found to minimize both chronic and acute photodamage when applied to the skin. Only the organic forms of vitamin E, tocotrienol and alpha-tocopherol reduce skin roughness, the lengths of facial lines, and the thickness of wrinkles when administered topically. Vitamin E administered topically improves the hydration and water-binding capability of the stratum corneum. Collagenase, a damaging collagen-degrading enzyme, is reduced by alpha-tocopherol, which regrettably rises with age. Vitamin E is an emollient as well as a free radical scavenger [205].

Triticum Vulgare (wheat germ) oil is high in vitamin E and has a lot of antioxidant potential in topical antiaging compositions. It also hydrates the skin and protects it from losing moisture. Extra virgin Corylus avellana (hazelnut) oil, as well as Helianthus annuus (sunflower) and Sesamum indicum (sesame) oils, are high in tocopherols [206].

Resveratrol

Stilbenes are a kind of polyphenolic substance that includes resveratrol. Resveratrol is a fat-soluble molecule that comes in two forms: *cis* and *trans*. Resveratrol is a polyphenolic phytoalexin that occurs naturally [207]. Resveratrol was discovered to have antioxidant and antimutagenic properties, as well as differentiation and anti-inflammatory effects in human promyelocytic leukaemia cells. It also reduced carcinogenesis in a mouse skin cancer model and the formation of preneoplastic lesions in carcinogen-treated mouse mammary glands in culture. Prior to UVB irradiation, resveratrol was applied topically to SKH-1 hairless mice, which resulted in a substantial reduction in UVB-generated H_2O_2, along with infiltration of leukocytes and suppression of skin edoema. Long-term research has shown that applying resveratrol to the skin (both pre- and post-treatment) decreases the chances of UVB-induced tumours and delays the initiation of skin carcinogenesis.

Cranberries, Grapes, grape juice, wine, peanuts, peanut products, and cranberry juice are the only foods known to contain resveratrol. The roots of the weed Polygonum cuspidatum are one of the greatest sources of resveratrol (2 960–3 770 ppm), according to Vastano *et al.* [208]. High quantities of resveratrol have also been found in Veratrum grandiflorum leaves, as well as Veratrum formosanum roots and rhizomes. For their medicinal characteristics, these latter 3 plants have been widely employed in Japanese and Chinese traditional medicine (laxative, anticancer, anti-arteriosclerosis) [209].

Alpha Lipoic Acid

An important antioxidant that may be obtained through food or supplementation is alpha lipoic acid. Brewer's yeast Spinach and broccoli are all good sources of alpha lipoic acid. Alpha Lipoic acid is known to stimulate cellular energy, boost immunity and muscular strength, and improve cognitive function, hence it plays an important role in cellular processes. While it was not identified as an antioxidant until 1989, it is now reported to enhance the activities of vitamins C and E, CoQ10, and glutathione [210]. Because of its tiny size, it easily penetrates cell membranes and passes through the nuclear envelope, allowing it to have an antioxidant effect not only in circulation but also in the cell membrane and cellular components. The anti-inflammatory and photoprotective characteristics of topical alpha lipoic acid at 3% have also been demonstrated, it reduces UV-induced skin problems [211].

Isothiocyanates

Isothiocyanates are sulfur-containing substances found in broccoli, cabbage, brussels sprouts, watercress, turnips, cauliflower, and radishes, among other crops. Isothiocyanates, which are known for their anti-carcinogenic characteristics, impede cancer cell growth and cause cancer cells to assault one another. Recent studies on broccoli sprout extract have revealed that it has strong sun protection properties [212]. The extract, unlike sunscreens, does not absorb UV rays and hence prevents them from entering the skin. Rather, the extract's sulforaphane, which is found in isothiocyanate-rich foods, operates within cells by increasing the creation of a network of protective enzymes that protects cells from various types of UV damage. As a result, the benefits are long-lasting; the protection lasts for many days, even after the extract has been removed from the skin. The decreases in UV-induced erythema ranged from 8% to 78 percent in the broccoli sprout extract trial, with a mean of 37.7% [213].

Beta-Glucan

Beta-glucan is a kind of carbohydrate found in foods including bran, barley, baker's yeast, oats, mushrooms, and wheat germ. Beta-glucan affects biological responses in a positive way. Because of its cell-stimulating properties, it can help with wound repair and skin irritation. Beta-glucan has been demonstrated to enter epidermal layers when given topically, where it is thought to mobilize growth factors that induce fibroblasts to manufacture collagen. In terms of photoprotection, beta-glucan has been shown to keep glutathione levels in cells stable following UV exposure. Beta-glucan has a unique capacity to repair and prevent UV-induced oxidative damage while having no phototoxic effects on the skin [214].

Polyphenols

Polyphenols, a collection of phytochemicals defined by the presence of more than one phenol unit or building block per molecule, is a developing field of research. Fruits, vegetables, and herbs all contain polyphenols. Our main source of polyphenols in food is liquids such as juices, wines, and teas. Polyphenols have gained popularity because of their beneficial and preventative effects on heart disease, infection, stroke, and cancer. Polyphenols, along with other dietary agents such as vitamin E, vitamin C, and carotenoids, protect the body's tissues and immune system against oxidative stress. The most powerful polyphenol is ellagic acid, which may be found in high concentrations in raspberries, brightly coloured fruits strawberries, and pomegranates berries, whole-grain cereals, nuts, vegetables, soybeans, tea (particularly green tea), red wine, red grapes, citrus fruits and onions. They are also good sources of polyphenols [215].

Essential Fatty Acids

EFAs (essential fatty acids) boost the immune system by strengthening the skin's barrier properties. They have antibacterial, antifungal, and antiviral properties, as well as anti-inflammatory properties due to their capacity to inhibit the synthesis of pro-inflammatory cellular components. According to one research, the omega-3 fatty acid eicosapentaenoic acid reduces UV-induced damage to the skin, making it a promising component for skin ageing prevention and therapy. While studies suggest that topical EFAs have no direct UV-absorbing properties, their photoprotection is thought to be mediated through their cell and cell membrane mending capacities. Durian is an Asian fruit that contains omega-3 EFAs and antioxidants that prevent collagen and elastin breakdown and control the activation of inflammatory mediators, reducing free-radical tissue damage [216].

Honokiol

Magnolia officinalis and other Magnolia genus plants contain honokiol, a small molecule hydroxylated biphenolic chemical. Its many pharmacological characteristics as antioxidant, antibacterial, anti-inflammatory, anticarcinogenic, and antiangiogenic, have only recently been recognised by western medicine. Honokiol has been shown to lessen inflammation caused by reactive oxygen species (ROS). In a mouse model, honokiol dramatically reduced UVB-induced production of inflammatory mediators such as COX2, IL-1, and IL-6, indicating that it may protect against UVR. In melanoma, Honokiol regulates the expression of cell cycle proteins, resulting in anti-neoplastic effects. UVR-induced immunosuppression plays a critical role in the progression of cutaneous carcinogenesis. Topical treatment of honokiol was recently discovered to counteract UV-induced immunosuppression, resulting in a substantial reduction in touch sensitivity suppression in CeH/HeN mice [217].

Sulforaphane

Broccoli contains the natural antioxidant sulforaphane, which has anticarcinogenic, antidiabetic, and antibacterial effects. Through the activation of Nrf2 and subsequent up-regulation of phase 2 antioxidant enzymes, sulforaphane extracts administered topically to mouse skin protected against UVR-induced inflammation and edoema. According to research, the activity of Nrf2 decreases as people age. Although the reasons for Nrf2's decreased activity are unknown, research suggests that Nrf2 loses its capacity to attach to the antioxidant response element (ARE) sequence in antioxidant genes. Importantly, Nrf2 agonists such as lipoic acid and sulforaphane appear to reverse Nrf2's capacity to bind to the *cis*-element. Sulforaphane has been demonstrated to restore Nrf2's transactivation capacity and give cytoprotection against UVB-induced damage in human lens epithelial cells, not only by raising phase 2 enzyme expression, but also by increasing the antioxidant enzyme catalase. The recovery of Nrf2 activity in aged cells and cells exposed to UVB proves that sulforaphane is a natural chemical with major preventive and therapeutic properties [218].

Ginseng

Ginseng is utilised as an active ingredient in herbal cosmetics and has a presence in the worldwide market as a health food. Ginseng's main active ingredients are ginsenosides, a varied collection of steroidal saponins that let ginseng target a wide range of tissues. Other active components in ginseng include phenolic compounds, polysaccharides, and proteins.Ginseng has been shown to reduce nitric oxide manufacturing and iNOS mRNA formation in HaCaT keratinocytes and human dermal fibroblasts, indicating that it has anti-inflammatory properties. Ginseng has also been shown to inhibit COX2 expression and TNF transcription in HaCaT keratinocyte cells when exposed to UVB. Atopic dermatitis (AD), a chronic and relapsing inflammatory skin disease, was recently found to be improved by ginseng extract. The mammalian target of rapamycin (mTOR)/p70 ribosomal protein S6 kinase (p70S6K) signalling pathway is known to be active in Atopic dermatitis [219, 220].

Propolis

Honeybees collect propolis, a plant resin. Propolis has been shown to provide UVR photoprotection and can be compounded to have an SPF rating comparable to several commercial agents [221]. Propolis' anti-inflammatory and antioxidant capabilities, in addition to its UV-absorbing characteristics, make it an appealing natural dermatologic solution. Propolis has been demonstrated to inhibit UVA-induced ROS generation and protect against UV-induced apoptosis in HaCaT cells [222]. Several studies using mouse and rat models have confirmed the photoprotective and anti-oxidant effects of propolis *in vivo* Propolis' anti-inflammatory properties have also been shown to be a helpful strategy for facilitating wound healing.

FUTURE DIRECTIONS

Many skin diseases, including skin cancer, are due to exposure to harmful radiation. The best sunblock should be economical, effective, and safe, with a considerable ability to block UV rays. The use of synthetic chemicals for radiation protection (oxybenzone, octinoxate, homosalate, nanoparticles, amino benzoic acid, Oxylisadimate, padimate O, roxadimate, *etc.*) could outcome in other toxic effects such as contact allergies, endocrine disruption, photoallergies, melanoma, reproductive toxicity, skin irritation, hormonal disruption, *etc.* These natural compounds have antioxidant, anti-inflammatory, anticancer and anti-aging activity to bring the homeostatic conditions to the intracellular level. Cosmetic industries are mainly focusing to trace the skin-loving products that protect our skin from harmful radiation without any side effects. Furthermore, sunscreen efficiency must be optimized by raising UV absorber skin accumulation with low absorption into the blood circulation. A thin sprayable gel comprising a film-forming polymer paired with emollients and cooling chemicals can be created to create an ideal cosmetic product. It is not impossible to identify naturally derived skincare products from natural sources, but it will take more concerted efforts.

CONCLUSION

In conclusion, the skin is the largest organ of the human body that faces environmental hazards like toxic substances, harmful radiation and eco-microbes. These agents are responsible for harmful internal fluctuations at keratinocytes like boosting ROS production, DNA damage, provoking the wrinkling of the skin, skin cancer skin allergies *via* skin-related metabolic pathways. So, nature provides a great niche for microbial as well as Phyto-based products, which have a great ability to fight against these changes without any side-effects. Researchers are seeking to develop tools for increasing the production of compounds that would be beneficial for mankind.

REFERENCES

[1]   Choi MS, Chae YJ, Choi JW, Chang JE. Potential therapeutic approaches through modulating the autophagy process for skin barrier dysfunction. Int J Mol Sci 2021; 22(15): 7869.
[http://dx.doi.org/10.3390/ijms22157869] [PMID: 34360634]

[2]   Lin TK, Zhong L, Santiago J. Anti-inflammatory and skin barrier repair effects of topical application of some plant oils. Int J Mol Sci 2017; 19(1): 70.
[http://dx.doi.org/10.3390/ijms19010070] [PMID: 29280987]

[3]   Yardman-Frank JM, Fisher DE. Skin pigmentation and its control: from ultraviolet radiation to stem cells. Exp Dermatol 2021; 30(4): 560-71.
[http://dx.doi.org/10.1111/exd.14260] [PMID: 33320376]

[4]   Ishaq AR, Younis T, Noor A, Jabeen F, Shouwen C, Eds. Natural polyphenols a new paradigm in treatment of various diseases. Polyphenols-based nanotherapeutics for cancer management. Singapore: Springer 2021; pp. 17-55.
[http://dx.doi.org/10.1007/978-981-16-4935-6_2]

[5]   Ashrafizadeh M, Ahmadi Z, Yaribeygi H, Sathyapalan T, Sahebkar A. Astaxanthin and Nrf2 signaling pathway: A novel target for new therapeutic approaches. Mini Rev Med Chem 2022; 22(2): 312-21.
[http://dx.doi.org/10.2174/1389557521666210505112834] [PMID: 33964864]

[6]   Melnikova VO, Ananthaswamy HN. Cellular and molecular events leading to the development of skin cancer. Mutat Res 2005; 571(1-2): 91-106.
[http://dx.doi.org/10.1016/j.mrfmmm.2004.11.015] [PMID: 15748641]

[7]   Duthie MS, Kimber I, Norval M. The effects of ultraviolet radiation on the human immune system. Br J Dermatol 1999; 140(6): 995-1009.
[http://dx.doi.org/10.1046/j.1365-2133.1999.02898.x] [PMID: 10354063]

[8]   Hussein MR. Ultraviolet radiation and skin cancer: molecular mechanisms. J Cutan Pathol 2005; 32(3): 191-205.
[http://dx.doi.org/10.1111/j.0303-6987.2005.00281.x] [PMID: 15701081]

[9]   Clydesdale GJ, Dandie GW, Muller HK. Ultraviolet light induced injury: Immunological and inflammatory effects. Immunol Cell Biol 2001; 79(6): 547-68.
[http://dx.doi.org/10.1046/j.1440-1711.2001.01047.x] [PMID: 11903614]

[10]   MacKie RM. Effects of ultraviolet radiation on human health. Radiat Prot Dosimetry 2000; 91(1): 15-8.
[http://dx.doi.org/10.1093/oxfordjournals.rpd.a033186]

[11]   Trautinger F. Mechanisms of photodamage of the skin and its functional consequences for skin ageing. Clin Exp Dermatol 2001; 26(7): 573-7.
[http://dx.doi.org/10.1046/j.1365-2230.2001.00893.x] [PMID: 11696060]

[12]   Heck DE, Gerecke DR, Vetrano AM, Laskin JD. Solar ultraviolet radiation as a trigger of cell signal transduction. Toxicol Appl Pharmacol 2004; 195(3): 288-97.
[http://dx.doi.org/10.1016/j.taap.2003.09.028] [PMID: 15020191]

[13]   Kulms D, Schwarz T. Molecular mechanisms of UV□induced apoptosis. Photodermatol Photoimmunol Photomed 2000; 16(5): 195-201.

[14]   Pattison DI, Davies MJ. Actions of ultraviolet light on cellular structures. EXS 2006; 96: 131-57.
[http://dx.doi.org/10.1007/3-7643-7378-4_6] [PMID: 16383017]

[15]   Horikoshi S, Sato T, Sakamoto K, Abe M, Serpone N. Microwave discharge electrodeless lamps (MDEL). Photochem Photobiol Sci 2011; 10(7): 1239-48.
[http://dx.doi.org/10.1039/c1pp05059a] [PMID: 21523270]

[16]   Oshimura E, Sakamoto K. Amino acids, peptides, and proteins. Cosmet Sci Technol Theor Princ Appl. 2017; pp. 285-303.

[17]   Kanofsky JR, Sima P. Singlet oxygen production from the reactions of ozone with biological molecules. J Biol Chem 1991; 266(14): 9039-42.
[http://dx.doi.org/10.1016/S0021-9258(18)31548-5] [PMID: 2026612]

[18]   Thiele J, Elsner P. Oxidants and antioxidants in cutaneous biology. Karger Medical and Scientific Publishers, 2001.

[19]   Youssef NA, Shaban SA, Ibrahim FA, Mahmoud AS. Degradation of methyl orange using Fenton catalytic reaction. Egypt J Pet 2016; 25(3): 317-21.
[http://dx.doi.org/10.1016/j.ejpe.2015.07.017]

[20]   Banerjee N, Chakraborty A, Lahiri A, Biswas K. Exclusive breast feeding reduces diarrhoeal episodes among children: Results from a cross-sectional study among the mothers of under-five children in Kolkata. Int J Commun Med Public Health 2019; 6(2): 733-7.
[http://dx.doi.org/10.18203/2394-6040.ijcmph20190199]

[21]   Yang GP, Zhao XK, Sun XJ, Lu XL. Oxidative degradation of diethyl phthalate by photochemically-enhanced Fenton reaction. J Hazard Mater 2005; 126(1-3): 112-8.
[http://dx.doi.org/10.1016/j.jhazmat.2005.06.014] [PMID: 16051432]

[22]   Pillai S, Oresajo C, Hayward J. Ultraviolet radiation and skin aging: roles of reactive oxygen species, inflammation and protease activation, and strategies for prevention of inflammation-induced matrix degradation : A review. Int J Cosmet Sci 2005; 27(1): 17-34.
[http://dx.doi.org/10.1111/j.1467-2494.2004.00241.x] [PMID: 18492178]

[23]   Takashima A, Bergstresser PR. Impact of UVB radiation on the epidermal cytokine network. Photochem Photobiol 1996; 63(4): 397-400.
[http://dx.doi.org/10.1111/j.1751-1097.1996.tb03054.x] [PMID: 8934748]

[24]   Clingen PH, Arlett CF, Roza L, Mori T, Nikaido O, Green MHL. Induction of cyclobutane pyrimidine dimers, pyrimidine(6-4)pyrimidone photoproducts, and Dewar valence isomers by natural sunlight in normal human mononuclear cells. Cancer Res 1995; 55(11): 2245-8.
[PMID: 7757971]

[25]   Tornaletti S, Pfeifer GP. UV damage and repair mechanisms in mammalian cells. BioEssays 1996; 18(3): 221-8.
[http://dx.doi.org/10.1002/bies.950180309] [PMID: 8867736]

[26]   Ichihashi M, Ueda M, Budiyanto A, *et al.* UV-induced skin damage. Toxicology 2003; 189(1-2): 21-39.
[http://dx.doi.org/10.1016/S0300-483X(03)00150-1] [PMID: 12821280]

[27]   Mouret S, Baudouin C, Charveron M, Favier A, Cadet J, Douki T. Cyclobutane pyrimidine dimers are predominant DNA lesions in whole human skin exposed to UVA radiation. Proc Natl Acad Sci USA 2006; 103(37): 13765-70.
[http://dx.doi.org/10.1073/pnas.0604213103] [PMID: 16954188]

[28]   Peak JG, Peak MJ. Induction of slowly developing alkali-labile sites in human P3 cell DNA by UVA and blue- and green-light photons: action spectrum. Photochem Photobiol 1995; 61(5): 484-7.
[http://dx.doi.org/10.1111/j.1751-1097.1995.tb02349.x] [PMID: 7770511]

[29]   Peak MJ, Peak JG. Cellular effects of UVA: DNA damages Photobiology. Springer 1991; pp. 855-9.

[30]   Cooke MS, Mistry N, Ladapo A, Herbert KE, Lunec J. Immunochemical quantitation of UV-induced oxidative and dimeric DNA damage to human keratinocytes. Free Radic Res 2000; 33(4): 369-81.
[http://dx.doi.org/10.1080/10715760000300911] [PMID: 11022846]

[31]   Dahle J, Kvam E. Induction of delayed mutations and chromosomal instability in fibroblasts after UVA-, UVB-, and X-radiation. Cancer Res 2003; 63(7): 1464-9.
[PMID: 12670891]

[32]   Erden Inal M, Kahraman A, Köken T. Beneficial effects of quercetin on oxidative stress induced by

ultraviolet A. Clin Exp Dermatol 2001; 26(6): 536-9.
[http://dx.doi.org/10.1046/j.1365-2230.2001.00884.x] [PMID: 11678884]

[33]   Afaq F, Mukhtar H. Photochemoprevention by botanical antioxidants. Skin Pharmacol Physiol 2002; 15(5): 297-306.
[http://dx.doi.org/10.1159/000064533] [PMID: 12239423]

[34]   Sander CS, Chang H, Hamm F, Elsner P, Thiele JJ. Role of oxidative stress and the antioxidant network in cutaneous carcinogenesis. Int J Dermatol 2004; 43(5): 326-35.
[http://dx.doi.org/10.1111/j.1365-4632.2004.02222.x] [PMID: 15117361]

[35]   Halliday GM. Inflammation, gene mutation and photoimmunosuppression in response to UVR-induced oxidative damage contributes to photocarcinogenesis. Mutat Res 2005; 571(1-2): 107-20.
[http://dx.doi.org/10.1016/j.mrfmmm.2004.09.013] [PMID: 15748642]

[36]   Pinnell SR. Cutaneous photodamage, oxidative stress, and topical antioxidant protection. J Am Acad Dermatol 2003; 48(1): 1-22.
[http://dx.doi.org/10.1067/mjd.2003.16] [PMID: 12522365]

[37]   Nishigori C, Hattori Y, Toyokuni S. Role of reactive oxygen species in skin carcinogenesis. Antioxid Redox Signal 2004; 6(3): 561-70.
[http://dx.doi.org/10.1089/152308604773934314] [PMID: 15130282]

[38]   Lipczynska-Kochany E, Sprah G, Harms S. Influence of some groundwater and surface waters constituents on the degradation of 4-chlorophenol by the Fenton reaction. Chemosphere 1995; 30(1): 9-20.
[http://dx.doi.org/10.1016/0045-6535(94)00371-Z] [PMID: 22454978]

[39]   Lee JL, Mukhtar H, Bickers DR, Kopelovich L, Athar M. Cyclooxygenases in the skin: pharmacological and toxicological implications. Toxicol Appl Pharmacol 2003; 192(3): 294-306.
[http://dx.doi.org/10.1016/S0041-008X(03)00301-6] [PMID: 14575647]

[40]   Mahns A, Wolber R, Stäb F, Klotz LO, Sies H. Contribution of UVB and UVA to UV-dependent stimulation of cyclooxygenase-2 expression in artificial epidermis. Photochem Photobiol Sci 2004; 3(3): 257-62.
[http://dx.doi.org/10.1039/b309067a] [PMID: 14993941]

[41]   Allanson M, Reeve VE. Ultraviolet A (320-400nm) modulation of ultraviolet B (290-320nm)-induced immune suppression is mediated by carbon monoxide. J Invest Dermatol 2005; 124(3): 644-50.
[http://dx.doi.org/10.1111/j.0022-202X.2005.23614.x] [PMID: 15737207]

[42]   Basu-Modak S, Lüscher P, Tyrrell RM. Lipid metabolite involvement in the activation of the human heme oxygenase-1 gene. Free Radic Biol Med 1996; 20(7): 887-97.
[http://dx.doi.org/10.1016/0891-5849(95)02182-5] [PMID: 8743975]

[43]   Tyrrell RM. Solar ultraviolet A radiation: an oxidizing skin carcinogen that activates heme oxygenase-1. Antioxid Redox Signal 2004; 6(5): 835-40.
[PMID: 15345143]

[44]   Hillebrand GG, Winslow MS, Benzinger MJ, Heitmeyer DA, Bissett DL. Acute and chronic ultraviolet radiation induction of epidermal ornithine decarboxylase activity in hairless mice. Cancer Res 1990; 50(5): 1580-4.
[PMID: 2302717]

[45]   Katiyar SK, Mukhtar H, Matsui MS. Ultraviolet-B exposure of human skin induces cytochromes P450 1A1 and 1B1. J Invest Dermatol 2000; 114(2): 328-33.
[http://dx.doi.org/10.1046/j.1523-1747.2000.00876.x] [PMID: 10651994]

[46]   Villard PH, Sampol E, Elkaim JL, *et al.* Increase of CYP1B1 transcription in human keratinocytes and HaCaT cells after UV-B exposure. Toxicol Appl Pharmacol 2002; 178(3): 137-43.
[http://dx.doi.org/10.1006/taap.2001.9335] [PMID: 11858729]

[47]   Grandjean-Laquerriere A, Le Naour R, Gangloff SC, Guenounou M. Differential regulation of TNF-α,

IL-6 and IL-10 in UVB-irradiated human keratinocytes *via* cyclic AMP/protein kinase A pathway. Cytokine 2003; 23(4-5): 138-49.
[http://dx.doi.org/10.1016/S1043-4666(03)00224-2] [PMID: 12967650]

[48]   Lavker RM, Gerberick GF, Veres D, Irwin CJ, Kaidbey KH. Cumulative effects from repeated exposures to suberythemal doses of UVB and UVA in human skin. J Am Acad Dermatol 1995; 32(1): 53-62.
[http://dx.doi.org/10.1016/0190-9622(95)90184-1] [PMID: 7822517]

[49]   Matsumura Y, Ananthaswamy HN. Toxic effects of ultraviolet radiation on the skin. Toxicol Appl Pharmacol 2004; 195(3): 298-308.
[http://dx.doi.org/10.1016/j.taap.2003.08.019] [PMID: 15020192]

[50]   Chamcheu JC, Walker AL, Noubissi FK. Natural and Synthetic Bioactives for Skin Health, Disease and Management. Multidisciplinary Digital Publishing Institute 2021; p. 4383.

[51]   Lee AY. Skin Pigmentation Abnormalities and Their Possible Relationship with Skin Aging. Int J Mol Sci 2021; 22(7): 3727.
[http://dx.doi.org/10.3390/ijms22073727] [PMID: 33918445]

[52]   Ito S, Wakamatsu K, Sarna T. Photodegradation of eumelanin and pheomelanin and its pathophysiological implications. Photochem Photobiol 2018; 94(3): 409-20.
[http://dx.doi.org/10.1111/php.12837] [PMID: 28873228]

[53]   Onkoksoong T, Jeayeng S, Poungvarin N, *et al.* Thai herbal antipyretic 22 formula (APF22) inhibits UVA-mediated melanogenesis through activation of Nrf2-regulated antioxidant defense. Phytother Res 2018; 32(8): 1546-54.
[http://dx.doi.org/10.1002/ptr.6083] [PMID: 29672960]

[54]   Nahhas AF, Abdel-Malek ZA, Kohli I, Braunberger TL, Lim HW, Hamzavi IH. The potential role of antioxidants in mitigating skin hyperpigmentation resulting from ultraviolet and visible light-induced oxidative stress. Photodermatol Photoimmunol Photomed 2019; 35(6): 420-8.
[http://dx.doi.org/10.1111/phpp.12423] [PMID: 30198587]

[55]   Solano F. Photoprotection and skin pigmentation: Melanin-related molecules and some other new agents obtained from natural sources. Molecules 2020; 25(7): 1537.
[http://dx.doi.org/10.3390/molecules25071537] [PMID: 32230973]

[56]   Solano F. Photoprotection *versus* photodamage: updating an old but still unsolved controversy about melanin. Polym Int 2016; 65(11): 1276-87.
[http://dx.doi.org/10.1002/pi.5117]

[57]   Tatalovich Z, Wilson JP, Mack T, Yan Y, Cockburn M. The objective assessment of lifetime cumulative ultraviolet exposure for determining melanoma risk. J Photochem Photobiol B 2006; 85(3): 198-204.
[http://dx.doi.org/10.1016/j.jphotobiol.2006.08.002] [PMID: 16963272]

[58]   Qureshi AA, Laden F, Colditz GA, Hunter DJ. Geographic variation and risk of skin cancer in US women. Differences between melanoma, squamous cell carcinoma, and basal cell carcinoma. Arch Intern Med 2008; 168(5): 501-7.
[http://dx.doi.org/10.1001/archinte.168.5.501] [PMID: 18332296]

[59]   Solano F. On the metal cofactor in the tyrosinase family. Int J Mol Sci 2018; 19(2): 633.
[http://dx.doi.org/10.3390/ijms19020633] [PMID: 29473882]

[60]   Lai X, Wichers HJ, Soler-López M, Dijkstra BW. Phenylthiourea binding to human tyrosinase-related protein 1. Int J Mol Sci 2020; 21(3): 915.
[http://dx.doi.org/10.3390/ijms21030915] [PMID: 32019241]

[61]   Xiao M, Chen W, Li W, *et al.* Elucidation of the hierarchical structure of natural eumelanins. J R Soc Interface 2018; 15(140): 20180045.
[http://dx.doi.org/10.1098/rsif.2018.0045] [PMID: 29514988]

[62]   Napolitano A, Panzella L, Monfrecola G, d'Ischia M. Pheomelanin-induced oxidative stress: bright
        and dark chemistry bridging red hair phenotype and melanoma. Pigment Cell Melanoma Res 2014;
        27(5): 721-33.
        [http://dx.doi.org/10.1111/pcmr.12262] [PMID: 24814217]

[63]   D'Orazio J, Jarrett S, Amaro-Ortiz A, Scott T. UV radiation and the skin. Int J Mol Sci 2013; 14(6):
        12222-48.
        [http://dx.doi.org/10.3390/ijms140612222] [PMID: 23749111]

[64]   Geoffrey K, Mwangi AN, Maru SM. Sunscreen products: Rationale for use, formulation development
        and regulatory considerations. Saudi Pharm J 2019; 27(7): 1009-18.
        [http://dx.doi.org/10.1016/j.jsps.2019.08.003] [PMID: 31997908]

[65]   Suh SS, Hwang J, Park M, *et al.* Anti-inflammation activities of mycosporine-like amino acids
        (MAAs) in response to UV radiation suggest potential anti-skin aging activity. Mar Drugs 2014;
        12(10): 5174-87.
        [http://dx.doi.org/10.3390/md12105174] [PMID: 25317535]

[66]   Davinelli S, Nielsen M, Scapagnini G. Astaxanthin in skin health, repair, and disease: A
        comprehensive review. Nutrients 2018; 10(4): 522.
        [http://dx.doi.org/10.3390/nu10040522] [PMID: 29690549]

[67]   Juturu V, Bowman J, Deshpande J. Overall skin tone and skin-lightening-improving effects with oral
        supplementation of lutein and zeaxanthin isomers: a double-blind, placebo-controlled clinical trial.
        Clin Cosmet Investig Dermatol 2016; 9: 325-32.
        [http://dx.doi.org/10.2147/CCID.S115519] [PMID: 27785083]

[68]   Murillo AG, Hu S, Fernandez ML. Zeaxanthin: Metabolism, properties, and antioxidant protection of
        eyes, heart, liver, and skin. Antioxidants 2019; 8(9): 390.
        [http://dx.doi.org/10.3390/antiox8090390] [PMID: 31514298]

[69]   Sun G, Mao JJ. Engineering dextran-based scaffolds for drug delivery and tissue repair. Nanomedicine
        2012; 7(11): 1771-84.
        [http://dx.doi.org/10.2217/nnm.12.149] [PMID: 23210716]

[70]   Bark BP, Gründe PO. Infusion rate and plasma volume expansion of dextran and albumin in the septic
        guinea pig. Acta Anaesthesiol Scand 2014; 58(1): 44-51.
        [http://dx.doi.org/10.1111/aas.12228] [PMID: 24251847]

[71]   Hudita A, Galateanu B, Costache M, *et al. In Vitro* cytotoxic protective effect of alginate-encapsulated
        capsaicin might improve skin side effects associated with the topical application of capsaicin.
        Molecules 2021; 26(5): 1455.
        [http://dx.doi.org/10.3390/molecules26051455] [PMID: 33800110]

[72]   Xing M, Cao Q, Wang Y, *et al.* Advances in research on the bioactivity of alginate oligosaccharides.
        Mar Drugs 2020; 18(3): 144.
        [http://dx.doi.org/10.3390/md18030144] [PMID: 32121067]

[73]   Pagano C, Puglia D, Luzi F, *et al.* Development and characterization of xanthan gum and alginate
        based bioadhesive film for pycnogenol topical use in wound treatment. Pharmaceutics 2021; 13(3):
        324.
        [http://dx.doi.org/10.3390/pharmaceutics13030324] [PMID: 33802607]

[74]   Pangestuti R, Kurnianto D. Green seaweeds-derived polysaccharides ulvan: occurrence, medicinal
        value and potential applications. In: Seaweed Polysaccharides. Elsevier 2017; pp. 205-21
        [http://dx.doi.org/10.1016/B978-0-12-809816-5.00011-6]

[75]   Papakonstantinou E, Roth M, Karakiulakis G. Hyaluronic acid: A key molecule in skin aging.
        Dermatoendocrinol 2012; 4(3): 253-8.
        [http://dx.doi.org/10.4161/derm.21923] [PMID: 23467280]

[76]   Sekhon Randhawa KK, Rahman PKSM. Rhamnolipid biosurfactants—past, present, and future

scenario of global market. Front Microbiol 2014; 5: 454.
[http://dx.doi.org/10.3389/fmicb.2014.00454] [PMID: 25228898]

[77]   Morita T, Fukuoka T, Imura T, Kitamoto D. Production of mannosylerythritol lipids and their application in cosmetics. Appl Microbiol Biotechnol 2013; 97(11): 4691-700.
[http://dx.doi.org/10.1007/s00253-013-4858-1] [PMID: 23584242]

[78]   Nitschke M, Costa SGVAO. Biosurfactants in food industry. Trends Food Sci Technol 2007; 18(5): 252-9.
[http://dx.doi.org/10.1016/j.tifs.2007.01.002]

[79]   Ueno Y, Hirashima N, Inoh Y, Furuno T, Nakanishi M. Characterization of biosurfactant-containing liposomes and their efficiency for gene transfection. Biol Pharm Bull 2007; 30(1): 169-72.
[http://dx.doi.org/10.1248/bpb.30.169] [PMID: 17202680]

[80]   Villeneuve P. Lipases in lipophilization reactions. Biotechnol Adv 2007; 25(6): 515-36.
[http://dx.doi.org/10.1016/j.biotechadv.2007.06.001] [PMID: 17681737]

[81]   Gupta PL, Rajput M, Oza T, Trivedi U, Sanghvi G. Eminence of microbial products in cosmetic industry. Nat Prod Bioprospect 2019; 9(4): 267-78.
[http://dx.doi.org/10.1007/s13659-019-0215-0] [PMID: 31214881]

[82]   Carrillo C, Teruel JA, Aranda FJ, Ortiz A. Molecular mechanism of membrane permeabilization by the peptide antibiotic surfactin. Biochim Biophys Acta Biomembr 2003; 1611(1-2): 91-7.
[http://dx.doi.org/10.1016/S0005-2736(03)00029-4] [PMID: 12659949]

[83]   Singh P, Patil Y, Rale V. Biosurfactant production: emerging trends and promising strategies. J Appl Microbiol 2019; 126(1): 2-13.
[http://dx.doi.org/10.1111/jam.14057] [PMID: 30066414]

[84]   Yildiz H, Karatas N. Microbial exopolysaccharides: resources and bioactive properties. Process Biochem 2018; 72: 41-6.
[http://dx.doi.org/10.1016/j.procbio.2018.06.009]

[85]   Wang Z, Wu J, Zhu L, Zhan X. Characterization of xanthan gum produced from glycerol by a mutant strain Xanthomonas campestris CCTCC M2015714. Carbohydr Polym 2017; 157: 521-6.
[http://dx.doi.org/10.1016/j.carbpol.2016.10.033] [PMID: 27987957]

[86]   Bilanovic D, Starosvetsky J, Armon RH. Preparation of biodegradable xanthan–glycerol hydrogel, foam, film, aerogel and xerogel at room temperature. Carbohydr Polym 2016; 148: 243-50.
[http://dx.doi.org/10.1016/j.carbpol.2016.04.058] [PMID: 27185137]

[87]   Kumar A, Rao KM, Han SS. Application of xanthan gum as polysaccharide in tissue engineering: a review. Carbohydr Polym 2018; 180: 128-44.
[http://dx.doi.org/10.1016/j.carbpol.2017.10.009] [PMID: 29103488]

[88]   Sze JH, Brownlie JC, Love CA. 2016.

[89]   Izawa N, Serata M, Sone T, Omasa T, Ohtake H. Hyaluronic acid production by recombinant Streptococcus thermophilus. J Biosci Bioeng 2011; 111(6): 665-70.
[http://dx.doi.org/10.1016/j.jbiosc.2011.02.005] [PMID: 21371932]

[90]   Del Valle EMM. Cyclodextrins and their uses: a review. Process Biochem 2004; 39(9): 1033-46.
[http://dx.doi.org/10.1016/S0032-9592(03)00258-9]

[91]   Buschmann H-J, Schollmeyer E. Applications of cyclodextrins in cosmetic products: a review. J Cosmet Sci 2002; 53(3): 185-91.
[PMID: 12053209]

[92]   Kato T, Horikoshi K. A new. GAMMA.-cyclodextrin forming enzyme produced by *Bacillus subtilis* No. 313. J Jap Soc Starch Sci 1986; 33(2): 137-43.
[http://dx.doi.org/10.5458/jag1972.33.137]

[93]   Kim MH, Sohn CB, Oh TK. Cloning and sequencing of a cyclodextrin glycosyltransferase gene from

Brevibacillus brevis CD162 and its expression in *Escherichia coli*. FEMS Microbiol Lett 1998; 164(2): 411-8.
[http://dx.doi.org/10.1111/j.1574-6968.1998.tb13117.x] [PMID: 9682490]

[94]   Mori S, Oya T, Kitahata S. Properties and applications of γ-cyclodextrin glucanotransferase from brevibacterium sp. No. 9605. J Appl Glycosci 1997; 44(2): 185-94.

[95]   Rajput KN, Patel KC, Trivedi UB. A novel cyclodextrin glucanotransferase from an alkaliphile Microbacterium terrae KNR 9: purification and properties. 3 Biotech 2016; 6(2): 168.
[http://dx.doi.org/10.1007/s13205-016-0495-6] [PMID: 28330240]

[96]   Martins RF, Hatti-Kaul R. A new cyclodextrin glycosyltransferase from an alkaliphilic Bacillus agaradhaerens isolate: purification and characterisation. Enzyme Microb Technol 2002; 30(1): 116-24.
[http://dx.doi.org/10.1016/S0141-0229(01)00461-6]

[97]   Lods LM, Dres C, Johnson C, Scholz DB, Brooks GJ. The future of enzymes in cosmetics. Int J Cosmet Sci 2000; 22(2): 85-94.
[http://dx.doi.org/10.1046/j.1467-2494.2000.00012.x] [PMID: 18503464]

[98]   Lin X, Lee CG, Casale ES, Shih JCH. Purification and characterization of a keratinase from a feather-degrading Bacillus licheniformis strain. Appl Environ Microbiol 1992; 58(10): 3271-5.
[http://dx.doi.org/10.1128/aem.58.10.3271-3275.1992] [PMID: 16348784]

[99]   Gherbawy YAMH, Maghraby TA, El-Sharony HM, Hussein MA. Diversity of keratinophilic fungi on human hairs and nails at four governorates in upper egypt. Mycobiology 2006; 34(4): 180-4.
[http://dx.doi.org/10.4489/MYCO.2006.34.4.180] [PMID: 24039495]

[100]   Secchi G. Role of protein in cosmetics. Clin Dermatol 2008; 26(4): 321-5.
[http://dx.doi.org/10.1016/j.clindermatol.2008.04.004] [PMID: 18691510]

[101]   R G, Q B, P L. Bacterial alkaline proteases: molecular approaches and industrial applications. Appl Microbiol Biotechnol 2002; 59(1): 15-32.
[http://dx.doi.org/10.1007/s00253-002-0975-y] [PMID: 12073127]

[102]   Watanabe K. Collagenolytic proteases from bacteria. Appl Microbiol Biotechnol 2004; 63(5): 520-6.
[http://dx.doi.org/10.1007/s00253-003-1442-0] [PMID: 14556041]

[103]   Robinson LR, Fitzgerald NC, Doughty DG, Dawes NC, Berge CA, Bissett DL. Topical palmitoyl pentapeptide provides improvement in photoaged human facial skin1. Int J Cosmet Sci 2005; 27(3): 155-60.
[http://dx.doi.org/10.1111/j.1467-2494.2005.00261.x] [PMID: 18492182]

[104]   Guiry MD. How many species of algae are there? J Phycol 2012; 48(5): 1057-63.
[http://dx.doi.org/10.1111/j.1529-8817.2012.01222.x] [PMID: 27011267]

[105]   Wang T, Tian X, Liu T, *et al.* A two-stage fed-batch heterotrophic culture of Chlorella protothecoides that combined nitrogen depletion with hyperosmotic stress strategy enhanced lipid yield and productivity. Process Biochem 2017; 60: 74-83.
[http://dx.doi.org/10.1016/j.procbio.2017.05.027]

[106]   Babitha S, Kim E-K. Effect of marine cosmeceuticals on the pigmentation of skin. In: Marine Cosmeceuticals: Trends and Prospects. Taylors and Francis 2016; p. 63.

[107]   Yang G, Cozad MA, Holland DA, Zhang Y, Luesch H, Ding Y. Photosynthetic production of sunscreen shinorine using an engineered cyanobacterium. ACS Synth Biol 2018; 7(2): 664-71.
[http://dx.doi.org/10.1021/acssynbio.7b00397] [PMID: 29304277]

[108]   Davis TE III, Kurtz PF, Gardner AW, Carman NB. Cognitive-behavioral treatment for specific phobias with a child demonstrating severe problem behavior and developmental delays. Res Dev Disabil 2007; 28(6): 546-58.
[http://dx.doi.org/10.1016/j.ridd.2006.07.003] [PMID: 16950598]

[109]   Heo SJ, Ko SC, Cha SH, et al. Effect of phlorotannins isolated from Ecklonia cava on melanogenesis

and their protective effect against photo-oxidative stress induced by UV-B radiation. Toxicol *In Vitro* 2009; 23(6): 1123-30.
[http://dx.doi.org/10.1016/j.tiv.2009.05.013] [PMID: 19490939]

[110] Hyun YJ, Piao MJ, Ko MH, *et al.* Photoprotective effect of Undaria crenata against ultraviolet B-induced damage to keratinocytes. J Biosci Bioeng 2013; 116(2): 256-64.
[http://dx.doi.org/10.1016/j.jbiosc.2013.02.003] [PMID: 23474096]

[111] Hur S, Lee H, Kim Y, Lee BH, Shin J, Kim TY. Sargaquinoic acid and sargachromenol, extracts of *Sargassum sagamianum,* induce apoptosis in HaCaT cells and mice skin: Its potentiation of UVB-induced apoptosis. Eur J Pharmacol 2008; 582(1-3): 1-11.
[http://dx.doi.org/10.1016/j.ejphar.2007.12.025] [PMID: 18243174]

[112] Bedoux G, Hardouin K, Burlot AS, Bourgougnon N. Bioactive components from seaweeds: cosmetic applications and future development. Adv Bot Res 2014; 71: 345-78.
[http://dx.doi.org/10.1016/B978-0-12-408062-1.00012-3]

[113] Henríquez V, Escobar C, Galarza J, Gimpel J. Carotenoids in microalgae. Subcell Biochem 2016; 79: 219-37.
[http://dx.doi.org/10.1007/978-3-319-39126-7_8] [PMID: 27485224]

[114] Rastogi RP, Incharoensakdi A. Characterization of UV-screening compounds, mycosporine-like amino acids, and scytonemin in the cyanobacterium *Lyngbya* sp. CU2555. FEMS Microbiol Ecol 2014; 87(1): 244-56.
[http://dx.doi.org/10.1111/1574-6941.12220] [PMID: 24111939]

[115] Kim S-K. Marine cosmeceuticals: trends and prospects. CRC Press 2011.

[116] Miko Enomoto T, Johnson T, Peterson N, Homer L, Walts D, Johnson N. Combination glutathione and anthocyanins as an alternative for skin care during external-beam radiation. Am J Surg 2005; 189(5): 627-31.
[http://dx.doi.org/10.1016/j.amjsurg.2005.02.001] [PMID: 15862509]

[117] Yoon NY, Eom TK, Kim MM, Kim SK. Inhibitory effect of phlorotannins isolated from Ecklonia cava on mushroom tyrosinase activity and melanin formation in mouse B16F10 melanoma cells. J Agric Food Chem 2009; 57(10): 4124-9.
[http://dx.doi.org/10.1021/jf900006f] [PMID: 19361156]

[118] Shen CT, Chen PY, Wu JJ, *et al.* Purification of algal anti-tyrosinase zeaxanthin from Nannochloropsis oculata using supercritical anti-solvent precipitation. J Supercrit Fluids 2011; 55(3): 955-62.
[http://dx.doi.org/10.1016/j.supflu.2010.10.003]

[119] Fitton J, Dell'Acqua G, Gardiner VA, Karpiniec S, Stringer D, Davis E. Topical benefits of two fucoidan-rich extracts from marine macroalgae. Cosmetics 2015; 2(2): 66-81.
[http://dx.doi.org/10.3390/cosmetics2020066]

[120] Bari E, Arciola C, Vigani B, *et al. In vitro* effectiveness of microspheres based on silk sericin and Chlorella vulgaris or Arthrospira platensis for wound healing applications. Materials (Basel) 2017; 10(9): 983.
[http://dx.doi.org/10.3390/ma10090983] [PMID: 28832540]

[121] Bak SS, Sung YK, Kim SK. 7-Phloroeckol promotes hair growth on human follicles *in vitro.* Naunyn Schmiedebergs Arch Pharmacol 2014; 387(8): 789-93.
[http://dx.doi.org/10.1007/s00210-014-0986-0] [PMID: 24833298]

[122] Shibata T, Ishimaru K, Kawaguchi S, Yoshikawa H, Hama Y, Eds. Antioxidant activities of phlorotannins isolated from Japanese Laminariaceae. Springer 2007.

[123] Wang HMD, Chen CC, Huynh P, Chang JS. Exploring the potential of using algae in cosmetics. Bioresour Technol 2015; 184: 355-62.
[http://dx.doi.org/10.1016/j.biortech.2014.12.001] [PMID: 25537136]

[124] Pimentel FB, Alves RC, Harnedy PA, FitzGerald RJ, Oliveira MBPP. Macroalgal-derived protein hydrolysates and bioactive peptides: Enzymatic release and potential health enhancing properties. Trends Food Sci Technol 2019; 93: 106-24.
[http://dx.doi.org/10.1016/j.tifs.2019.09.006]

[125] Ariede MB, Candido TM, Jacome ALM, Velasco MVR, de Carvalho JCM, Baby AR. Cosmetic attributes of algae - A review. Algal Res 2017; 25: 483-7.
[http://dx.doi.org/10.1016/j.algal.2017.05.019]

[126] Blackwell M. The Fungi: 1, 2, 3 … 5.1 million species? Am J Bot 2011; 98(3): 426-38.
[http://dx.doi.org/10.3732/ajb.1000298] [PMID: 21613136]

[127] Kumari M, Survase SA, Singhal RS. Production of schizophyllan using *Schizophyllum commune* NRCM. Bioresour Technol 2008; 99(5): 1036-43.
[http://dx.doi.org/10.1016/j.biortech.2007.02.029] [PMID: 17446065]

[128] Gautier S, Xhauflaire-Uhoda E, Gonry P, Piérard GE. Chitin-glucan, a natural cell scaffold for skin moisturization and rejuvenation. Int J Cosmet Sci 2008; 30(6): 459-69.
[http://dx.doi.org/10.1111/j.1468-2494.2008.00470.x] [PMID: 19099547]

[129] Jiang MY, Feng T, Liu JK. *N-Containing* compounds of macromycetes. Nat Prod Rep 2011; 28(4): 783-808.
[http://dx.doi.org/10.1039/c0np00006j] [PMID: 21305063]

[130] Prasad R, Koul A, Mukherjee PK, Ghannoum MA. Lipids of *Candida albicans* lipids of pathogenic fungi. CRC Press 2017; pp. 105-38.

[131] Rampler E, Criscuolo A, Zeller M, *et al.* A novel lipidomics workflow for improved human plasma identification and quantification using RPLC-MSn methods and isotope dilution strategies. Anal Chem 2018; 90(11): 6494-501.
[http://dx.doi.org/10.1021/acs.analchem.7b05382] [PMID: 29708737]

[132] Hyde KD, Bahkali AH, Moslem MA. Fungi—an unusual source for cosmetics. Fungal Divers 2010; 43(1): 1-9.
[http://dx.doi.org/10.1007/s13225-010-0043-3]

[133] Wilkerson EC, Goldberg DJ. Poly-L-lactic acid for the Improvement of photodamage and rhytids of the décolletage. J Cosmet Dermatol 2018; 17(4): 606-10.
[http://dx.doi.org/10.1111/jocd.12447] [PMID: 29119683]

[134] Dubost NJ, Beelman RB, Royse DJ. Influence of selected cultural factors and postharvest storage on ergothioneine content of common button mushroom *Agaricus bisporus* (J. Lge) Imbach (Agaricomycetideae). Int J Med Mushrooms 2007; 9(2): 163-76.
[http://dx.doi.org/10.1615/IntJMedMushr.v9.i2.70]

[135] Fang SH, Rao YK, Tzeng YM. Anti-oxidant and inflammatory mediator's growth inhibitory effects of compounds isolated from Phyllanthus urinaria. J Ethnopharmacol 2008; 116(2): 333-40.
[http://dx.doi.org/10.1016/j.jep.2007.11.040] [PMID: 18187278]

[136] Ventura J, Belmares R, Aguilera-Carbo A, Gutiérrez-Sanchez G, Rodríguez-Herrera R, Aguilar CN. Fungal biodegradation of tannins from creosote bush (*Larrea tridentata*) and tar bush (*Fluorensia cernua*) for gallic and ellagic acid production. Food Technol Biotechnol 2008; 46(2): 213-7.

[137] Dweck A. Herbal medicine for the skin.Their chemistry and effects on skin and mucous membranes. J Appl Cosmetol 2002; 20(1): 83.

[138] Barcroft A, Myskja A. Aloe vera: Nature's silent healer. AlasdairAloeVera; 2003.

[139] Gil MI, Tomás-Barberán FA, Hess-Pierce B, Holcroft DM, Kader AA. Antioxidant activity of pomegranate juice and its relationship with phenolic composition and processing. J Agric Food Chem 2000; 48(10): 4581-9.
[http://dx.doi.org/10.1021/jf000404a] [PMID: 11052704]

[140] Syed DN, Malik A, Hadi N, Sarfaraz S, Afaq F, Mukhtar H. Photochemopreventive effect of pomegranate fruit extract on UVA-mediated activation of cellular pathways in normal human epidermal keratinocytes. Photochem Photobiol 2006; 82(2): 398-405.
[http://dx.doi.org/10.1562/2005-06-23-RA-589] [PMID: 16613491]

[141] Afaq F, Malik A, Syed D, Maes D, Matsui MS, Mukhtar H. Pomegranate fruit extract modulates UV-B-mediated phosphorylation of mitogen-activated protein kinases and activation of nuclear factor kappa B in normal human epidermal keratinocytes paragraph sign. Photochem Photobiol 2005; 81(1): 38-45.
[http://dx.doi.org/10.1562/2004-08-06-RA-264.1] [PMID: 15493960]

[142] Hora JJ, Maydew ER, Lansky EP, Dwivedi C. Chemopreventive effects of pomegranate seed oil on skin tumor development in CD1 mice. J Med Food 2003; 6(3): 157-61.
[http://dx.doi.org/10.1089/10966200360716553] [PMID: 14585180]

[143] Mantena SK, Meeran SM, Elmets CA, Katiyar SK. Orally administered green tea polyphenols prevent ultraviolet radiation-induced skin cancer in mice through activation of cytotoxic T cells and inhibition of angiogenesis in tumors. J Nutr 2005; 135(12): 2871-7.
[http://dx.doi.org/10.1093/jn/135.12.2871] [PMID: 16317135]

[144] Singh T, Katiyar SK. Green tea polyphenol, (−)-epigallocatechin-3-gallate, induces toxicity in human skin cancer cells by targeting β-catenin signaling. Toxicol Appl Pharmacol 2013; 273(2): 418-24.
[http://dx.doi.org/10.1016/j.taap.2013.09.021] [PMID: 24096034]

[145] Janjua R, Munoz C, Gorell E, *et al.* A two-year, double-blind, randomized placebo-controlled trial of oral green tea polyphenols on the long-term clinical and histologic appearance of photoaging skin. Dermatol Surg 2009; 35(7): 1057-65.
[http://dx.doi.org/10.1111/j.1524-4725.2009.01183.x] [PMID: 19469799]

[146] Heinrich U, Moore CE, De Spirt S, Tronnier H, Stahl W. Green tea polyphenols provide photoprotection, increase microcirculation, and modulate skin properties of women. J Nutr 2011; 141(6): 1202-8.
[http://dx.doi.org/10.3945/jn.110.136465] [PMID: 21525260]

[147] Raab WP, Tronnier H, Wiskemann A. Photoprotection and skin coloring by oral carotenoids. Dermatology 1985; 171(5): 371-3.
[http://dx.doi.org/10.1159/000249456] [PMID: 3935496]

[148] Alemzadeh R, Feehan T. Variable effects of beta-carotene therapy in a child with erythropoietic protoporphyria. Eur J Pediatr 2004; 163(9): 547-9.
[http://dx.doi.org/10.1007/s00431-004-1453-6] [PMID: 15241683]

[149] Rizwan M, Rodriguez-Blanco I, Harbottle A, Birch-Machin MA, Watson REB, Rhodes LE. Tomato paste rich in lycopene protects against cutaneous photodamage in humans *in vivo*: a randomized controlled trial. Br J Dermatol 2011; 164(1): 154-62.
[http://dx.doi.org/10.1111/j.1365-2133.2010.10057.x] [PMID: 20854436]

[150] Carini M, Aldini G, Orioli M, Facino RM. Antioxidant and photoprotective activity of a lipophilic extract containing neolignans from Krameria triandra roots. Planta Med 2002; 68(3): 193-7.
[http://dx.doi.org/10.1055/s-2002-23167] [PMID: 11914952]

[151] Jańczyk A, Garcia-Lopez MA, Fernandez-Peñas P, *et al.* A Polypodium leucotomos extract inhibits solar-simulated radiation-induced TNF-? and iNOS expression, transcriptional activation and apoptosis. Exp Dermatol 2007; 16(10): 823-9.
[http://dx.doi.org/10.1111/j.1600-0625.2007.00603.x] [PMID: 17845214]

[152] Torricelli P, Fini M, Fanti PA, Dika E, Milani M. Protective effects of *Polypodium leucotomos* extract against UVB-induced damage in a model of reconstructed human epidermis. Photodermatol Photoimmunol Photomed 2017; 33(3): 156-63.
[http://dx.doi.org/10.1111/phpp.12297] [PMID: 28140474]

[153] An S-M, Lee S-J, Park K-M, Koh J-S, Boo Y-C. Effects of plant extract containing creams on UVB radiation-induced inflammatory responses in mice. J Soc Cosmeti Sci Korea 2010; 36(4): 271-80.

[154] Gupta VK, Sharma SK. Plants as natural antioxidants. Indian J Nat Prod Res 2014; 5(4): 326-34.

[155] Prakash YG, Ilango K, Kumar S, Elumalai A. *In vitro* antioxidant activity of *Luffa cylindrica* seed oil. J Global Pharma Technol 2009; 2(3): 93-7.

[156] Mahran GH, Kadry HA, Thabet CK, *et al.* GC/MS analysis of volatile oil of fruits of Anethum graveolens. Int J Pharmacogn 1992; 30(2): 139-44.

[157] Nadkarni K, Nadkarni AK. Indian Materia Medica. Popular Prakashan Pvt. Ltd, Bombay 1976; 1: 799.

[158] Mishra AK, Mishra A, Chattopadhyay P. Herbal cosmeceuticals for photoprotection from ultraviolet B radiation: a review. Trop J Pharm Res 2011; 10(3).
[http://dx.doi.org/10.4314/tjpr.v10i3.7]

[159] Naik GH. Radioprotecting ability and phytochemical analysis of an Indian medicinal plant: *Terminalia chebula*. BARC Newsletter 2003; 221-6.

[160] Balachandran P, Govindarajan R. Cancer—an ayurvedic perspective. Pharmacol Res 2005; 51(1): 19-30.
[http://dx.doi.org/10.1016/j.phrs.2004.04.010] [PMID: 15519531]

[161] Koul I, Kapil A. Evaluation of the liver protective potential of piperine, an active principle of black and long peppers. Planta Med 1993; 59(5): 413-7.
[http://dx.doi.org/10.1055/s-2006-959721] [PMID: 8255933]

[162] Fujii T, Wakaizumi M, Ikami T, Saito M. Amla (*Emblica officinalis Gaertn.*) extract promotes procollagen production and inhibits matrix metalloproteinase-1 in human skin fibroblasts. J Ethnopharmacol 2008; 119(1): 53-7.
[http://dx.doi.org/10.1016/j.jep.2008.05.039] [PMID: 18588964]

[163] Yokozawa T, Kim HY, Kim HJ, *et al.* Amla (*Emblica officinalis Gaertn.*) attenuates age-related renal dysfunction by oxidative stress. J Agric Food Chem 2007; 55(19): 7744-52.
[http://dx.doi.org/10.1021/jf072105s] [PMID: 17715896]

[164] Anila L, Vijayalakshmi NR. Flavonoids from *Emblica officinalis* and *Mangifera indica* effectiveness for dyslipidemia. J Ethnopharmacol 2002; 79(1): 81-7.
[http://dx.doi.org/10.1016/S0378-8741(01)00361-0] [PMID: 11744299]

[165] Kim J, Hwang JS, Cho YK, Han Y, Jeon YJ, Yang KH. Protective effects of (-)-epigallocatechi--3-gallate on UVA- and UVB-induced skin damage. Skin Pharmacol Physiol 2001; 14(1): 11-9.
[http://dx.doi.org/10.1159/000056329] [PMID: 11174086]

[166] Abdullaev FI. Biological effects of saffron. Biofactors 1993; 4(2): 83-6.
[PMID: 8347278]

[167] Salomi MJ, Nair SC, Panikkar KR. Inhibitory effects of Nigella sativa and saffron (Crocus sativus) on chemical carcinogenesis in mice. Nutr Cancer 1991; 16(1): 67-72.
[http://dx.doi.org/10.1080/01635589109514142] [PMID: 1923908]

[168] Lin JK, Wang CJ. Protection of crocin dyes on the acute hepatic damage induced by aflatoxin B$_1$ and dimethylnitrosamine in rats. Carcinogenesis 1986; 7(4): 595-9.
[http://dx.doi.org/10.1093/carcin/7.4.595] [PMID: 2870820]

[169] Das I, Chakrabarty RN, Das S. Saffron can prevent chemically induced skin carcinogenesis in Swiss albino mice. Asian Pac J Cancer Prev 2004; 5(1): 70-6.
[PMID: 15075009]

[170] O'Brien P, Carrasco-Pozo C, Speisky H. Boldine and its antioxidant or health-promoting properties. Chem Biol Interact 2006; 159(1): 1-17.
[http://dx.doi.org/10.1016/j.cbi.2005.09.002] [PMID: 16221469]

[171] Griffiths HR, Mistry P, Herbert KE, Lunec J. Molecular and cellular effects of ultraviolet light-induced genotoxicity. Crit Rev Clin Lab Sci 1998; 35(3): 189-237.
[http://dx.doi.org/10.1080/10408369891234192] [PMID: 9663376]

[172] Hidalgo ME, Gonzalez I, Toro F, Fernandez E, Speisky H, Jimenez I. Boldine as a sunscreen. Formulat Sun 2006; 129-36.

[173] Rancan F, Rosan S, Boehm K, *et al.* Protection against UVB irradiation by natural filters extracted from lichens. J Photochem Photobiol B 2002; 68(2-3): 133-9.
[http://dx.doi.org/10.1016/S1011-1344(02)00362-7] [PMID: 12468208]

[174] Lee MJ, Kim MJ, Song YS, Song YO, Moon GS. Bamboo culm extract supplementation elevates HDL-cholesterol and ameliorates oxidative stress in C57BL/6 mice fed atherogenic diet. J Med Food 2008; 11(1): 69-77.
[http://dx.doi.org/10.1089/jmf.2007.009] [PMID: 18361740]

[175] Zhang Y, Yao X, Bao B, Zhang Y. Anti-fatigue activity of a triterpenoid-rich extract from Chinese bamboo shavings (*Caulis bamfusae* in taeniam). Phytother Res 2006; 20(10): 872-6.
[http://dx.doi.org/10.1002/ptr.1965] [PMID: 16886233]

[176] Seok JK, Kwak JY, Seo HH, Suh HJ, Boo YC. Effects of Bambusae caulis in Taeniam Extract on the UVB-induced cell death, oxidative stress and matrix metalloproteinase 1 expression in keratinocytes. J Soc Cosmet Sci Korea 2015; 41(1): 9-20.
[http://dx.doi.org/10.15230/SCSK.2015.41.1.9]

[177] Jianjun J, Huiru D. Preparation of high-purity baicalein from *Scutellaria baicalensis* Georgi. Nat Prod Res 2008; 22(16): 1410-2.
[http://dx.doi.org/10.1080/14786410701823967] [PMID: 19023802]

[178] Choi W, No RH, Kwon HS, Lee HY. Enhancement of skin anti-inflammatory activities of *Scutellaria baicalensis* extract using a nanoencapsulation process. J Cosmet Laser Ther 2014; 16(6): 271-8.
[http://dx.doi.org/10.3109/14764172.2014.946051] [PMID: 25046235]

[179] Silva-Carvalho R, Baltazar F, Almeida-Aguiar C. Propolis: A complex natural product with a plethora of biological activities that can be explored for drug development. Evid Based Complement Alternat Med 2015; 2015: 206439.
[http://dx.doi.org/10.1155/2015/206439] [PMID: 26106433]

[180] Cole N, Sou PW, Ngo A, *et al.* Topical 'Sydney' propolis protects against UV-radiation-induced inflammation, lipid peroxidation and immune suppression in mouse skin. Int Arch Allergy Immunol 2010; 152(2): 87-97.
[http://dx.doi.org/10.1159/000265530] [PMID: 20016191]

[181] Kitamura H. Effects of propolis extract and propolis-derived compounds on obesity and diabetes: knowledge from cellular and animal models. Molecules 2019; 24(23): 4394.
[http://dx.doi.org/10.3390/molecules24234394] [PMID: 31805752]

[182] Karapetsas A, Voulgaridou GP, Konialis M, *et al.* Propolis extracts inhibit UV-induced photodamage in human experimental *in vitro* skin models. Antioxidants 2019; 8(5): 125.
[http://dx.doi.org/10.3390/antiox8050125] [PMID: 31075866]

[183] Dinkova-Kostova AT, Fahey JW, Benedict AL, *et al.* Dietary glucoraphanin-rich broccoli sprout extracts protect against UV radiation-induced skin carcinogenesis in SKH-1 hairless mice. Photochem Photobiol Sci 2010; 9(4): 597-600.
[http://dx.doi.org/10.1039/b9pp00130a] [PMID: 20354656]

[184] Murapa P, Dai J, Chung M, Mumper RJ, D'Orazio J. Anthocyanin-rich fractions of blackberry extracts reduce UV-induced free radicals and oxidative damage in keratinocytes. Phytother Res 2012; 26(1): 106-12.
[http://dx.doi.org/10.1002/ptr.3510] [PMID: 21567508]

[185] Kapoor LD. CRC handbook of Ayurvedic medicinal plants. CRC press 2018.

[http://dx.doi.org/10.1201/9781351070997]

[186] El-Seedi HR, Burman R, Mansour A, *et al.* The traditional medical uses and cytotoxic activities of sixty-one Egyptian plants: Discovery of an active cardiac glycoside from Urginea maritima. J Ethnopharmacol 2013; 145(3): 746-57.
[http://dx.doi.org/10.1016/j.jep.2012.12.007] [PMID: 23228916]

[187] Nadkarni KM, Nadkarni AK. Indian Materia Medica. Bombay, India: Popular Prakashan Private Limited 1976; Vol. I & II.

[188] Smijs T, Pavel S. Titanium dioxide and zinc oxide nanoparticles in sunscreens: focus on their safety and effectiveness. Nanotechnol Sci Appl 2011; 4: 95-112.
[http://dx.doi.org/10.2147/NSA.S19419] [PMID: 24198489]

[189] Bensouilah J, Buck P. Aromadermatology: aromatherapy in the treatment and care of common skin conditions. Radcliffe Publishing 2006.

[190] Saewan N, Jimtaisong A. Natural products as photoprotection. J Cosmet Dermatol 2015; 14(1): 47-63.
[http://dx.doi.org/10.1111/jocd.12123] [PMID: 25582033]

[191] Nichols JA, Katiyar SK. Skin photoprotection by natural polyphenols: anti-inflammatory, antioxidant and DNA repair mechanisms. Arch Dermatol Res 2010; 302(2): 71-83.
[http://dx.doi.org/10.1007/s00403-009-1001-3] [PMID: 19898857]

[192] Brown MW, Hamilton LG, Long SP. Antioxidants: What is their significance in sun protection? SÖFW J 2003; 129(7): 2-12.

[193] Tsuda T, Horio F, Osawa T. The role of anthocyanins as an antioxidant under oxidative stress in rats. Biofactors 2000; 13(1-4): 133-9.
[http://dx.doi.org/10.1002/biof.5520130122] [PMID: 11237172]

[194] Tsuda T, Horio F, Osawa T. Dietary cyanidin 3-O-β-d-glucoside increases *ex vivo* oxidation resistance of serum in rats. Lipids 1998; 33(6): 583-8.
[http://dx.doi.org/10.1007/s11745-998-0243-5] [PMID: 9655373]

[195] Noda Y, Kneyuki T, Igarashi K, Mori A, Packer L. Antioxidant activity of nasunin, an anthocyanin in eggplant peels. Toxicology 2000; 148(2-3): 119-23.
[http://dx.doi.org/10.1016/S0300-483X(00)00202-X] [PMID: 10962130]

[196] Korać R, Khambholja K. Potential of herbs in skin protection from ultraviolet radiation. Pharmacogn Rev 2011; 5(10): 164-73.
[http://dx.doi.org/10.4103/0973-7847.91114] [PMID: 22279374]

[197] Choquenet B, Couteau C, Paparis E, Coiffard LJM. Quercetin and rutin as potential sunscreen agents: determination of efficacy by an *in vitro* method. J Nat Prod 2008; 71(6): 1117-8.
[http://dx.doi.org/10.1021/np7007297] [PMID: 18512988]

[198] Widyarini S, Spinks N, Husband AJ, Reeve VE. Isoflavonoid compounds from red clover (Trifolium pratense) protect from inflammation and immune suppression induced by UV radiation. Photochem Photobiol 2001; 74(3): 465-70.
[http://dx.doi.org/10.1562/0031-8655(2001)074<0465:ICFRCT>2.0.CO;2] [PMID: 11594062]

[199] Saraf S, Kaur CD. Phytoconstituents as photoprotective novel cosmetic formulations. Pharmacogn Rev 2010; 4(7): 1-11.
[http://dx.doi.org/10.4103/0973-7847.65319] [PMID: 22228936]

[200] Kumar A, Shamim H, Nagaraju U. Premature graying of hair: Review with updates. Int J Trichology 2018; 10(5): 198-203.
[http://dx.doi.org/10.4103/ijt.ijt_47_18] [PMID: 30607038]

[201] Murdock KA, Schauss AG. Jucara and Açai fruit-based dietary supplements. Google Patents; 2009

[202] Baliga MS, Katiyar SK. Chemoprevention of photocarcinogenesis by selected dietary botanicals. Photochem Photobiol Sci 2006; 5(2): 243-53.

[http://dx.doi.org/10.1039/b505311k] [PMID: 16465310]

[203] Dayan N. Skin aging handbook: an integrated approach to biochemistry and product development. William Andrew; 2008.

[204] Fryer MJ. Evidence for the photoprotective effects of vitamin E. Photochem Photobiol 1993; 58(2): 304-12.
[http://dx.doi.org/10.1111/j.1751-1097.1993.tb09566.x] [PMID: 8415922]

[205] Kerscher M, Williams S, Trüeb RM. Topische Dermatokosmetika. Dermatokosmetik 2009; pp. 85-126.
[http://dx.doi.org/10.1007/978-3-7985-1739-4_6]

[206] Kapoor S, Saraf S. Assessment of viscoelasticity and hydration effect of herbal moisturizers using bioengineering techniques. Pharmacogn Mag 2010; 6(24): 298-304.
[http://dx.doi.org/10.4103/0973-1296.71797] [PMID: 21120032]

[207] Baumann LS, Baumann L. Cosmetic dermatology. McGraw-Hill Professional Publishing; 2009.

[208] Counet C, Callemien D, Collin S. Chocolate and cocoa: New sources of *trans*-resveratrol and trans-piceid. Food Chem 2006; 98(4): 649-57.
[http://dx.doi.org/10.1016/j.foodchem.2005.06.030]

[209] Soleas GJ, Diamandis EP, Goldberg DM. Resveratrol: A molecule whose time has come? And gone? Clin Biochem 1997; 30(2): 91-113.
[http://dx.doi.org/10.1016/S0009-9120(96)00155-5] [PMID: 9127691]

[210] Murad H. 2004. Antioxidants: Nutritive Effects on the Skin. In: Noah Worcester Meeting, January 2004.

[211] Hansen J, Hammann M. Risk in Science Instruction. Sci Educ 2017; 26(7-9): 749-75.
[http://dx.doi.org/10.1007/s11191-017-9923-1]

[212] Amagase H, Nance DM. A randomized, double-blind, placebo-controlled, clinical study of the general effects of a standardized Lycium barbarum (Goji) Juice, GoChi. J Altern Complement Med 2008; 14(4): 403-12.
[http://dx.doi.org/10.1089/acm.2008.0004] [PMID: 18447631]

[213] Talalay P, Fahey JW, Healy ZR, et al. Sulforaphane mobilizes cellular defenses that protect skin against damage by UV radiation. Proc Natl Acad Sci USA 2007; 104(44): 17500-5.
[http://dx.doi.org/10.1073/pnas.0708710104] [PMID: 17956979]

[214] Zulli F, Suter F, Biltz H, Nissen HP. Improving skin function with CM-glucan, a biological response modifier from yeast. Int J Cosmet Sci 1998; 20(2): 79-86.
[http://dx.doi.org/10.1046/j.1467-2494.1998.171740.x] [PMID: 18505493]

[215] Scalbert A, Williamson G. Dietary intake and bioavailability of polyphenols. J Nutr 2000; 130(8) (Suppl.): 2073S-85S.
[http://dx.doi.org/10.1093/jn/130.8.2073S] [PMID: 10917926]

[216] Danno K, Ikai K, Imamura S. Anti-inflammatory effects of eicosapentaenoic acid on experimental skin inflammation models. Arch Dermatol Res 1993; 285(7): 432-5.
[http://dx.doi.org/10.1007/BF00372139] [PMID: 8304784]

[217] Costa A, Facchini G, Pinheiro ALTA, et al. Honokiol protects skin cells against inflammation, collagenolysis, apoptosis, and senescence caused by cigarette smoke damage. Int J Dermatol 2017; 56(7): 754-61.
[http://dx.doi.org/10.1111/ijd.13569] [PMID: 28229451]

[218] Thimmulappa RK, Mai KH, Srisuma S, Kensler TW, Yamamoto M, Biswal S. Identification of Nrf2-regulated genes induced by the chemopreventive agent sulforaphane by oligonucleotide microarray. Cancer Res 2002; 62(18): 5196-203.
[PMID: 12234984]

[219] Kubo E, Chhunchha B, Singh P, Sasaki H, Singh DP. Sulforaphane reactivates cellular antioxidant defense by inducing Nrf2/ARE/Prdx6 activity during aging and oxidative stress. Sci Rep 2017; 7(1): 14130.
[http://dx.doi.org/10.1038/s41598-017-14520-8] [PMID: 29074861]

[220] Guillermo-Lagae R, Deep G, Ting H, Agarwal C, Agarwal R. Silibinin enhances the repair of ultraviolet B-induced DNA damage by activating p53-dependent nucleotide excision repair mechanism in human dermal fibroblasts. Oncotarget 2015; 6(37): 39594-606.
[http://dx.doi.org/10.18632/oncotarget.5519] [PMID: 26447614]

[221] Gregoris E, Fabris S, Bertelle M, Grassato L, Stevanato R. Propolis as potential cosmeceutical sunscreen agent for its combined photoprotective and antioxidant properties. Int J Pharm 2011; 405(1-2): 97-101.
[http://dx.doi.org/10.1016/j.ijpharm.2010.11.052] [PMID: 21134430]

[222] Batista CM, Alves AVF, Queiroz LA, *et al.* The photoprotective and anti-inflammatory activity of red propolis extract in rats. J Photochem Photobiol B 2018; 180: 198-207.
[http://dx.doi.org/10.1016/j.jphotobiol.2018.01.028] [PMID: 29454853]

CHAPTER 2

Natural Products and Burns: A Tough Case to Crack

Samar Thiab[1,*], **Safa Daoud**[1], **Rana Abutaima**[2], **Muna Barakat**[1] and **May Abu Taha**[1]

[1] *Faculty of Pharmacy, Applied Science Private University, Amman, Jordan*

[2] *Faculty of Pharmacy, Zarqa University, Zarqa, Jordan*

Abstract: Burns are a type of skin injury that occurs due to close contact with a heat source or corrosive chemicals. The use of natural products to treat burns dates back to ancient civilizations. This chapter discusses naturally derived products from plants, animals and fungi sources. The natural origin, chemical composition, burn healing mechanisms, clinical studies, and used pharmaceutical formulation are also covered.

Keywords: *Aloe vera, Areca catechu, Arnebia euchroma,* Berberis, *Boswellia carterii,* Burns, *Centella asiatica, Cinnamomum camphora,* Healing mechanism, Honey, *Hypercium perforaturm, Lawsonia inermis, Malva sylvestris, Melaleuca alternifolia, Myrtus communis, Olea europaea, Plantago major,* Propolis, Sacchachitin, *Sesamum indicum.*

INTRODUCTION

According to recent reports from the American Burn Association (ABA), more than 400,000 United States (US) residents have suffered from burn injuries, and require medical treatment annually [1]. Around 70% of burns occur at home, and children are more exposed to burns than adults [1]. Similarly, the World Health Organization (WHO) and Centers for Disease Control and Prevention (CDC) disclosed that the mortality rate associated with burns is around 10,000 deaths per year in the US, mainly due to burn-related infections [2, 3]. Unfortunately, higher rates were documented in low- and middle-income countries [2, 3], which shed light on the need for proper awareness, prevention, diagnosis and treatment approaches.

* **Corresponding author Samar Thiab:** Department of Pharmaceutical Chemistry and Pharmacognosy, Faculty of Pharmacy, Applied Science Private University, Al Arab St., P.O. Box 166, Amman 11931, Jordan; Tel: +96265609999, Ext. 1505; E-mail: s_thiab@asu.edu.jo

Heba Abd El-Sattar El-Nashar, Mohamed El-Shazly & Nouran Mohammed Fahmy (Eds.)

The World Health Organization (WHO) defines burns as an injury to the skin or other organic tissue primarily caused by heat or due to radiation, radioactivity, electricity, friction or contact with chemicals. Thermal (heat) burns occur when some or all of the cells in the skin or other tissues are destroyed by hot liquids (scalds), hot solids (contact burns), or flames (flame burns) [2]. Burn classifications are usually subcategorized based on many classification systems such as skin integrity and depth of injury using the old system (*i.e.*, degrees) or new (*i.e.*, partial *vs.* full-thickness injuries) [4, 5]. Factors that aggravate burn injuries include the temperature of the causative agent, exposure duration, number of involved skin layers (*e.g.*, epidermis and dermis) and blood supply to the injured area [5]. Fig. (**1**) summarizes the burn classifications based on the old and new systems. Unfortunately, it is not always easy to determine the depth of burn during the first incidence period (*e.g.*, the first 48 to 72 hours). The tolerance for heat on different body surface areas is not the same, *i.e.*, the tolerance of heat on the palms of the hands, soles of the feet, and back can bear high temperatures for a long time, as compared to the eyelids [5]. The skin of children and the elderly is thinner than adults, and less tolerable to injuries [4].

New system (old system)	Superficial (first degree)	Superficial partial-thickness (second degree)	Deep partial-thickness (second degree)	Full-thickness (third degree)	Full-thickness (fourth degree)
Etiology	Ultraviolet light, very short flash flame exposure	Scald (spill or splash), short flash	Scald (spill), flame, oil, grease	Scald (immersion), flame, steam, oil, grease, chemical, high-voltage electricity	Cause as for deep partial-thickness burns
Histology	Epidermis only	Epidermis and papillary dermis, skin appendages intact	Epidermis and reticular dermis, most skin appendages destroyed	Epidermis and dermis; all skin appendages destroyed	Involves fascia and muscle and/or bone
Clinical presentation	Erythema, dry and pink or red; blanches with pressure	Erythema, blisters; moist, red and weeping; blanches with pressure	Blisters, wet or waxy dry; variable color (patchy to cheesy white to red); does not blanch with pressure	Waxy white to leathery gray to charred and black; dry and inelastic; does not blanch with pressure	Black (dry, dull, and charred)
Sensation	Painful	Painful to air and temperature	Perceptive of pressure only	Deep pressure only (insensate)	Deep pressure only (insensate)
Healing time/ Scaring	3 to 6 days/None	7 to 20 days/Unusual$	>21 days/Severe	Never*/Very severe	Never*/Eschar tissue

Fig. (1). Classifications of burns based on the wound-depth using the old and new systems. This figure has been adapted from Abazari *et al.* [4] (***Note***: *No spontaneous healing. $Potential pigmentary changes, moist, elastic. Eschar tissue (hard and inelastic)).

Accordingly, a different classification system was released by the American Burn Association (ABA) based on severity, which subcategories the burns into three types (minor, moderate, and major). This system depends on the degree of injury, which is presented as a percentage of the total body surface area (%TBSA) involved in the burn [5], considering the patients' age and complications. However, superficial (first-degree) burns are not included in the percentage TBSA burn assessment. The ABA clarified that the most common method to estimate the second and more profound degrees of burn is by using the "Rule of Nines." As demonstrated in Fig. (2), the adults' distinct anatomic regions represent approximately 9% or a multiple thereof of the TBSA. While, in the infant or child, the "Rule" deviates because of the large surface area of the child's head and the smaller surface area of the lower extremities [5, 6]. Finally, the classification of burns is pivotal for the appropriate management of the burns, the required time for healing, and the anticipation of consequences such as infections [6, 7].

Burn Healing Mechanism

The healing process of skin burns can primarily go through four stages that involve coagulation which resembles the homeostasis phase, followed by the inflammatory process that is led by mononuclear cell infiltration, and then cellular proliferation that would be in the form of tissue epithelialization, fibroplasia, angiogenesis, and granulation tissue formation [8]. The final phase would be the scar formation or collagen protein deposits at the burned site [8].

Immediately after a burn occurs, the infiltration of dendritic cells, which are considered a major part of innate and antigen-specific immunity, would occur to support the process of burn healing *via* protecting the wound from being infected and promoting cellular proliferation [9]. This process includes the activation of keratinocytes, fibroblasts, and endothelial cell proliferation that will mediate new skin formation *via* re-epithelialization, collagen secretion to constitute a new extracellular matrix, and new blood vessel formation, *i.e.*, angiogenesis, respectively [9]. In a murine burn model, dendritic cells played a significant role in transforming growth factor β (TGF-β) to release early following a burn injury to support cell proliferation [9].

Historical Treatments of Burns

The earliest descriptions of burn injuries and treatments were found in cave drawings [10], but the entire knowledge of burn treatments comes from the old medicine of the Egyptians, Greeks, Romans, and other peoples of Asia, which is limited but applicable [11].

Before 2500 BC, burns were treated with the milk of mothers who had given birth. Writing inventions enabled ancient Egyptian doctors to write their observations down on papyrus scrolls [11, 12]. Treatment recommendations were found in ancient Egyptian writings, known as the Smith and Ebers papyri, dating to about 1500 BC [10, 12]. One of the oldest burn treatment records was described in the Egyptian Smith papyrus, advocating resin and honey salve for treating burns [13]. The Ebers papyrus comprises an important section entitled "Beginning of the remedies for a burn" [11] which suggests the use of a series of diverse remedies to treat burn wounds which include applying black mud, excrement of small cattle, resin of acacia, barley dough, carob, wax, oil, cooked unwritten papyrus, red ochre, *khes* part of *theima* tree (an unknown tree), and copper flakes [11, 13]. It also described the application of lemon stripes on burn wounds topically [12].

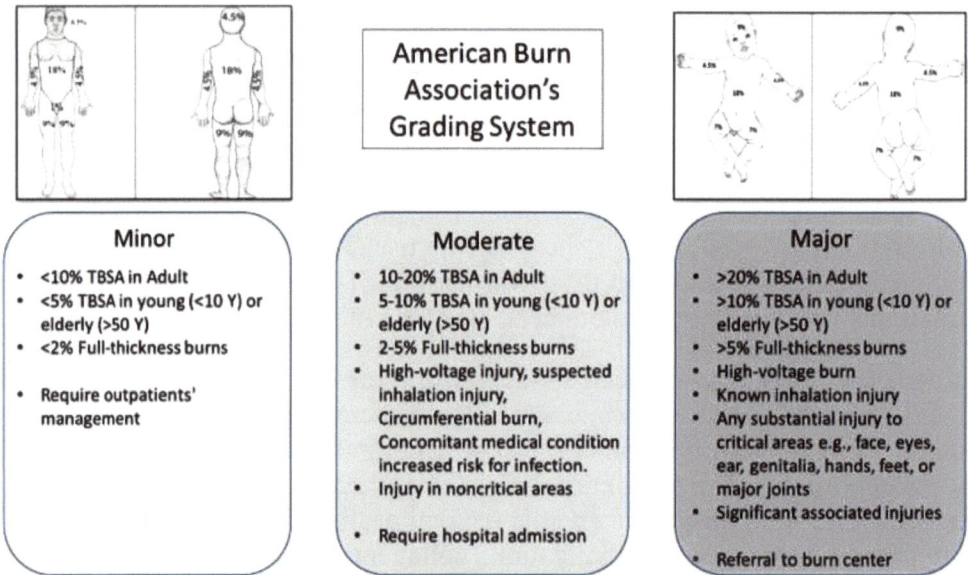

American Burn Association's Grading System

Minor
- <10% TBSA in Adult
- <5% TBSA in young (<10 Y) or elderly (>50 Y)
- <2% Full-thickness burns

- Require outpatients' management

Moderate
- 10-20% TBSA in Adult
- 5-10% TBSA in young (<10 Y) or elderly (>50 Y)
- 2-5% Full-thickness burns
- High-voltage injury, suspected inhalation injury, Circumferential burn, Concomitant medical condition increased risk for infection.
- Injury in noncritical areas

- Require hospital admission

Major
- >20% TBSA in Adult
- >10% TBSA in young (<10 Y) or elderly (>50 Y)
- >5% Full-thickness burns
- High-voltage burn
- Known inhalation injury
- Any substantial injury to critical areas e.g., face, eyes, ear, genitalia, hands, feet, or major joints
- Significant associated injuries

- Referral to burn center

Fig. (2). American Burn Association's (ABA) Grading System based on severity and TBSA calculations. TBSA stands for total body surface area. Concomitant medical conditions such as Diabetes mellitus increase the risk for infection, and significant associated injuries, such as major trauma. This figure has been adapted from American Burn Association.

In the Hearst papyrus, which is a collection of medical prescriptions, tannic acid obtained from Acacia herb seeds and fruits was used to treat burns. Dressings of willow leaf wraps, moldy bread, honey, and garlic could lower the risk of infection as well as the use of copper salts and wine solutions for antisepsis. Additionally, opium, thyme, and belladonna were utilized to relieve pain. Finally, in the Ipsinger papyrus, cedar oil was used as an antiseptic. Red-hot metal was applied to the burn if the patient was severely injured to stop bleeding. *Aloe vera* was also used for the treatment of burns [11].

Hippocrates, the most famous Greek doctor in the 4th century BC, recommended different treatment options for burns according to his writings. Treatment options included pig fat-impregnated dressings, resin alternated with warm vinegar-impregnated dressings, and balms made from oak bark [10 - 13]. Hippocrates also used bitumen mixed with resin to treat advanced cases of burns [12]. In addition, burns treated locally by applying slices of lemon, formulations of several oils, and blends of tea leaves were in practice around 430 BC [11].

In ancient Rome, writings by Aulus Cornelius Celsus proposed various topical remedies for the treatment of burns, such as using a mixture of honey and bran [10 - 12]. With the Roman expansion, treating war injuries drew many physicians' interest. Gaius Plinius Secundus counseled using garlic on burn wounds [12]. Pedanios Dioscurides, a Greek physician in the Roman army, described honey as the treatment of choice for treating rotten and hollow ulcers and recommended the dressings be changed frequently. He also used a conch shell and burned leather from shoes as treatments for burn wounds and wrote down various recipes of cattle droppings for the treatment of purulent burns, which were used with rose oil and honey for inflamed burn wounds [12]. Additionally, Dioscorides wrote about treating burn wounds with pine bark, grinded blossoms of the *Cistus creticus,* and pickled olives to avoid blistering. Furthermore, he differentiated between deep and superficial burn wounds and suggested putting figs together with barley flour on sunburns [12].

In the 6th century BC, Chinese medicine described the use of tea leaf extracts and tinctures for burns [10, 13]. Traditional Chinese medicine records gave two recipes for burn treatment used in ancient times: the first recommended dressings with a mixture of vegetable oils, and the second one had mature forms of sponges from *Calcarea sulphurica* or lard boiled with willow bark. Impregnated bandages with the described mixture decreased the probability of wound infection [11].

Ayurvedic records of Charaka and Sushruta used honey in their dressing to clean sores and promote the healing of wounds and burns [11].

Arabian doctors used ice-cold water, which was first advocated by Muhammad ibn Zakariya al-Razi in the ninth century AC [10, 13]. Ibn Sina (980-1037 AD), known in the West as Avicenna, was a famous Persian physician who wrote the Canon of Medicine (al-Qanun-fi-al-tibb). In his second book of Canon, he searched for burn remedies, and 28 simple herbal drugs were described. Ibn Sina defined burn treatment as following two goals: prevention of blistering and the treatment of the burn wound after blister formation. He considered cold drugs as appropriate for the first goal and detergent and dry drugs moderated in cold and hot qualities as better for the second goal. That is, when a burn wound happened, a herbal remedy by cold temperament like *Myrtus communis* L. or *Malva sylves-*

tris L. must be used, and when the wound has more discharge, it is better to use herbal drugs by dryness temperament and so on [14].

Physicians have investigated and formulated a variety of burn treatments over the centuries. There was an exponential increase in medical research and knowledge from the 18th to early 20th century in burn care. Nevertheless, this was not reflected in increasing survival, and many patients with burns died [13].

Even though the knowledge and medical treatment of burns have developed and advanced, natural remedies are still popular and common. In the following sections, naturally-derived products from plant, animal, and fungal origins with burn-treatment benefits have been described.

Substances of Plant Origin

Aloe Vera

Aloe vera (*Aloe barbadensis Miller*) is a perennial succulent belonging to the family Asphodelaceae (Liliaceae) [15]. It is a tropical plant that is easily grown in hot and dry climates and widely distributed in Asia, Africa, and other tropical areas [16]. The gel extract of *Aloe vera* has been reported to promote wound and burn healing [17]. Diverse compounds have been isolated from *Aloe vera*, including glycoproteins, anthraquinones, chromones, saccharides, lipids, enzymes, vitamins, salicylic acid, amino acids, and proteins [15, 18, 19]. *Aloe vera* extracts contain mannose-6-phosphate and other polysaccharides, which are considered enhancers of fibroblast replication through cytokines release [20]. *in vitro* neovascularization was enhanced following the *Aloe vera* application of mouse Matrigel due to the presence of β-sitosterol [21]. Additionally, *Aloe vera* extracts are helpful for burn and wound healing because of their anti-inflammatory, anti-histamine, and bradykinin destruction properties that are mainly ascribed to the presence of aloin A and B (Fig. **3**) [22].

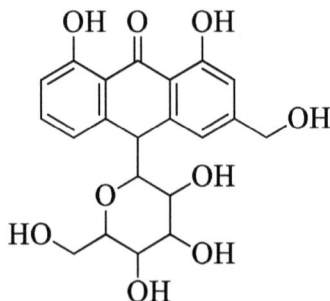

Fig. (3). The chemical structure of aloin.

Extracts of *Aloe vera* in different preparations, such as gel, cream, and ointment, have shown variable wound and burn healing properties [23]. This could be attributed to the instability of its main components that are susceptible to biological degradation [23]. However, the gel and cream showed promising results in improving skin epithelialization and anti-inflammatory properties in treating first and second-degree burns in addition to retarding the burn progression [23]. Furthermore, *Aloe vera* gel was investigated in an *in vivo* trial that deployed rats to examine burn healing properties in combination with honey and milk, as it enhances the epidermal cell proliferation and re-epithelialization of burns, especially when it is applied with the described combination [24]. Various clinical trials were conducted on humans to test the efficacy of *Aloe vera* for burn wound healing, and the clinical evidence obtained supports the fact that *Aloe vera* can enhance wound healing for first to second-degree burns [17, 25, 26]. Topical application of *Aloe vera* can cause some side effects, including redness, burning, and stinging sensation in addition to the possibly of causing allergic reactions mostly due to the presence of anthraquinones [27].

Areca Catechu

Areca catechu (*Areca catechu Linn.*) is a medicinal plant that belongs to the family Palmaceae [28]. The seed is the main part of *A. catechu,* which is used in medicine, and it is commonly known as "areca nut" [29]. It is widely distributed in southern and southeast Asia, including China, India, Indonesia, Malaysia, Philippines, and New Guinea [30]. This species contains catechins, tannins, gallic acid, fat, gum, and alkaloids [31]. The four major alkaloids isolated in the arecanut are arecoline, arecaidine, guvacoline and guvacine (Fig. **4**) [28]. The formerly mentioned phytochemicals are well-established antioxidants which are one of the predominant mechanisms of burn healing [32 - 35].

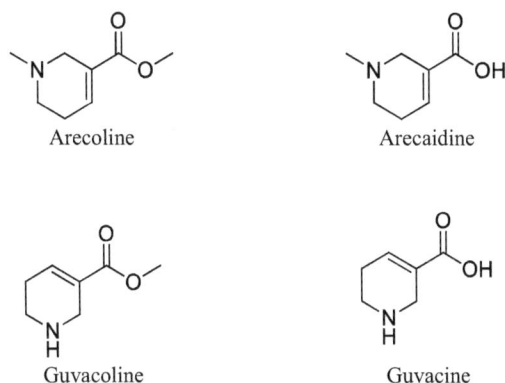

Arecoline   Arecaidine

Guvacoline   Guvacine

Fig. (4). Alkaloids identified in *Areca catechu.*

In animal studies, the alcoholic extract of *A. catechu* showed an improvement in burn healing that could be mediated through the increase in the period of epithelialization following the treatment of a burn rat model until day 15 of a 2% *A. catechu* treatment [36]. In one study, the percentage of wound contraction and epithelialization period were investigated using a burned rat model following treatment with 2% ethyl acetate extract of *A. catechu* (Betel nut) in the form of a gel compared to *Salaccazalacca* (snake fruit) extract [37]. Significant improvement was observed in the percentage of wound contraction between day 12 and 14 of the study following treatment with betel nut gel by 55.56% compared to the control group, which received the gel base only [37]. Traditionally, *A. catechu* is used for burns and wound healing in combination with coconut oil and the stem juice of *Canna indica* [38]. There is supporting clinical evidence that arecoline also has wound-healing properties that can help in wound healing [38, 39].

Arnebia Euchroma

Arnebia euchroma, belonging to the family Boraginaceae, is distributed in Asia and the drier regions of northern Africa [40]. *A. euchroma* (Royle) Johnst is traditionally used to treat various skin disorders [41]. The major pharmacological constituents in *A. euchroma* (Royle) Johnst. are naphthoquinone pigments, among which shikonin and β, β'-dimethylacrylshikonin (Fig. **5**) are chosen as "marker compounds" in the chemical standardization of *A. euchroma* and its products [42].

In an *in vivo* study in rats to investigate the efficacy of *A. euchroma* extract for burn treatment that continued for 28 days, both 10% and 20% extracts enhanced granulation tissue formation *via* re-epithelization, fibroblasts proliferation, neovascularization, and collagen synthesis [43]. Additionally, *A. euchroma* showed an anti-inflammatory effect that was comparable to a traditional burn treatment of silver sulfadiazine ointment, where 10% extract was superior to that 20% [43]. Furthermore, different diethyl ether extract preparations of *A. euchroma* in combination with goat lipid and cold cream were used on induced burn Wistar rat models and then compared to other treatments. A significant reduction in the burned area at day 16 ($p < 0.001$) was reported for the extract preparations [41]. According to the histopathological assessment, the goat lipid preparation with *A. euchroma* demonstrated increased wound contraction through re-epithelization and collagen synthesis that induced burn healing [41]. Additionally, *A. euchroma* showed anti-microbial activity against methicillin-resistant *Staphylococcus aureus* (MRSA) and vancomycin-resistant enterococci, which could help in treating burn-induced infections [44]. Similar results were obtained with humans in a randomized clinical trial where patients treated with

A. euchroma ointment showed significantly shorter healing time when compared with the group treated with silver sulfadiazine cream [45].

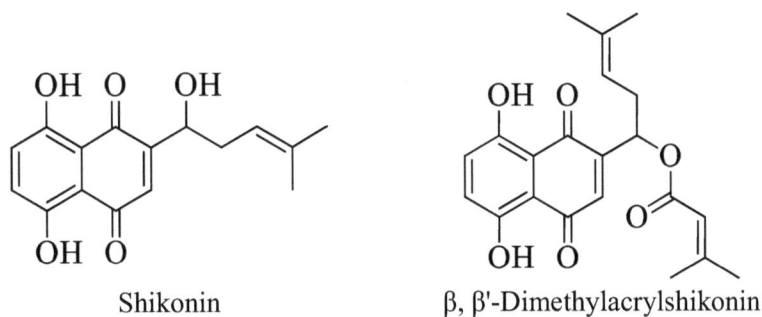

Fig. (5). Naphthoquinone pigments identified in *Arnebia euchroma.*

Berberis

The genus *Berberis* from the family Berberidaceae includes about 500 species that are commonly distributed in most areas of central and southern Europe, the northeastern region of the US, and South Asia, including the northern area of Pakistan [46]. The plant contains a number of important phytochemicals, including berberine and berbamine alkaloids (Fig. **6**) and other bioactive constituents like triterpenes, tannins, flavonoids, and phenolic compounds [47, 48].

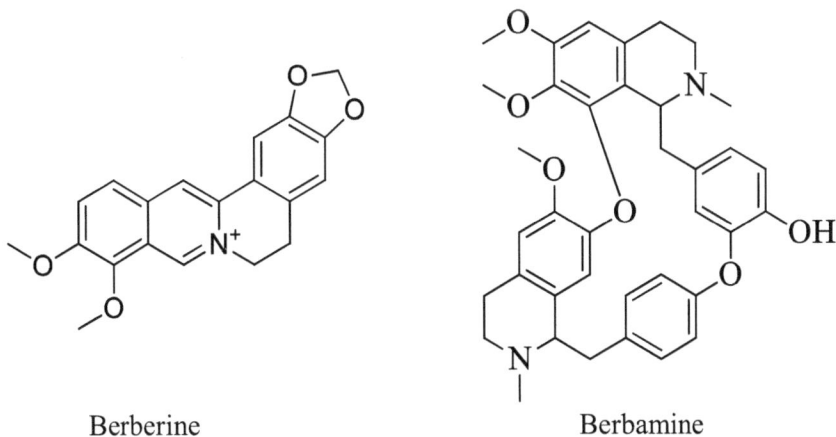

Fig. (6). Alkaloids identified in *Berberis.*

The main alkaloid berberine, which is an isoquinolone, is believed to be responsible for the pharmacological effect of Berberis in wound healing. When used in combination with sterols such as beta-sitosterol, which is a phytosterol, it was non-inferior to silver sulfadiazine in treating burns [46, 49]. A 15%(w/w) in petroleum jelly ointment of *Berberis aristata* supported minimal modification of cellular proliferation during the wound healing process when applied to a burned rat model [50]. *B. aristata* is one of the plants that is used in Ayurvedic medicine for wound healing, usually in combination with other local herbs, but there is limited evidence to support its wound activity [50, 51].

Boswellia Carterii

Boswellia carterii is one of 43 species in the genus *Boswellia* of the family Burseraceae [52]. *B. carterii* is a traditional plant distributed in east Africa and China [53]. The commercial oil of this plant, Frankincense oil, has wound-healing properties [54]. The olibanum resin produced by *B. carterii* is rich in mono-, sesqui-, di-, and tri-terpenoic constituents. The triterpenic acid constituents, boswellic acids (Fig. **7**), have been identified as the main components responsible for pharmaceutical activity [55].

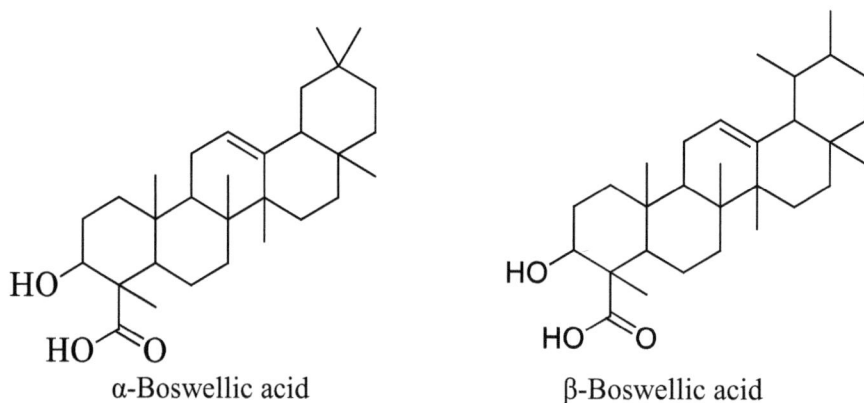

α-Boswellic acid   β-Boswellic acid

Fig. (7). Boswellic acids in *Boswellia carterii*.

That is, boswellic acid could potentially be the agent for the anti-inflammatory activity of *B. carterii* [56, 57]. *Boswellia* gum, in combination with moxifloxacin, chitosan, acetic acid, and ethylenediaminetetraacetic acid (EDTA), was investigated in a novel topical gel formula for its antimicrobial activity to eradicate methicillin-resistant *Staphylococcus aureus* in an *ex vivo* burn rat model and murine burn model [58]. The novel formula improved the wound contraction significantly compared to an untreated control group with no pus formation until day 12 of infection [58]. Moreover, the gel-induced re-epithelialization and collagen synthesis were observed at day 12 [58]. An *in vivo* model that deployed rabbits with induced thermal injury investigated the efficacy of another *Boswellia* species, *Boswellia serrata*-dextrin-glycerin formula. It exhibited the tumor necrosis factor-α (TNF-α) and vascular endothelial growth factor (VEGF), which support the improvement of an inflammatory response, tissue granulation, and collagen synthesis [59].

Centella Asiatica

Centella Asiatica, also known asgotu kola or tiger grass, belongs to the family Apiaceae. It grows in Asia, mainly in India, Pakistan, Madagascar, equatorial Africa, Central America, and the tropical region of Oceania [60]. The primary active constituents of *C. asiatica* are asiaticoside and madecassoside, which are both saponins in which a tri-saccharide moiety is linked to the aglycone asiatic acid and madecassic acid, respectively (Fig. **8**) [61].

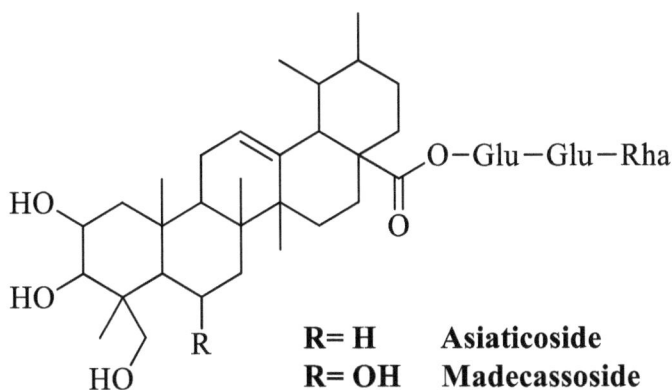

O—Glu—Glu—Rha

R= H   Asiaticoside
R= OH   Madecassoside

Fig. (8). The primary constituents of *Centella asiatica*.

Asiaticoside and madecassoside themselves, rather than their corresponding metabolites, are recognized as the main active constituents of *C. asiatica* herbs responsible for burn wound healing [62]. In a murine model, madecassoside played a major role in tissue remodeling through collagen synthesis and angiogenesis, besides its antioxidant activity that decreased nitric oxide levels and malondialdehyde species concentrations in the burned skin while increasing the number of glutathione [63]. Extracts of *C. asiatica* in hexane, ethyl acetate, and methanol extracts of *C. asiatica* extracts promoted wound contraction as well as epithelialization on day 14 following burn induction in rats [64]. The efficacy of both asiaticoside and madecassoside was investigated following oral administration of the formerly mentioned compounds to a burn mice model, and the levels of matrix metalloproteinase-1 (MMP-1) and transforming growth factor-beta 1 (TGF-β1) were examined [62]. Both compounds significantly enhanced collagen type I and III syntheses *via* TGF-β1 that promotes fibroblast differentiation [62, 65]. In a clinical trial using a cream containing *C. asiatica* and *Pinus sylvestris* and where all the patients responded to the study, 57.1% of the burns completely disappeared after 8 weeks of the treatment, 46.7% of the scars got smaller by more than 50%, and the color of the burns and scars improved [66]. Asiaticoside inducedcell-cycle progression, proliferation, and collagen synthesis in human dermal fibroblasts [67].

Cinnamomum Camphora

Cinnamomum camphora, belonging to the family Lauraceae, is an evergreen broad-leaf tree indigenous to southern China and Japan [68]. It is commonly known as the camphor tree [69]. It has been reported that *C. camphora* contains alkaloids, tannins, flavonoids, saponins, and essential oil, mainly camphor (Fig. **9**) [70, 71].

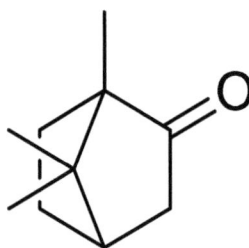

Fig. (9). The chemical structure of camphor.

In vitro analysis of silver nanoparticles formulated from a *C. camphora* leaf extract reported antimicrobial activity against several types of bacteria such as *Staphylococcus aureus*, *Bacillus subtilis*, *Escherichia coli*, *Pseudomonas aeruginosa*, and *Candida albicans* [72, 73]. An ethyl acetate soluble fraction of *C. camphora* leaf extract improved tissue granulation, collagen, and elastin synthesis when administered orally to burn wounded rats [71]. An improved degree of wound contraction, epithelialization, and tissue granulation that is manifested by the enhanced production of hydroxyproline, elastin, and collagen was observed on day 16 following treatment with an ethanolic extract of *C. camphora* leaves at a dose of 100 mg/kg/day in rats with a wound reduction percentage of 95 compared to 84 in the control group [74]. *C. camphora*, known in Arabic as *kafoor* and *mashtak*, was used in Unani medicine due to its cold, antimicrobial, and anti-inflammatory properties [75].

Hypericum Perforatum

Known to most as *St. John's wort*, *Hypericum perforatum* belongs to the family Hypericaceae. It has shown potential as an antidepressant [49], and its extract is the most widely prescribed antidepressant in Germany [76]. Moreover, this species has traditionally been utilized as an external anti-inflammatory and healing remedy for the treatment of swellings, wounds, and burns [77]. These medicinal properties are attributed in part to its naphtodianthrones (hypericin and pseudohypericin), phloroglucinols (hyperforin and adhyperforin) (Fig. **10**), phenolics, and polyphenols metabolites, including flavanoids, tannins, and xanthones [78, 79].

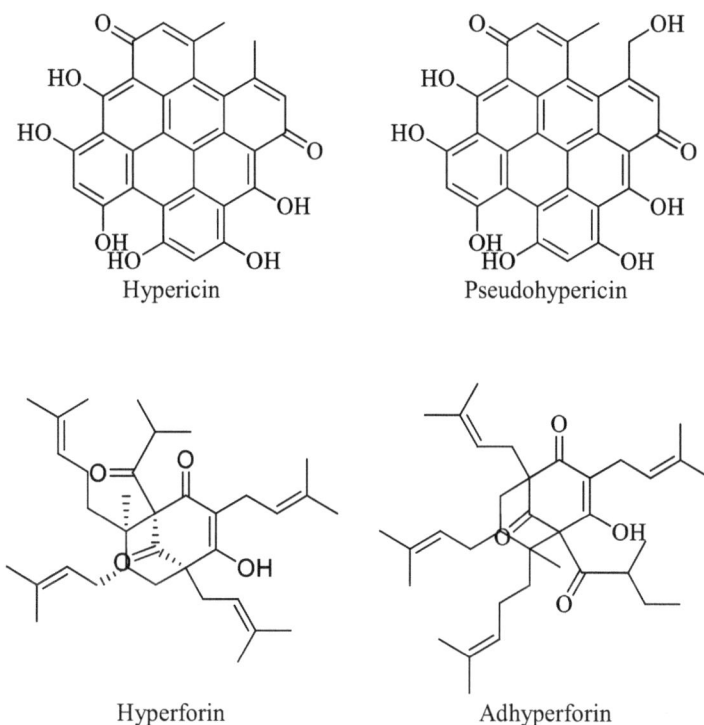

Fig. (10). Characteristic phytochemicals in *Hypericum perforatum.*

Hyperforin has an anti-inflammatory effect *via* the inhibition caused by natural compounds cyclooxygenase-1 (COX-1) and lipoxygenase-5 (LOX-5), which interfere with prostaglandin synthesis as well as the inhibition of T-lymphocyte proliferation [80, 81]. Reduced congestion and edema that result from burn induction were observed following treatment with *H. perforatum*. Also, improved tissue re-epithelization and collagen synthesis were reported [82]. *H. perforatum* oil topical administration was investigated on rats 24 hours post-induced burns for 20 days [83]. Fibroblast proliferation and angiogenesis were enhanced by the treatment. Keratinocytes differentiation was noticed as a result of Transient Receptor Potential Cation Channel Subfamily C Member 6(TRPC6) channel activation following hyperforin treatment [83]. Topical administration of *H.*

perforatum four times daily in the first 24 hours of induced thermal burn increased epidermal thickness and angiogenesis which indicate proper tissue remodeling [84]. In another study, an ointment of *H. perforatum* oil was investigated on an animal model for its efficacy in burn wound healing. The results revealed that the ointment was capable of inducing wound closure starting from day 6 of treatment and significantly improved closure by day 9 ($p < 0.0001$) compared to the control groups which received the ointment base or no treatment [82].

Lawsonia Inermis Linn.

Lawsonia inermis Linn., commonly known as henna, belongs to the family Lythraceae [85]. It is generally considered a native of Africa and Asia. However, the plant is now widely cultivated in tropical regions as an ornamental and dye plant [86]. Lawsone is the principal coloring matter of henna (Fig. **11**) along with other phytochemicals, including gallic acid, tannins, flavonoids, coumarins, essential oils, glucose, mannitol, fats, resin, mucilage, and traces of an alkaloid [87].

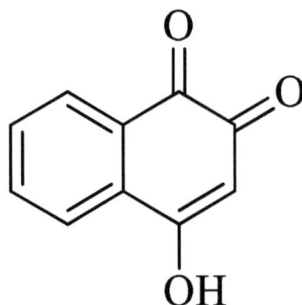

Fig. (11). The chemical structure of Lawsone.

Anti-microbial activity from an ethanolic extract of *L. inermis* was reported against the primary invaders of burn wounds: *Escherichia coli, Staphylococcus aureus, Bacillus subtilis, Salmonella typhi, Klebsiella,* and *Pseudomonas aeruginosa.* Additionally, the extract resulted in improved wound contraction (71% reduction, $p<0.001$), tissue epithelialization, and granulation when applied to an induced burn rodent model at a concentration of 200 mg/kg/day [88]. Anti-inflammatory activity of *L. inermis* following the application of gelatin-oxidized starch-henna has also been observed [89].

The oil extract of *L. inermis* has shown an ability to promote re-epithelialization in addition to collagen synthesis in rats by day 11 of treatment ($p=0.002$) [90]. *L. inermis* oil contains a significant amount of polyunsaturated fatty acids, such as oleic, linoleic, and linolenic acids, that play a major role in the inflammatory response during wound healing by enhancing new blood vessels formation, fibroblast differentiation, and tissue remodeling [90].

In vivo investigation into the ability of *L. inermis* hydrogel film in combination with chitosan showed an improvement in wounds through angiogenesis expression, fibroblasts, macro-phages and collagen formation ($p<0.001$) [91].The natural extract of *L. inermis,* when used in ointment formulation alone and in combination with *Punica granatum* and *Commiphora,* was found to promote wound contraction in percentages reaching 98.5% [92].

Malva Sylvestris

Malva sylvestris, belonging to the family Malvaceae and usually known as common mallow, is a native plant to Europe, North Africa, and Asia. It is traditionally used, especially in Iran, to treat various skin disorders, including cut wounds, dermal infected wounds, and eczema, and for its antimicrobial and anti-inflammatory activities [41, 93]. Phytochemical reports revealed the presence of malvone A, a naphthoquinone (Fig. **12**), and different known monoterpenes and diterpenes. Additionally, vitamin C, vitamin E, β-carotene, flavonoids, polyphenols, and mucilage polysaccharides have been reported [94, 95].

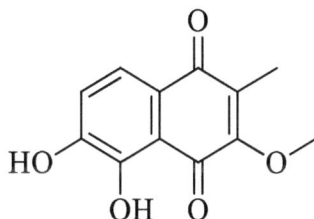

Fig. (12). The chemical structure of malvone A.

A 5% and 10% *M. sylvestris* cream were investigated *in vivo* for their ability to enhance burn wound healing [96]. The results showed that the wound size decreased significantly by day 15 compared to the control groups that were treated with 1% silver sulfadiazine and cold cream base ($p=0.001$), especially after the 10% *M. sylvestris* cream application [96]. Wound contraction was almost complete after the 30th day of 10% *M. sylvestris* cream application. On the other hand, re-epithelialization that is manifested by the degree of epidermal and granular cell layer thickness and squamous cell differentiation and keratinocytes disposition showed comparable results in 5% and 10% treated groups at day 8 [96]. Generally, the extent of re-epithelialization, tissue granulation, and new dermal tissue formation was comparable between the animal groups treated with either a 5% or 10% *M. sylvestris* cream. Malvone A was suggested to contribute to the anti-oxidant as well as anti-inflammatory activity of *Malva* extract [41, 96].

Furthermore, a combination of *M. sylvestris* and *A. euchroma* in the form of an ointment was found to accelerate burn wound healing [41].

Myrtus Communis

Myrtus communis, common myrtle belonging to the family Myrtaceae, is native to southern Europe, north Africa, and west Asia. Now, it is distributed in South America, the northwestern Himalayas, and Australia and is widespread in the Mediterranean region. It is also cultivated in gardens, especially in the north-west Indian region, for its fragrant flowers [97]. A wide range of biologically active compounds, such as tannins, flavonoids, coumarins, fixed oil, fibers, sugars, citric acid, malic acid, caffeic acids, antioxidants, and essential oil, are present in the plant. Although the components of essential oil are highly variable, terpenoid compounds are the major constituents found in myrtle essential oil [98].

Several studies have described the efficacy of *M. communis* leaves as anti-inflammatory and antioxidant [99 - 101]. The potential mechanism of *M. communis* antioxidant activity could be the free radical scavenging ability of the essential oils of the leaves and flowers [100]. Essential oils could disrupt the lipid oxidation that might be initiated through enzymatic or non-enzymatic free radical reactions [100]. Topical administration of 5% (w/w) ointment as well as oral administration at a dose of 100 mg/kg of *M. communis* leaves extract to induced thermal burns in rats showed a significant increase in glutathione, catalase, tissue factor III (coagulation factor), and superoxide dismutase levels compared to the control group ($p < 0.05$) [102, 103]. Conversely, malondialdehyde levels subsided following treatment with either topical or oral extract of *M. communis* leaves ($p < 0.05$) [102, 103]. The anti-inflammatory effect was revealed *via* the reduction of TNF-α besides the reduction of IL-6 and neutrophils at the wound site [102, 104].

Olea Europaea

Olive, Olea europaea, known as *zaytoun* in Arabic, is an evergreen tree belonging to the family Oleaceae. *Olea europaea* preparations have been used widely in folk medicine in the European Mediterranean area, Arabian Peninsula, India, and other tropical and subtropical regions. Furthermore, olive oil represents an important component of the Mediterranean diet [105]. Nowadays, the major producers of olives and olive oil are Spain, Italy, and Greece [106]. The nutritional properties of *Olea europaea* are due to the presence of high levels of fatty acids, oleic acid in particular, as well as other valuable components like phenolics, phytosterols, tocopherols, and squalene [106]. A number of variable phenolic compounds have been identified, including oleuropeosides, oleuropein, verbascoside, flavonoids, tyrosol, hydroxytyrosol, vanillin, vanillic acid, and caffeic acid. Oleuropein (Fig.

13) is the most important component from a quantitative point of view. It is a secoiridoid glucoside that contains both a monoterpenic and orhto-diphenolic unit [107, 108].

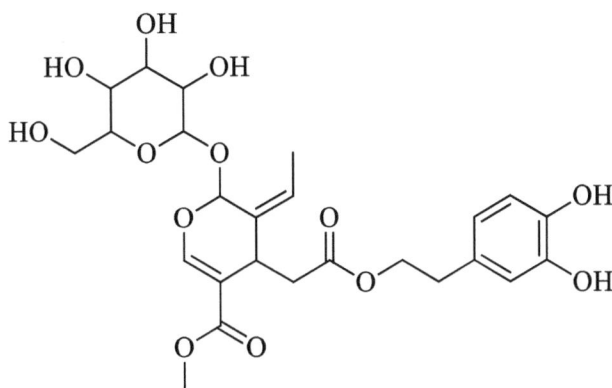

Fig. (13). The chemical structure of Oleuropein.

An aqueous extract of *O. europaea* leaves and fruits enhanced wound contraction by 87.1% by day 12 ($p<0.001$), as well as antioxidant activity in animals subjected to induced thermal injuries [109]. Tissue epithelialization, collagen, and fibroblasts synthesis were enhanced following the treatment of wounded animals with the aqueous extract of *O. europaea* leaves [109]. These pharmacological effects could be attributed to oleuropein, the main active ingredient of *O. europaea* [109]. Additionally, wound contraction was observed following the treatment of diabetic and normal rats with the leaf extract [110]. Animals treated with ointment of *O. europaea* in combination with shea butter showed anti-microbial activity against MRSA [110]. Additionally, scavenging of 2,2-diphenyl-1-picrylhydrazyl (DPPH) free radicals was observed [110]. All the formerly mentioned processes have a significant effect upon wound healing of burns.

Plantago Major

Plantago major is a perennial medicinal plant that belongs to the family of Plantaginaceae. *P. major* and is known by a number of common names around the world: 'common plantain' (English), 'Plantain majeur' (French), 'Breitwegerich' (German), 'Tanchagem-maior' (Portuguese), 'llantén' (Spanish), 'Lisan Al-hamal' (Arabic) and 'Groblad' (Swedish) meaning healing leaves. The plant is native to most of Europe and northern and central Asia but has widely naturalized elsewhere in the world [111]. It is popular in traditional medicine for wound healing as well as for treating diseases related to the skin [112]. Phytochemical studies of *P. major* have determined the presence of various bioactive compounds, including flavonoids, alkaloids, terpenoids, phenolic compounds (caffeic acid derivatives), iridoid glycosides, fatty acids, sterols, polysaccharides, mucilage, and vitamins [113].

The wound-healing property of the leaf extract of *P. major* was confirmed in an *ex vivo* porcine wound-healing model [114]. A solution of *P. major* (50%) promoted healing of induced burns in rats after 21 days of treatment with significant improvement in tissue epithelization, granulation, and formation of spindled fibroblasts (*p*= 0.05) [115]. Additionally, newly formed capillaries were observed which indicates angiogenesis and mild anti-inflammatory activity was also observed with a decrease in the number of inflammatory cells [115, 116]. The flavonoid content of the leaf and seed extract showed antioxidant activity [113]. However, the wound healing activity is mainly attributed to polyphenols, especially plantamajoside (Fig. **14**) [113].

A mixture of cabbage, *Punica granatum*, and *P. major* ointment was investigated on rats and showed significant effect over burn healing 12 days following treatment (*p*<0.027) [117, 118]. Another mixture of 5% of both *P. major* and *Aloe vera* gel showed superior and significant wound healing compared to a gel base treatment group in rats (*p*<0.05). Tissue remodeling manifested *via* the improvement of the density of collagen bundles in addition to neovascularization which was the proposed mechanisms for wound healing [119]. Other studies indicated some antioxidant and anti–inflammatory activity as well as cell proliferation enhancement activities of *P. major* extracts during wound healing [115, 119]. Furthermore, the plant's aqueous extract has antimicrobial activity against *Staphylococcus aureus* [120], and the methanolic extract has inhibitory effects on lipopolysaccharide-induced interleukin-1β and interleukin-6 in addition to COX-2 mRNA expression in mouse macrophage cells [121].

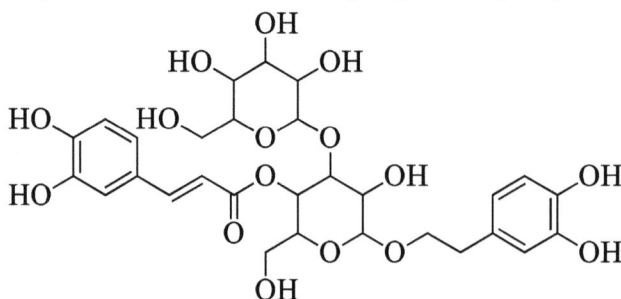

Fig. (14). The chemical structure of Plantamajoside.

Sesamum Indicum

Sesamum indicum, commonly called sesame, is an annual shrub that belongs to the family Pedaliaceae [122]. It is one of the oldest crops in the world that is mainly grown for its oil rich edible seeds. The crop has early origins in east Africa and India and has been under cultivation in Asia for over 5,000 years [123]. Traditionally, sesame seeds are used in the treatment of wounds, especially burn wounds [124]. A number of chemical compounds have been isolated from sesame seeds and leaves: sesamin, sesamol, and sesamolin (Fig. **15**), which are lignan compounds that have revealed many therapeutic potentials for this plant [125].

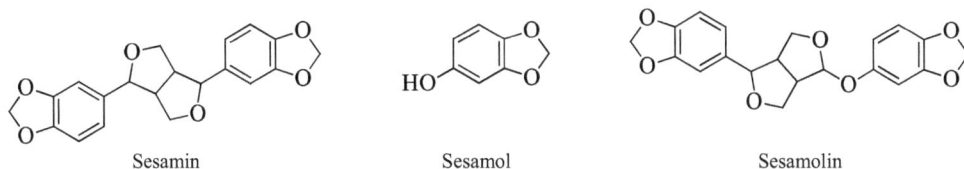

Sesamin   Sesamol   Sesamolin

Fig. (15). Lignans identified in *Sesamum indicum.*

Also, the phytochemical screening of *S. indicum* indicates the presence of proteins, carbohydrates, alkaloids, flavonoids, saponins, terpenoids, steroids, anthraquinones, and tannins [126]. Sesame has been found to be a high source of minerals; potassium was the highest, followed in descending order by phosphorus, magnesium, calcium, and sodium [127].

Sesamol has antioxidant properties [128 - 130], and its intraperitoneal administration to rats played a significant role in wound contraction improvement ($p<0.05$) by day 7 of treatment with a 50 mg/kg dose [128]. Histopathological examination following treatment with sesamol showed enhanced collagen fiber and fibroblast formations and lower inflammatory cell infiltrations to the wound site [128]. Epithelization and wound contraction improved in a murine model following topical treatment with a combination of *S. indicum, Pistacia atlantica, Cannabis sativa*, and *Juglans regia L.* twice daily, in which full tissue remodeling was observed at day 21 [131]. The use of *S. indicum* seed extract on rats confirmed enhanced tissue epithelization and wound contraction [132].

Melaleuca Alternifolia

Tea tree oil is a pale-yellow essential oil extracted from the leaves of the *Melaleuca alternifolia* plant, which belongs to the family Myrtaceae. This native shrub grows on the northeastern Australian coast, often alongside bodies of water [133]. It has been demonstrated to be effective in a variety of skin infections, skin cancer, and the management of immune disorders that affect the skin [134]. Tea tree oil consists of terpene hydrocarbons, mainly monoterpenes, sesquiterpenes, and their associated alcohols. It has a minimum content of 30% of terpinen-4-ol and a maximum content of 15% of 1,8-cineole (Fig. **16**). The former is the major component and exhibits medicinal properties, whereas the latter is the one which shows an undesirable allergen in tea tree oil products [134, 135].

Despite the antimicrobial activity of tea tree oil, its use in burns treatment is not advised [136, 137]. This was ascribed to tea tree oil as one of the components in a commercially available cream, Burnaid™ (*Aloe vera*, saliva, and tea tree oil). This cream inversely affects the process of burn wound healing due to its toxicity against fibroblasts and epithelial cells [136, 138].

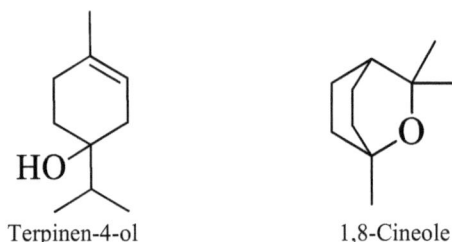

Terpinen-4-ol   1,8-Cineole

Fig. (16). Characteristic phytochemicals in tea tree oil.

Substances of Animal Origin

Honey

Honey has been used as a traditional medicine for the treatment of burns and chronic wounds. Owing to the fact that honey is produced *via* bees from different medicinal plant flower nectars, honey could possess some therapeutic effects due to the presence of phytochemicals that are transmitted from the original plants [139]. Consequently, the therapeutic effect of honey might vary according to the source of flower nectar. Manuka (*Leptospermum scoparium*) and Revamil® source (RS) honey, produced under standardized conditions in greenhouses, showed antimicrobial as well as anti-oxidant properties that help in the treatment of infections, ulcers, burns, and other dermatological complications [139, 140]. As a result, both are the most used therapeutic honeys [141, 142]. Factors that are responsible for the antimicrobial activity of honey are the presence of high sugar concentration, hydrogen peroxide, methylglyoxal, antimicrobial peptide defensin-1, and low pH [143].

Despite the different types of honey, all contain phenolic compounds with variable concentrations depending on the honey color, darkness, and degree [139]. The phenolic contents of honey contribute to its antioxidant activity which is one of the main burn healing mechanisms [139]. Flavonoids are the main class of polyphenols and are present mainly as aglycone in a honey matrix [144]. Simple phenolic compounds are also identified in honey, such as caffeic acid, chlorogenic acid, cinnamic acid, ellagic acid, ferulic acid, and gallic acid. Additionally, honey contains about 180 types of different compounds, including water, sugars, free aminoacids, proteins, enzymes, essential minerals, vitamins, and various phytochemicals [145].

Honey dressings aid in reducing the healing time of wounds, including burns [146, 147]. The main pathway was found to be through wound contraction improvement, epithelialization, promoting granulation, collagen synthesis, and angiogenesis [146]. It was also found to induce burn healing due to the presence of saponins as a main component and which helps to promote new blood vessel formations and blood circulation improvement to the application area, in other words, angiogenesis as well as granulation and epithelialization [24, 148]. In addition, honey could induce fibroblast and monocyte differentiation and proliferation as well as connective tissue regeneration [24, 149]. Several observational studies showed that the use of honey for wound healing was efficacious and could accelerate partial thickness burn healing [150]. However, controlled clinical trials showed modest efficacy [151 - 153].

Propolis

Propolis, or bee glue, is a natural wax-like resinous substance found in beehives where it is used by honeybees as cement to seal cracks or open spaces. The best sources of propolis are species of poplar, willow, birch, elm, alder, beech, conifer, and horse-chestnut trees [154]. Propolis has been used as an antiseptic and wound healer since ancient times [155]. More than 180 compounds, mainly polyphenols, have been identified as constituents of propolis. The major polyphenols are flavonoids, accompanied by phenolic acids and esters. Other compounds in propolis are volatile oils, aromatic acids, waxes, resins, balms, and pollen grains, which are rich sources of essential elements such as magnesium, nickel, calcium, iron, and zinc. However, the composition of propolis is highly variable depending on the site of its collection [156].

Previous studies showed a significant effect of propolis in scavenging reactive oxygen species (ROS) that result from the burn wound [157]. Furthermore, propolis enhanced collagen type I and III synthesis during the granulation phase of wound healing and could inhibit MMP enzymes that interfere with new extracellular matrix formation through fibronectin catabolism [157]. Additionally, it was suggested propolis has the ability to promote glycosaminoglycan synthesis, especially, chondroitin/dermatan sulphate, during burn wound healing and that could be attributed to its flavonoid content that is capable of preventing cell necrosis [157]. It was previously reported that caffeic acid phenethyl ester, a component of propolis, is responsible for the anti-inflammatory as well as antimicrobial activity of propolis during the wound healing process [158]. Flavonoids and phenolic phytochemicals of propolis exert an antioxidant activity through lipid peroxidation inhibition *via* free radical scavenging, thus promoting burn wound healing [159]. Unfortunately, information regarding the dose, side effects, and clinical effectiveness for humans of propolis is still insufficient [160].

Substances of Fungal Origin

Sacchachitin

Sacchachitin is a skin wound-healing membrane made of the residual fruiting body of *Ganoderma tsugae* (Ganodermataceae) [161]. This mushroom belongs to basidiomycete white rot fungus, and it has been used as a medicinal mushroom in China and other Asian countries, including Japan and Korea [162]. The name of sacchachitin was from the combination of polysaccharide and chitin because it contains almost equal parts of both components [163]. It is a copolymer of β-1,3-glucan (~60%) and *N*-acetylglucosamine (~40%) [164]. Terpenes and sterols are also identified in sacchachitin [162].

Both *in vitro* and *in vivo* analysis of sacchachitin reported its ability to induce burn wound healing *via* enhancement of cell proliferation in addition to inhibition of proteolysis [165]. A dressing composed of 10% sacchachitinin combination with 5% carboxymethyl cellulose sodium salt was tested on Wistar rats induced thermal burns and resulted in improving cell proliferation and skin remodeling *via* increasing the level of PDGF, TGF-946;1, and VEGF growth factors MMP-9 and presumed MMP-2 suppression [166]. A sacchachitin membrane which is composed of β-1,3-glucan (ca 60%) and *N*-acetylglucosamine (ca 40%), was capable of inducing cell proliferation *via* fibroblast migration on day 9 after burning induction on animal models [167 - 169].

CONCLUDING REMARKS

The process of burn healing is complicated, and different factors are involved in the process. For example, oxidative damage to tissues and over-inflammation can interfere with burn healing. Natural products from different sources, especially those possessing antioxidant and inflammatory activities, are useful in enhancing the healing process. Several studies have identified natural products that are effective for accelerating burn healing and reducing scarring, yet others still need further investigation and research.

REFERENCES

[1]   American Burn Association (ABA). National Burn Awareness Week 2021. Available from: https://ameriburn.org/national-burn-awareness-week-2021/ (Updated 5th February 2021; cited: 30th August 2022).

[2]   World Health Organization (WHO). World Health Organization (WHO). Burns. Available from: https://www.who.int/en/news-room/fact-sheets/detail/burns (Updated 6th March 2018; cited 30th August 2022).

[3]   Centers for Disease Control and Prevention (CDC). Burns. Available from: https://www.cdc.gov/masstrauma/factsheets/public/burns.pdf (cited: 30th August 2022).

[4]   Abazari M, Ghaffari A, Rashidzadeh H, Badeleh SM, Maleki Y. A systematic review on classification, identification, and healing process of burn wound healing. Int J Low Extrem Wounds 2022; 21(1): 18-30.
[http://dx.doi.org/10.1177/1534734620924857] [PMID: 32524874]

[5]   Advanced burn life support course: provider manual 2018 Update. American Burn Association; 2018. Available from: https://ameriburn.org/wp-content/uploads/2019/08/2018-abls-providermanual.pdf (Updated 2018; cited 30th August 2022).

[6]   Wald DA. An Introduction to Clinical Emergency Medicine. 2nd. New York: Cambridge University Press 2012; pp. 1-884.

[7]   Warby R, Maani CV. Burn Classification BTI - StatPearls. StatPearls Publishing 2020.

[8]   Shpichka A, Butnaru D, Bezrukov EA, *et al.* Skin tissue regeneration for burn injury. Stem Cell Res Ther 2019; 10(1): 94.
[http://dx.doi.org/10.1186/s13287-019-1203-3] [PMID: 30876456]

[9]   Vinish M, Cui W, Stafford E, *et al.* Dendritic cells modulate burn wound healing by enhancing early proliferation. Wound Repair Regen 2016; 24(1): 6-13.
[http://dx.doi.org/10.1111/wrr.12388] [PMID: 26609910]

[10]   El Khatib A, Jeschke MG. Contemporary aspects of burn care. Medicina 2021; 57(4): 386.
[http://dx.doi.org/10.3390/medicina57040386] [PMID: 33923571]

[11]   Pećanac M, Janjić Z, Komarcević A, Pajić M, Dobanovački D, Misković SS. Burns treatment in ancient times. Med Pregl 2013; 66(5-6): 263-7.
[PMID: 23888738]

[12]   Wallner C, Moormann E, Lulof P, Drysch M, Lehnhardt M, Behr B. Burn care in the Greek and Roman antiquity. Medicina (Kaunas) 2020; 56(12): 657.
[http://dx.doi.org/10.3390/medicina56120657] [PMID: 33260533]

[13]   Lee KC, Joory K, Moiemen N. History of burns: the past, present and the future. Burns Trauma 2014; 2(4): 2321-3868.143620.

[14]   Aliasl J, Khoshzaban F. Traditional herbal remedies for burn wound healing in canon of Avicenna. Jundishapur J Nat Pharm Prod 2013; 8(4): 192-6.
[http://dx.doi.org/10.17795/jjnpp-11686]

[15]   Choi S, Chung MH. A review on the relationship between *Aloe vera* components and their biologic effects. Semin Integr Med 2003; 1(1): 53-62.
[http://dx.doi.org/10.1016/S1543-1150(03)00005-X]

[16]   Feily A, Namazi MR. *Aloe vera* in dermatology: a brief review. G Ital Dermatol Venereol 2009; 144(1): 85-91.
[PMID: 19218914]

[17]   Maenthaisong R, Chaiyakunapruk N, Niruntraporn S, Kongkaew C. The efficacy of *Aloe vera* used for burn wound healing: a systematic review. Burns 2007; 33(6): 713-8.

[18]   Hamman J. Composition and applications of *Aloe vera* leaf gel. Molecules 2008; 13(8): 1599-616.
[http://dx.doi.org/10.3390/molecules13081599] [PMID: 18794775]

[19]   Hu Y, Xu J, Hu Q. Evaluation of antioxidant potential of *Aloe vera* (*Aloe barbadensis* miller) extracts. J Agric Food Chem 2003; 51(26): 7788-91.
[http://dx.doi.org/10.1021/jf034255i] [PMID: 14664546]

[20]   Davis RH, Donato JJ, Hartman GM, Haas RC. Anti-inflammatory and wound healing activity of a growth substance in *Aloe vera.* J Am Podiatr Med Assoc 1994; 84(2): 77-81.
[http://dx.doi.org/10.7547/87507315-84-2-77] [PMID: 8169808]

[21]   Moon EJ, Lee YM, Lee OH, *et al.* A novel angiogenic factor derived from *Aloe vera* gel: β-sitosterol,

a plant sterol. Angiogenesis 1999; 3(2): 117-23.
[http://dx.doi.org/10.1023/A:1009058232389] [PMID: 14517429]

[22]   Ebadi M. Pharmacodynamic basis of herbal medicine. 2nd ed. CRC press 2006; pp. 1-699.
[http://dx.doi.org/10.1201/9781420006452]

[23]   Bunyapraphatsara N, Jirakulchaiwong S, Thirawarapan S, Manonukul J. The efficacy of *Aloe vera* cream in the treatment of first, second and third degree burns in mice. Phytomedicine 1996; 2(3): 247-51.
[http://dx.doi.org/10.1016/S0944-7113(96)80050-X] [PMID: 23194624]

[24]   Farzadinia P, Jofreh N, Khatamsaz S, *et al.* Anti-inflammatory and wound healing activities of *Aloe vera*, honey and milk ointment on second-degree burns in rats. Int J Low Extrem Wounds 2016; 15(3): 241-7.
[http://dx.doi.org/10.1177/1534734616645031] [PMID: 27217089]

[25]   Hekmatpou D, Mehrabi F, Rahzani K, Aminiyan A. The effect of *Aloe vera* clinical trials on prevention and healing of skin wound: a systematic review. Iran J Med Sci 2019; 44(1): 1-9.
[PMID: 30666070]

[26]   Khorasani G, Hosseinimehr SJ, Azadbakht M, Zamani A, Mahdavi MR. Aloe *versus* silver sulfadiazine creams for second-degree burns: A randomized controlled study. Surg Today 2009; 39(7): 587-91.
[http://dx.doi.org/10.1007/s00595-008-3944-y] [PMID: 19562446]

[27]   Surjushe A, Vasani R, Saple DG. *Aloe vera*: A short review. Indian J Dermatol 2008; 53(4): 163-6.
[http://dx.doi.org/10.4103/0019-5154.44785] [PMID: 19882025]

[28]   Amudhan MS, Begum VH, Hebbar K. A review on phytochemical and pharmacological potential of *Areca catechu L.* seed. Int J Pharm Sci 2012; 3(11): 4151-7.

[29]   Salehi B, Konovalov DA, Fru P, *et al.* Areca catechu-From farm to food and biomedical applications. Phytother Res 2020; 34(9): 2140-58.
[http://dx.doi.org/10.1002/ptr.6665] [PMID: 32159263]

[30]   Peng W, Liu YJ, Wu N, *et al. Areca catechu L. (Arecaceae):* A review of its traditional uses, botany, phytochemistry, pharmacology and toxicology. J Ethnopharmacol 2015; 164: 340-56.
[http://dx.doi.org/10.1016/j.jep.2015.02.010] [PMID: 25681543]

[31]   Bharat M, Verma DK, Shanbhag V, Rajput RS, Nayak D, Amuthan A. Ethanolic extract of oral Areca catechu promotes burn wound healing in rats. Int J Pharm Sci Rev Res 2014; 25(2): 145-8.

[32]   Hamsar MN, Ismail S, Mordi MN, Ramanathan S, Mansor SM. Antioxidant activity and the effect of different parts of *Areca catechu* extracts on glutathione-*S*-transferase activity *in vitro*. Free Radic Antioxid 2011; 1(1): 28-33.
[http://dx.doi.org/10.5530/ax.2011.1.6]

[33]   Sari EF, Prayogo GP, Loo YT, Zhang P, McCullough MJ, Cirillo N. Distinct phenolic, alkaloid and antioxidant profile in betel quids from four regions of Indonesia. Sci Rep 2020; 10(1): 16254.
[http://dx.doi.org/10.1038/s41598-020-73337-0] [PMID: 33004929]

[34]   Wetwitayaklung P, Phaechamud T, Limmatvapirat C, Keokitichai S. The study of antioxidant capacity in various parts of Areca catechu L. Naresuan Univ J Sci Technol 2013; 14(1): 1-14.

[35]   Hu M, Peng W, Liu Y, *et al.* Optimum extraction of polysaccharide from Areca catechu using response surface methodology and its Antioxidant Activity. J Food Process Preserv 2017; 41(1): e12798.
[http://dx.doi.org/10.1111/jfpp.12798]

[36]   Verma DK, Bharat M, Nayak D, Shanbhag T, Shanbhag V, Rajput RS, *et al.* Areca catechu: Effect of topical ethanolic extract on burn wound healing in albino rats. Int J Pharmacol Clin Sci 2012; 1(3)

[37]   Sherliana F, Girsang E, Nasution AN, Lister IN. Comparison of burn wound healing ability between

ethyl acetate extract gel of betel nut (*Areca catechu*) and snake Fruit seed (*Salacca zalacca*) in rats. Am Acad Sci Res J Eng Technol Sci 2020; 68(1): 210-5.

[38]   Ayyanar M, Ignacimuthu S. Herbal medicines for wound healing among tribal people in Southern India: Ethnobotanical and Scientific evidences. Int J Appl Res 2009; 2(3): 29-42.

[39]   Padmaja P, Bairy K, Kulkarni D. Pro-healing effect of betel nut and its polyphenols. Fitoterapia 1994; 65(4): 298-300.

[40]   Aliasl J, Barikbin B, Khoshzaban F, *et al.* Effect of *Arnebia euchroma* ointment on post-laser wound healing in rats. J Cosmet Laser Ther 2015; 17(1): 41-5.
         [http://dx.doi.org/10.3109/14764172.2014.968583] [PMID: 25260137]

[41]   Pirbalouti AG, Yousefi M, Nazari H, Karimi I, Koohpayeh A. Evaluation of burn healing properties of *Arnebia euchroma* and *Malva sylvestris*. Electron J Biotechnol 2009; 5(3): 62-6.

[42]   Xiao Y, Wang Y, Gao S, *et al.* Determination of the active constituents in *Arnebia euchroma* (Royle) Johnst. by ionic liquid-based ultrasonic-assisted extraction high-performance liquid chromatography. J Chromatogr B Analyt Technol Biomed Life Sci 2011; 879(20): 1833-8.
         [http://dx.doi.org/10.1016/j.jchromb.2011.05.009] [PMID: 21606007]

[43]   Ashkani-Esfahani S, Imanieh MH, Khoshneviszadeh M, *et al.* The healing effect of *Arnebia euchroma* in second degree burn wounds in rat as an animal model. Iran Red Crescent Med J 2012; 14(2): 70-4.
         [PMID: 22737558]

[44]   Shen CC, Syu WJ, Li SY, Lin CH, Lee GH, Sun CM. Antimicrobial activities of naphthazarins from *Arnebia euchroma*. J Nat Prod 2002; 65(12): 1857-62.
         [http://dx.doi.org/10.1021/np010599w] [PMID: 12502328]

[45]   Nasiri E, Hosseinimehr SJ, Zaghi Hosseinzadeh A, Azadbakht M, Akbari J, Azadbakht M. The effects of *Arnebia euchroma* ointment on second-degree burn wounds: A randomized clinical trial. J Ethnopharmacol 2016; 189: 107-16.
         [http://dx.doi.org/10.1016/j.jep.2016.05.029] [PMID: 27180881]

[46]   Saeidnia S, Gohari AR, Kurepaz-Mahmoodabadi M, Mokhber-Dezfuli N. Phytochemistry and pharmacology of berberis species. Pharmacogn Rev 2014; 8(15): 8-15.
         [http://dx.doi.org/10.4103/0973-7847.125517] [PMID: 24600191]

[47]   Potdar D, Hirwani RR, Dhulap S. Phyto-chemical and pharmacological applications of Berberis aristata. Fitoterapia 2012; 83(5): 817-30.
         [http://dx.doi.org/10.1016/j.fitote.2012.04.012] [PMID: 22808523]

[48]   Zovko Končić M, Kremer D, Karlović K, Kosalec I. Evaluation of antioxidant activities and phenolic content of Berberis vulgaris L. and Berberis croatica Horvat. Food Chem Toxicol 2010; 48(8-9): 2176-80.
         [http://dx.doi.org/10.1016/j.fct.2010.05.025] [PMID: 20488218]

[49]   Vujanovic S, Vujanovic J. Bioresources in the pharmacotherapy and healing of burns: a mini-review. Burns 2013; 39(6): 1031-8.
         [http://dx.doi.org/10.1016/j.burns.2013.03.016] [PMID: 23642293]

[50]   Biswas TK, Mukherjee B. Plant medicines of Indian origin for wound healing activity: a review. Int J Low Extrem Wounds 2003; 2(1): 25-39.
         [http://dx.doi.org/10.1177/1534734603002001006] [PMID: 15866825]

[51]   Bahramsoltani R, Farzaei MH, Rahimi R. Medicinal plants and their natural components as future drugs for the treatment of burn wounds: an integrative review. Arch Dermatol Res 2014; 306(7): 601-17.
         [http://dx.doi.org/10.1007/s00403-014-1474-6] [PMID: 24895176]

[52]   Su S, Hua Y, Wang Y, *et al.* Evaluation of the anti-inflammatory and analgesic properties of individual and combined extracts from *Commiphora myrrha*, and *Boswellia carterii.* J Ethnopharmacol 2012; 139(2): 649-56.

[http://dx.doi.org/10.1016/j.jep.2011.12.013] [PMID: 22178177]

[53]   Chevrier MR, Ryan AE, Lee DY, Zhongze M, Wu-Yan Z, Via CS. *Boswellia carterii* extract inhibits TH1 cytokines and promotes TH2 cytokines *in vitro*. Clin Diagn Lab Immunol 2005; 12(5): 575-80.
[PMID: 15879017]

[54]   Faraji A, Aghdaki M, Hessami K, *et al.* Episiotomy wound healing by *Commiphora myrrha* (Nees) Engl. and *Boswellia carteri* Birdw. in primiparous women: a randomized controlled trial. J Ethnopharmacol 2021; 264: 113396.
[http://dx.doi.org/10.1016/j.jep.2020.113396] [PMID: 32971163]

[55]   Basar S, Koch A, König WA. A verticillane-type diterpene from *Boswellia carterii* essential oil. Flavour Fragrance J 2001; 16(5): 315-8.
[http://dx.doi.org/10.1002/ffj.992]

[56]   Banno N, Akihisa T, Yasukawa K, *et al.* Anti-inflammatory activities of the triterpene acids from the resin of Boswellia carteri. J Ethnopharmacol 2006; 107(2): 249-53.
[http://dx.doi.org/10.1016/j.jep.2006.03.006] [PMID: 16621377]

[57]   Jahandideh M, Hajimehdipoor H, Mortazavi SA, Dehpour A, Hassanzadeh G. A wound healing formulation based on Iranian traditional medicine and its HPTLC fingerprint. Iran J Pharm Res 2016; 15 (Suppl.): 149-57.
[PMID: 28228812]

[58]   Chhibber T, Gondil VS, Sinha VR. Development of chitosan-based hydrogel containing antibiofilm agents for the treatment of *Staphylococcus aureus* infected burn wound in mice. AAPS PharmSciTech 2020; 21(2): 43.
[http://dx.doi.org/10.1208/s12249-019-1537-2] [PMID: 31897806]

[59]   Khalil AM, Abd AH, Hussein BF. The use of methanolic extract of *Boswellia serrata* in combination with dextrin and glycerin for treatment of experimentally induced thermal injuries in rabbits. Iraqi J Med Sci 2016; 14(3)

[60]   Bylka W, Znajdek-Awiżeń P, Studzińska-Sroka E, Brzezińska M. Centella asiatica in cosmetology. Postepy Dermatol Alergol 2013; 1(1): 46-9.
[http://dx.doi.org/10.5114/pdia.2013.33378] [PMID: 24278045]

[61]   Gohil K, Patel J, Gajjar A. Pharmacological review on *Centella asiatica*: a potential herbal cure-all. Indian J Pharm Sci 2010; 72(5): 546-56.
[http://dx.doi.org/10.4103/0250-474X.78519] [PMID: 21694984]

[62]   Wu F, Bian D, Xia Y, Gong Z, Tan Q, Chen J, *et al.* Identification of major active ingredients responsible for burn wound healing of *Centella asiatica* herbs. Evid-based Complement Altern Med. 2012.

[63]   Liu M, Dai Y, Li Y, *et al.* Madecassoside isolated from *Centella asiatica* herbs facilitates burn wound healing in mice. Planta Med 2008; 74(8): 809-15.
[http://dx.doi.org/10.1055/s-2008-1074533] [PMID: 18484522]

[64]   Somboonwong J, Kankaisre M, Tantisira B, Tantisira MH. Wound healing activities of different extracts of Centella asiatica in incision and burn wound models: an experimental animal study. BMC Complement Altern Med 2012; 12(1): 103.
[http://dx.doi.org/10.1186/1472-6882-12-103] [PMID: 22817824]

[65]   Hossain ML, Rahman MA, Siddika A, *et al.* Burn and wound healing using radiation sterilized human amniotic membrane and centella asiatica derived gel: a review. Regen Eng Transl Med 2020; 6(3): 347-57.
[http://dx.doi.org/10.1007/s40883-019-00122-5]

[66]   Romo EM, Fundora FP, Albajes CR, López LE, Hana Z. The effectiveness of cream with *Centella Asiatica* and *Pinus Sylvestris* to treat scars and burns. Clinical Trial. Dermatologia Klin 2012; 14(3): 105-10.

[67]   Lu L, Ying K, Wei S, *et al.* Asiaticoside induction for cell-cycle progression, proliferation and collagen synthesis in human dermal fibroblasts. Int J Dermatol 2004; 43(11): 801-7.
[http://dx.doi.org/10.1111/j.1365-4632.2004.02047.x] [PMID: 15533060]

[68]   Chen C, Zheng Y, Zhong Y, *et al.* Transcriptome analysis and identification of genes related to terpenoid biosynthesis in *Cinnamomum camphora*. BMC Genomics 2018; 19(1): 550.
[http://dx.doi.org/10.1186/s12864-018-4941-1] [PMID: 30041601]

[69]   Wu L, Xiong W, Hu JW, *et al.* Secondary metabolites from the twigs of *Cinnamomum camphora*. Chem Nat Compd 2019; 55(2): 345-7.
[http://dx.doi.org/10.1007/s10600-019-02686-8]

[70]   Lee HJ, Hyun EA, Yoon WJ, *et al. In vitro* anti-inflammatory and anti-oxidative effects of *Cinnamomum camphora* extracts. J Ethnopharmacol 2006; 103(2): 208-16.
[http://dx.doi.org/10.1016/j.jep.2005.08.009] [PMID: 16182479]

[71]   Sen PK, Garg S. Wound repair and regenerating effect of ethyl acetate soluble fraction of ethanolic extract of *Cinnamomum camphora* leaves in wistar albino rats. J Drug Deliv Ther 2019; 9(4-s): 1173-6.

[72]   Li W, Qu F, Chen Y, *et al.* Antimicrobial activity of sliver nanoparticles synthesized by the leaf extract of *Cinnamomum camphora*. Biochem Eng J 2021; 172: 108050.
[http://dx.doi.org/10.1016/j.bej.2021.108050]

[73]   Abouzeid A, Reham A, Sarah H, Khaled M. Potential antimicrobial activity of different types of Libyan honeys. Egypt J Plant Prot Res Inst 2019; 2(4): 617-723.

[74]   Sen PK, Garg S. Influence of *Cinnamomum camphora* ethanolic extract on biophysical and biochemical parameters of cutaneous wounds in rats. J Drug Deliv Ther 2019; 9(4-s): 1169-72.

[75]   Sharma N, Yadevendra Y, Vipin K, Chand SK. Folkare and modern pharmacology of camphor (*Cinnamomum camphora* Nees & Eberm). Sch Int J Tradit Complement Med 2021; 4(7): 128-35.

[76]   Fahmi M, Huang C, Schweitzer I. A case of mania induced by hypericum. World J Biol Psychiatry 2002; 3(1): 58-9.
[http://dx.doi.org/10.3109/15622970209150602] [PMID: 12479089]

[77]   ciccarelli D, andreucci AC, pagni AM. The" black nodules" of Hypericurn perforaturn L. subsp. perforaturn: Morphological, anatomical, and histochemical studies during the course of ontogenesis. Isr J Plant Sci 2001; 49: 33-40.

[78]   Butterweck VSt. John's Wort: quality issues and active compounds. Botanical Medicine. From Bench to Bedside 2009; pp. 70-91.

[79]   Maffi L, Camoni L, Fornasiero RB, Bianchi A. Morphology and development of secretory structures in Hypericum perforatum and H. richeri. Nord J Bot 2003; 23(4): 453-61.
[http://dx.doi.org/10.1111/j.1756-1051.2003.tb00419.x]

[80]   Koeberle A, Rossi A, Bauer J, *et al.* Hyperforin, an anti-inflammatory constituent from St. John's wort, inhibits microsomal prostaglandin E2 synthase-1 and suppresses prostaglandin E2 formation *in vivo*. Front Pharmacol 2011; 2: 7.
[http://dx.doi.org/10.3389/fphar.2011.00007] [PMID: 21687502]

[81]   Kotsiou A, Tesseromatis C. Hypericum perforatum for experimental skin burns treatment in rats in comparison to nitrofurazone. Faslnamah-i Giyahan-i Daruyi 2020; 8(4): 227-31.

[82]   Prisăcaru AI, Andrițoiu CV, Andriescu C, *et al.* Evaluation of the wound-healing effect of a novel Hypericum perforatum ointment in skin injury. Rom J Morphol Embryol 2013; 54(4): 1053-9.
[PMID: 24399001]

[83]   Seyhan N. Evaluation of the healing effects of hypericum perforatum and curcumin on burn wounds in rats. Evid-based Complement Altern Med 2020.
[http://dx.doi.org/10.1155/2020/6462956]

[84]   Kıyan S. Investigation of acute effects of *Hypericum perforatum* (Kantaron) treatment in experimental thermal burns and comparison with silver sulfadiazine treatment. ulus travma acil cerrahi derg 2015.

[85]   Chaudhary G, Goyal S, Poonia P. *Lawsonia inermis* Linnaeus: a phytopharmacological review. Int J Pharm Sci Drug Res 2010; 2(2): 91-8.

[86]   Al-Snafi AE. A review on *Lawsonia inermis*: A potential medicinal plant. Int J Curr Pharm Res 2019; 11(5): 1-13.
       [http://dx.doi.org/10.22159/ijcpr.2019v11i5.35695]

[87]   Borade AS, Kale BN, Shete RV. A phytopharmacological review on *Lawsonia inermis* (Linn.). Int J Pharm Life Sci 2011; 2(1): 536-41.

[88]   Nayak BS, Isitor G, Davis EM, Pillai GK. The evidence based wound healing activity of *Lawsonia inermis* Linn. Phytother Res 2007; 21(9): 827-31.
       [http://dx.doi.org/10.1002/ptr.2181] [PMID: 17533628]

[89]   Hadisi Z, Nourmohammadi J, Nassiri SM. The antibacterial and anti-inflammatory investigation of *Lawsonia inermis* -gelatin-starch nano-fibrous dressing in burn wound. Int J Biol Macromol 2018; 107(Pt B): 2008-19.

[90]   Rekik DM, Ben Khedir S, Daoud A, Ksouda Moalla K, Rebai T, Sahnoun Z. Wound healing effect of *Lawsonia inermis*. Skin Pharmacol Physiol 2019; 32(6): 295-306.
       [http://dx.doi.org/10.1159/000501730] [PMID: 31466077]

[91]   Khan BA, Khan A, Khan MK, Braga VA. Preparation and properties of High sheared Poly(Vinyl Alcohol)/Chitosan blended Hydrogels films with *Lawsonia inermis* extract as wound dressing. J Drug Deliv Sci Technol 2021; 61: 102227.
       [http://dx.doi.org/10.1016/j.jddst.2020.102227]

[92]   Elzayat EM, Auda SH, Alanazi FK, Al-Agamy MH. Evaluation of wound healing activity of henna, pomegranate and myrrh herbal ointment blend. Saudi Pharm J 2018; 26(5): 733-8.
       [http://dx.doi.org/10.1016/j.jsps.2018.02.016] [PMID: 29991918]

[93]   Nasiri E, Hosseinimehr SJ, Azadbakht M, Akbari J, Enayati-Fard R, Azizi S. Effect of *Malva sylvestris* cream on burn injury and wounds in rats. Avicenna J Phytomed 2015; 5(4): 341-54.
       [PMID: 26909337]

[94]   Razavi SM, Zarrini G, Molavi G, Ghasemi G. Bioactivity of *Malva sylvestris* L., a medicinal plant from iran. Iran J Basic Med Sci 2011; 14(6): 574-9.
       [PMID: 23493458]

[95]   Barros L, Carvalho AM, Ferreira ICFR. Leaves, flowers, immature fruits and leafy flowered stems of *Malva sylvestris* : A comparative study of the nutraceutical potential and composition. Food Chem Toxicol 2010; 48(6): 1466-72.
       [http://dx.doi.org/10.1016/j.fct.2010.03.012] [PMID: 20233600]

[96]   Pirbalouti AG, Koohpyeh A. Wound healing activity of extracts of *Malva sylvestris* and *Stachys lavandulifolia*. Int J Biol 2011; 3(1): 174.

[97]   Afshar M, Ravarian B, Zardast M, Moallem SA, Fard MH, Valavi M. Evaluation of cutaneous wound healing activity of *Malva sylvestris* aqueous extract in BALB/c mice. Iran J Basic Med Sci 2015; 18(6): 616-22.
       [PMID: 26221487]

[98]   Sumbul S, Ahmad MA, Asif M, Akhtar M. *Myrtus communis* Linn. - a review. Indian J Nat Prod Resour 2011; 2(4): 395-402.

[99]   Alipour G, Dashti S, Hosseinzadeh H. Review of pharmacological effects of *Myrtus communis* L. and its active constituents. Phytother Res 2014; 28(8): 1125-36.
       [http://dx.doi.org/10.1002/ptr.5122] [PMID: 24497171]

[100] Hayder N, Abdelwahed A, Kilani S, *et al.* Anti-genotoxic and free-radical scavenging activities of

extracts from (Tunisian) Myrtus communis. Mutat Res Genet Toxicol Environ Mutagen 2004; 564(1): 89-95.
[http://dx.doi.org/10.1016/j.mrgentox.2004.08.001] [PMID: 15474415]

[101]   Miguel MG. Antioxidant and anti-inflammatory activities of essential oils: a short review. Molecules 2010; 15(12): 9252-87.
[http://dx.doi.org/10.3390/molecules15129252] [PMID: 21160452]

[102]   Raeiszadeh M, Esmaeili-Tarzi M, Bahrampour-Juybari K, *et al.* Evaluation the effect of *Myrtus communis* L. extract on several underlying mechanisms involved in wound healing: An *in vitro* study. S Afr J Bot 2018; 118: 144-50.
[http://dx.doi.org/10.1016/j.sajb.2018.07.006]

[103]   Ozcan O, Ipekci H, Alev B, *et al.* Protective effect of Myrtle (*Myrtus communis*) on burn induced skin injury. Burns 2019; 45(8): 1856-63.
[http://dx.doi.org/10.1016/j.burns.2019.07.015] [PMID: 31383607]

[104]   Ozcan O, Ipekci H, Alev B, *et al.* The effect of *Myrtus communis* L. ethanol extract on the small intestine and lungs in experimental thermal burn injury. J Therm Biol 2020; 93: 102685.
[http://dx.doi.org/10.1016/j.jtherbio.2020.102685] [PMID: 33077111]

[105]   Sen A, Kurkçuoglu M, Yıldırım A, Dogan A, Bitis L, Baser KHC. Chemical and biological profiles of essential oil from different parts of *Myrtus communis* L. subsp. communis from Turkey. ACS Agric Conspec Sci 2020; 85(1): 71-8.

[106]   Khan Y, Panchal S, Vyas N, Butani A, Kumar V. *Olea europaea*: a phyto-pharmacological review. Pharmacogn Rev 2007; 1(1): 114-8.

[107]   Romani A, Ieri F, Urciuoli S, *et al.* Health effects of phenolic compounds found in extra-virgin olive oil, by-products, and leaf of *Olea europaea* L. Nutrients 2019; 11(8): 1776.
[http://dx.doi.org/10.3390/nu11081776] [PMID: 31374907]

[108]   Bianco A, Ramunno A. The chemistry of *Olea europaea.* Stud Nat Prod Chem 2006; 33: 859-903.
[http://dx.doi.org/10.1016/S1572-5995(06)80042-6]

[109]   El SN, Karakaya S. Olive tree *(Olea europaea)* leaves: potential beneficial effects on human health. Nutr Rev 2009; 67(11): 632-8.
[http://dx.doi.org/10.1111/j.1753-4887.2009.00248.x] [PMID: 19906250]

[110]   Koca U, Süntar I, Akkol EK, Yılmazer D, Alper M. Wound repair potential of *(Olea europaea)* L. leaf extracts revealed by *in vivo* experimental models and comparative evaluation of the extracts' antioxidant activity. J Med Food 2011; 14(1-2): 140-6.
[http://dx.doi.org/10.1089/jmf.2010.0039] [PMID: 21128831]

[111]   Elnahas RA, Elwakil BH, Elshewemi SS, Olama ZA. Egyptian *(Olea europaea)* leaves bioactive extract: antibacterial and wound healing activity in normal and diabetic rats. J Tradit Complement Med 2021; 11(5): 427-34.
[http://dx.doi.org/10.1016/j.jtcme.2021.02.008] [PMID: 34522637]

[112]   Adom MB, Taher M, Mutalabisin MF, *et al.* Chemical constituents and medical benefits of *Plantago major.* Biomed Pharmacother 2017; 96: 348-60.
[http://dx.doi.org/10.1016/j.biopha.2017.09.152] [PMID: 29028587]

[113]   Hussan F, Mansor AS, Hassan SN, *et al.* Anti-inflammatory property of Plantago major leaf extract reduces the inflammatory reaction in experimental acetaminophen-induced liver injury. Evid-based Complement. Altern Med 2015; pp. 1-7.

[114]   Najafian Y, Hamedi SS, Kaboli Farshchi M, Feyzabadi Z. Plantago major in traditional persian medicine and modern phytotherapy: a narrative review. Electron Physician 2018; 10(2): 6390-9.
[http://dx.doi.org/10.19082/6390] [PMID: 29629064]

[115]   Zubair M, Nybom H, Lindholm C, Brandner JM, Rumpunen K. Promotion of wound healing by *Plantago major* L. leaf extracts – *ex-vivo* experiments confirm experiences from traditional medicine.

Nat Prod Res 2016; 30(5): 622-4.
[http://dx.doi.org/10.1080/14786419.2015.1034714] [PMID: 25898918]

[116] Amini M, Kherad M, Mehrabani D, Azarpira N, Panjehshahin MR, Tanideh N. Effect of Plantago major on burn wound healing in rat. J Appl Anim Res 2010; 37(1): 53-6.
[http://dx.doi.org/10.1080/09712119.2010.9707093]

[117] Ismayilnajadteymurabadi H, Farahpour MR, Amniattalab A. Histological evaluation of *Plantago lanceolata* L. extract in accelerating wound healing. J Med Plants Res 2012; 6(34): 4844-7.

[118] Bazafkan MH, Hardani A, Afzal Zadeh MR, *et al.* Wound healing effect of an ointment made from a mixture of brassica *Oleracea var*, *Punica granatum*, and *Plantago major* L. extracts in rats. Jentashapir J Health Res 2014; 5(4).

[119] Ashkani-Esfahani S, Khoshneviszadeh M, Noorafshan A, *et al.* The healing effect of *Plantago major* and *Aloe vera* mixture in excisional full thickness skin wounds: stereological study. World J Plast Surg 2019; 8(1): 51-7.
[http://dx.doi.org/10.29252/wjps.8.1.51] [PMID: 30873362]

[120] Velasco-Lezama R, Tapia-Aguilar R, Román-Ramos R, Vega-Avila E, Pérez-Gutiérrez MS. Effect of Plantago major on cell proliferation *in vitro*. J Ethnopharmacol 2006; 103(1): 36-42.
[http://dx.doi.org/10.1016/j.jep.2005.05.050] [PMID: 16226858]

[121] Ghezavat K, Sani AM, Yavarmanesh M. Assessment of the Plantago major extract for antimicrobial activities. Biotechnol 2014; 105

[122] Zhou Q, Lu W, Niu Y, *et al.* Identification and quantification of phytochemical composition and anti-inflammatory, cellular antioxidant, and radical scavenging activities of 12 Plantago species. J Agric Food Chem 2013; 61(27): 6693-702.
[http://dx.doi.org/10.1021/jf401191q] [PMID: 23767948]

[123] Chakraborthy G, Sharma G, Kaushik K. Sesamum indicum: a review. J Herb Med Toxicol 2008; 2(2): 15-9.

[124] Pham TD, Thi Nguyen T-D, Carlsson AS, Bui TM. Morphological evaluation of sesame *('Sesamum indicum' L.)* varieties from different origins. Aust J Crop Sci 2010; 4(7): 498-504.

[125] Kiran K, Asad M. Wound healing activity of *Sesamum indicum* L. seed and oil in rats. 2008; 46: 777-82.

[126] Amoo S, Okorogbona A, Du Plooy C, Venter S. *Sesamum indicum* medicinal spices and vegetables from Africa. Elsevier 2017; pp. 549-79.
[http://dx.doi.org/10.1016/B978-0-12-809286-6.00026-1]

[127] Sani I, Sule FA, Warra AA, Bello F, Fakai IM, Abdulhamid A. Phytochemicals and mineral elements composition of white *Sesamum indicum* L. seed oil. Int J Trad Nat Med 2013; 2(2): 118-30.

[128] Nzikou J, Matos L, Bouanga-Kalou G, *et al.* Chemical composition on the seeds and oil of sesame *(Sesamum indicum L.)* grown in Congo-Brazzaville. Adv J Food Sci Technol 2009; 1(1): 6-11.

[129] Shenoy RR, Sudheendra AT, Nayak PG, Paul P, Kutty NG, Rao CM. Normal and delayed wound healing is improved by sesamol, an active constituent of *Sesamum indicum (L.)* in albino rats. J Ethnopharmacol 2011; 133(2): 608-12.
[http://dx.doi.org/10.1016/j.jep.2010.10.045] [PMID: 21035533]

[130] Nagori BP, Solanki R. Role of medicinal plants in wound healing. Res J Med Plant 2011; 5(4): 392-405.
[http://dx.doi.org/10.3923/rjmp.2011.392.405]

[131] Anilakumar KR, Pal A, Khanum F, Bawa AS. Nutritional, medicinal and industrial uses of sesame *(Sesamum indicum L.)* seeds-an overview. ACS Agric Conspec Sci 2010; 75(4): 159-68.

[132] Mehrabani M, Seyyedkazemi SM, Nematollahi MH, *et al.* Accelerated burn wound closure in mice with a new formula based on traditional medicine. Iran Red Crescent Med J 2016; 18(11): e26613.

[http://dx.doi.org/10.5812/ircmj.26613] [PMID: 28191338]

[133] Somwanshi SB, Hiremath SN. *In-vivo* evaluation of the wound healing activity of the *Sesamum indicum* l. seed extract in novel ethosomal vesicular system. J Drug Deliv Ther 2018; 8(5): 411-20.
[http://dx.doi.org/10.22270/jddt.v8i5.1895]

[134] Larson D, Jacob SE. Tea tree oil. Dermatitis 2012; 23(1): 48-9.
[http://dx.doi.org/10.1097/DER.0b013e31823e202d] [PMID: 22653070]

[135] Pazyar N, Yaghoobi R, Bagherani N, Kazerouni A. A review of applications of tea tree oil in dermatology. Int J Dermatol 2013; 52(7): 784-90.
[http://dx.doi.org/10.1111/j.1365-4632.2012.05654.x] [PMID: 22998411]

[136] Carson CF, Hammer KA, Riley TV. *Melaleuca alternifolia* (Tea Tree) oil: a review of antimicrobial and other medicinal properties. Clin Microbiol Rev 2006; 19(1): 50-62.
[http://dx.doi.org/10.1128/CMR.19.1.50-62.2006] [PMID: 16418522]

[137] Woollard AC, Tatham KC, Barker S. The influence of essential oils on the process of wound healing: a review of the current evidence. J Wound Care 2007; 16(6): 255-7.
[http://dx.doi.org/10.12968/jowc.2007.16.6.27064] [PMID: 17722522]

[138] Faoagali J, George N, Leditschke JF. Does tea tree oil have a place in the topical treatment of burns? Burns 1997; 23(4): 349-51.
[http://dx.doi.org/10.1016/S0305-4179(96)00130-1] [PMID: 9248647]

[139] Cuttle L, Kempf M, Kravchuk O, *et al.* The efficacy of *Aloe vera*, tea tree oil and saliva as first aid treatment for partial thickness burn injuries. Burns 2008; 34(8): 1176-82.
[http://dx.doi.org/10.1016/j.burns.2008.03.012] [PMID: 18603378]

[140] Alvarez-Suarez J, Gasparrini M, Forbes-Hernández T, Mazzoni L, Giampieri F. The composition and biological activity of honey: a focus on Manuka honey. Foods 2014; 3(3): 420-32.
[http://dx.doi.org/10.3390/foods3030420] [PMID: 28234328]

[141] Patel S, Cichello S. Manuka honey: an emerging natural food with medicinal use. Nat Prod Bioprospect 2013; 3(4): 121-8.
[http://dx.doi.org/10.1007/s13659-013-0018-7]

[142] Majtan J. Honey: An immunomodulator in wound healing. Wound Repair Regen 2014; 22(2): 187-92.
[http://dx.doi.org/10.1111/wrr.12117] [PMID: 24612472]

[143] Lusby PE, Coombes A, Wilkinson JM. Honey. J Wound Ostomy Continence Nurs 2002; 29(6): 295-300.
[http://dx.doi.org/10.1097/00152192-200211000-00008] [PMID: 12439453]

[144] Kwakman PHS, Zaat SAJ. Antibacterial components of honey. IUBMB Life 2012; 64(1): 48-55.
[http://dx.doi.org/10.1002/iub.578] [PMID: 22095907]

[145] Battino M, Giampieri F, Cianciosi D, *et al.* The roles of strawberry and honey phytochemicals on human health: A possible clue on the molecular mechanisms involved in the prevention of oxidative stress and inflammation. Phytomedicine 2021; 86: 153170.
[http://dx.doi.org/10.1016/j.phymed.2020.153170] [PMID: 31980299]

[146] Cianciosi D, Forbes-Hernández T, Afrin S, *et al.* Phenolic compounds in honey and their associated health benefits: A review. Molecules 2018; 23(9): 2322.
[http://dx.doi.org/10.3390/molecules23092322] [PMID: 30208664]

[147] Al-Waili N, Salom K, Al-Ghamdi AA. Honey for wound healing, ulcers, and burns; data supporting its use in clinical practice. Sci World J 2011; 11: 766-87.
[http://dx.doi.org/10.1100/tsw.2011.78] [PMID: 21479349]

[148] Roshangar L, Soleimani RJ, Kheirjou R, Reza RM, Ferdowsi KA. Skin burns: review of molecular mechanisms and therapeutic approaches. Wounds 2019; 31(12): 308-15.
[PMID: 31730513]

[149] Molan PC. Potential of honey in the treatment of wounds and burns. Am J Clin Dermatol 2001; 2(1): 13-9.
[http://dx.doi.org/10.2165/00128071-200102010-00003] [PMID: 11702616]

[150] Al-Waili NS, Salom K, Butler G, Al Ghamdi AA. Honey and microbial infections: a review supporting the use of honey for microbial control. J Med Food 2011; 14(10): 1079-96.
[http://dx.doi.org/10.1089/jmf.2010.0161] [PMID: 21859350]

[151] Saikaly SK, Khachemoune A. Honey and wound healing: an update. Am J Clin Dermatol 2017; 18(2): 237-51.
[http://dx.doi.org/10.1007/s40257-016-0247-8] [PMID: 28063093]

[152] Medhi B, Puri A, Upadhyay S, Kaman L. Topical application of honey in the treatment of wound healing: a metaanalysis. JK Sci 2008; 10(4): 166-9.

[153] Lee DS, Sinno S, Khachemoune A. Honey and wound healing: an overview. Am J Clin Dermatol 2011; 12(3): 181-90.
[http://dx.doi.org/10.2165/11538930-000000000-00000] [PMID: 21469763]

[154] Molan PC. The evidence supporting the use of honey as a wound dressing. Int J Low Extrem Wounds 2006; 5(1): 40-54.
[http://dx.doi.org/10.1177/1534734605286014] [PMID: 16543212]

[155] Kuropatnicki AK, Szliszka E, Krol W. Historical aspects of propolis research in modern times. Evid-based Complement Altern Med 2013; pp. 1-11.

[156] Salatino A, Teixeira ÉW, Negri G, Message D. Origin and chemical variation of Brazilian propolis. Evid Based Complement Alternat Med 2005; 2(1): 33-8.
[http://dx.doi.org/10.1093/ecam/neh060] [PMID: 15841276]

[157] Castaldo S, Capasso F. Propolis, an old remedy used in modern medicine. Fitoterapia 2002; 73 (Suppl. 1): S1-6.
[http://dx.doi.org/10.1016/S0367-326X(02)00185-5] [PMID: 12495704]

[158] Olczyk P, Komosinska-Vassev K, Wisowski G, Mencner L, Stojko J, Kozma EM. Propolis modulates fibronectin expression in the matrix of thermal injury. BioMed Res Int 2014; 2014: 1-10.
[http://dx.doi.org/10.1155/2014/748101] [PMID: 24738072]

[159] Han M, Durmus A, Karabulut E, Yaman I. Effects of Turkish propolis and silver sulfadiazine on burn wound healing in rats. Rev Med Vet 2005; 156(12): 624.

[160] Mohd KS, Nafi NEM, Khadar ASA, Mohd AA. Traditional uses, phytochemical composition and pharmacological properties. Int J Eng Technol 2018; 7: 78-82.

[161] Oryan A, Alemzadeh E, Moshiri A. Potential role of propolis in wound healing: Biological properties and therapeutic activities. Biomed Pharmacother 2018; 98: 469-83.
[http://dx.doi.org/10.1016/j.biopha.2017.12.069] [PMID: 29287194]

[162] Hung WS, Fang CL, Su CH, Lai WFT, Chang YC, Tsai YH. Cytotoxicity and immunogenicity of sacchachitin and its mechanism of action on skin wound healing. J Biomed Mater Res 2001; 56(1): 93-100.
[http://dx.doi.org/10.1002/1097-4636(200107)56:1<93::AID-JBM1072>3.0.CO;2-B]   [PMID: 11309795]

[163] Chuang CM, Wang HE, Chang CH, *et al.* Sacchachitin, a novel chitin-polysaccharide conjugate macromolecule present in *Ganoderma lucidum* : Purification, composition, and properties. Pharm Biol 2013; 51(1): 84-95.
[http://dx.doi.org/10.3109/13880209.2012.711840] [PMID: 23043530]

[164] Hung WS, Fang CL, Su CH, Lai WF, Chang YC, Tsai YH. Cytotoxicity and immunogenicity of SACCHACHITIN and its mechanism of action on skin wound healing J Biomed Mater Res 2001; 56(1): 93-100.

[165] Araújo D, Ferreira IC, Torres CAV, Neves L, Freitas F. Chitinous polymers: extraction from fungal sources, characterization and processing towards value-added applications. J Chem Technol Biotechnol 2020; 95(5): 1277-89.
[http://dx.doi.org/10.1002/jctb.6325]

[166] Chen RN, Lee LW, Chen LC, *et al.* Wound-healing effect of micronized sacchachitin (mSC) nanogel on corneal epithelium. Int J Nanomed 2012; 7: 4697-706.
[PMID: 22956870]

[167] Li C, Chen C. Mode of action on sacchachitin P10 for traumatic and burn wound of pets. Thesis, 2005. Available from: http://www.scirus.com/srsapp/sciruslink?src=ndl&url=http%3A%2F%2Fwww.cetd.com.tw%2Fec%2Fthesisdetail.aspx%3Fetdun%3DU0007-1704200714545916

[168] Su CH, Sun CS, Juan SW, Hu CH, Ke WT, Sheu MT. Fungal mycelia as the source of chitin and polysaccharides and their applications as skin substitutes. Biomaterials 1997; 18(17): 1169-74.
[http://dx.doi.org/10.1016/S0142-9612(97)00048-3] [PMID: 9259514]

[169] Suarato G, Bertorelli R, Athanassiou A. Borrowing from nature: biopolymers and biocomposites as smart wound care materials. Front Bioeng Biotechnol 2018; 6: 137.
[http://dx.doi.org/10.3389/fbioe.2018.00137] [PMID: 30333972]

CHAPTER 3

Wounds and Natural Remedies: A Long Way of Effective Treatment

Gang Chen[1], **Xue Li**[1], **Jingsong Yan**[1] and **Ning Li**[1,*]

[1] *School of Traditional Chinese Materia Medica, Shenyang Pharmaceutical University, Shenyang, China*

Abstract: Wound healing is quite a complicated process in the human body, consisting of the action of constricting injured blood vessels, activating the immune system, angiogenesis, remodeling, *etc*. Under intensive mechanical stress, a fibrotic scar, which is unfavorable with respect to the beauty of the skin, can be formed to patch the wound. Moreover, chronic wounds due to the disruption in wound healing are another clinical problem for patients with diabetes or vascular diseases. Of note is that natural remedies, especially natural products, are demonstrated to elicit certain positive effects on many aspects of wound healing. In this chapter, global mechanisms, the role of natural remedies and newly emerging therapeutic targets regarding wound healing are presented, and the remaining hurdle for the natural product-based treatment in wound healing is also introduced.

Keywords: Non-coding RNAs, Diabetes, Fibrotic scar, Natural products, Skin, Wound healing.

INTRODUCTION

Skin is the first barrier protecting mammals from a wide array of external detrimental factors, such as bacteria and toxins. However, skin is susceptible to trauma, which impairs its protective effect and makes mammals vulnerable to environmental toxins. Therefore, maintaining the integrity of the skin is quite important. Generally, wound healing, which is a spontaneous self-repairing process, is initiated after wounding to restore the integrity of the injured skin without creating any "marks" on skin surface, while under certain stressful circumstances, a fibrotic scar is formed in a short period to patch the wound and thereby maintain the skin integrity. Just as every coin has two sides, the fibrotic scar is unfavorable for the beauty of the skin, and therefore elimination of skin

---

* **Corresponding author Ning Li:** School of Traditional Chinese Materia Medica, Shenyang Pharmaceutical University, Shenyang, China; Tel: 86-24-43520739; E-mail: liningsypharm@163.com

Heba Abd El-Sattar El-Nashar, Mohamed El-Shazly & Nouran Mohammed Fahmy (Eds.)

scars caused by mechanical stress, especially those induced by physical surgeries, has always been the attention-attracting research field [1].

To successfully complete skin wound healing, a quite complicated process comprising hemostasis, inflammation, angiogenesis, re-epithelialization, and remodeling is implemented through synchronizing various cell types with different roles (Fig. **1**). Disrupting any section of the wound healing process will lead to delayed wounding healing or chronic wounds. For example, for patients with other chronic diseases, such as diabetes, ectopic expression of some cytokines due to the nature of the disease in cells participating in wound healing evidently suppresses wound healing and makes it quite an intricate process [2].

Natural remedies, including therapies based on herbal medicines and natural products, have been used for the treatment of human ailments for generations. For the treatment of wound healing, some traditional natural therapies, such as honey, especially stingless bee honey [3], have been adopted since ancient times. Meanwhile, modern scientific studies have demonstrated that a variety of natural products also have positive effects on wound healing. For example, curcumin is proven to be able to enhance granulation tissue formation, collagen deposition, tissue remodeling, *etc.* [4]. Therefore, in this chapter, the mechanism of wound healing and the role of natural remedies in every phase of wound healing are presented. Moreover, the newly-emerging therapeutic targets and hurdles for natural products becoming an effective treatment for wound healing are also discussed.

THE MECHANISM OF WOUNDING HEALING: A COMPLICATED AND SYNERGETIC PROCESS

Once the wound is inflicted, hemostasis is initiated in the first place by contracting the injured blood vessels and forming a fibrin clot. Briefly, in the hemostasis phase, vasoconstrictors are released by injured cells to contract the smooth muscle and thereby provisionally suppress bleeding. However, the contracture of the smooth muscle itself is not sufficient enough for the complete stoppage of bleeding under most circumstances, and thereby the formation of a thrombus is crucial for hemostasis. Generally, the subendothelial matrix is exposed due to the rupture of blood vessels, triggering the initiation of thrombus formation. Platelets, whose aggregation and anti-thrombotic agents like nitric oxide inhibit attachment to the endothelial lining under normal circumstance, can either bind to the subendothelial matrix or aggregate through G protein-coupled receptors, integrins and glycoproteins. Meanwhile, platelets produce von Willebrand factor (vWF) that can also bind to the subendothelial matrix, and platelets can also bind to the vWF attached to the subendothelial matrix through their surface receptors to form a structurally heightened complex on the subendothelial matrix. In addition, blood coagulation Factor X, which is a vitamin K-dependent serine protease that plays an essential role in blood clotting, can be activated and lead to the cleavage of fibrinogen to fibrin, and the cross-linked fibrin can capture platelets aggregated to each other to form a thrombus. All these aforementioned processes collectively induce a complete stoppage of bleeding.

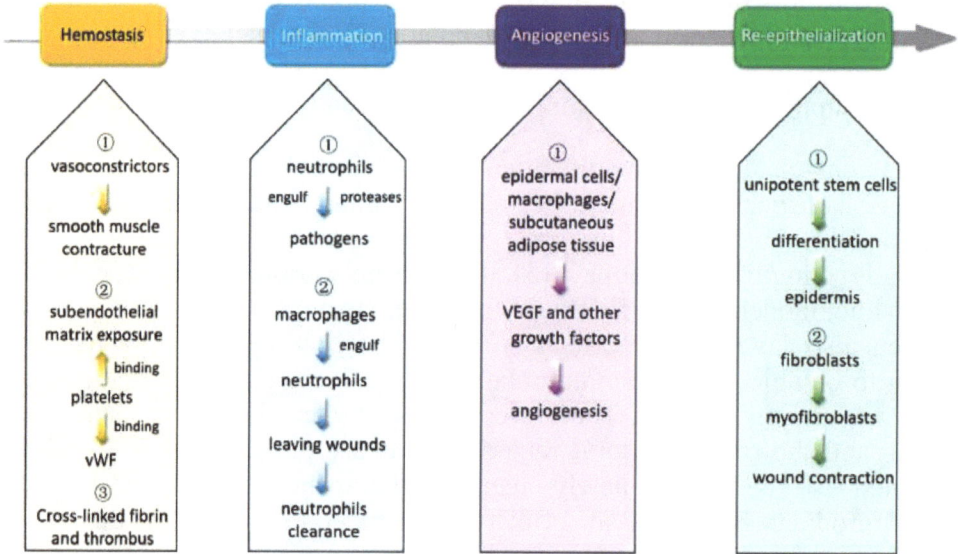

Fig. (1). Key stages of wounding healing regarding the closure of acute and/or chronic wounds.

Inflammation is another crucial phase of wound healing. Inflammatory cells, especially neutrophils, can be recruited to the wound due to a set of factors produced by resident cells instantaneously after the moment when the wound occurs, including calcium waves, hydrogen, lipid mediators, *etc*. The recruited neutrophils at the wound site can prevent the invasion of pathogens by releasing proteases, producing neutrophil extracellular traps, and forming a phagocytic cup that can engulf antigens. Meanwhile, in the phase of inflammation, macrophages can produce pro-inflammatory factors, such as IL-6, IL-1β, and TNF-α, to combat infection. However, on the contrary, a prolonged phase of inflammation is detrimental to wound healing, such as the uncontrolled cutaneous neutrophilic inflammation in pyoderma gangrenosum [5]. Thus, clearance of neutrophils is also important for wound healing. To achieve the resolution of inflammation, neutrophils can either be engulfed by macrophages through efferocytosis or leave the wound through the reverse-migration process.

New vessel formation is crucial for the growth phase of wound healing. To initiate angiogenesis, a few growth factors and enzymes produced by adjoining cells (epidermal cells, macrophages, *etc.*), including VEGF, FGF, PDGF-β, TGF-α, proteolytic enzymes, *etc.*, are required so that endothelial cells of injured vessels can proliferate, migrate, and interact with adjoining perivascular cells to form new capillaries through mechanisms of sprouting, intussusception and looping. Subsequently, pro-angiogenic macrophages can fuse newly-formed capillaries and complete the formation of new vessels. Besides, there are also other factors affecting the angiogenesis of the wound. To be specific, it is also acknowledged that the interaction between leukocytes and microvascular cells and the regulation of vascular permeability are two important processes in angiogenesis. Therefore, cytokines like surface markers ICAM-1, VCAM-1, and E-selectin that affect cell-cell interactions with leukocytes are also therapeutic targets for wound healing with respect to angiogenesis.

Re-epithelialization phase is responsible for the closure of acute and/or chronic wounds. In this phase, through the Wnt/β-catenin pathway, the dermal papilla fibroblast can signal unipotent stem cells located in the hair follicle, which subsequently migrate in a linear manner and differentiate into a variety of types of epidermal cells. Additionally, interfollicular stem cells located in the basement membrane of the epidermis can differentiate and proliferate to generate keratinocytes without cell-cell tight junctions, which subsequently migrate towards the wound to form the epithelial tongue. Therefore, the migration of stem cells and keratinocytes into the wound results in the re-epithelialization and closure of the wound.

Generally, the closure of acute and/or chronic wounds is viewed as the endpoint for wound healing (Fig. **1**). However, the post-closure phase of wound healing is also important, especially for scar formation and the relapse of wound. Actually, the post-closure phase of wound healing refers to remodeling or tissue maturation, which can last for several months or even years. Since remodeling or tissue maturation is quite complicated, we only present two key processes related to scar formation in this chapter. The first key process is the apoptosis of myofibroblasts. After the closure of the wounds, myofibroblasts are supposed to undergo mediated apoptosis within granulation tissues, and it is reported that delayed or suppressed myofibroblast apoptosis can result in the formation of hypertrophic scars [6]. Second, the signaling between macrophages and fibroblasts. Macrophages can exert the fibrinolytic function, thereby degrading the extracellular matrix and engulfing the debris of the extracellular matrix and the apoptotic cell like aforementioned apoptotic myofibroblasts to prevent scar formation. However, under certain pathological conditions, the "wrong" signal of CD47 released by the myofibroblast is "conveyed" to the macrophage, inhibiting the macrophage from engulfing the apoptotic myofibroblasts, which, as a result, will lead to the formation of hypertrophic scars.

NATURAL REMEDIES IN WOUND HEALING: THE PERSPECTIVE OF TRADITIONAL APPLICATION AND MODERN SCIENTIFIC ADVANCES

Generally, there have been many reports of natural remedies in wound healing, including those of whole-plant extraction and natural products. In this chapter, a few typical examples of effective natural remedies for wound healing are introduced.

Traditional Natural Remedies

In the first place, we would introduce some famous traditional natural remedies that have been clinically proven effective in wound healing. Of note is that many traditional natural remedies are still used in modern cosmetics, such as *Aloe vera*.

Aloe Vera

Aloe vera, a traditional medicinal plant, has been used since 1500 BC in many countries such as Greece and China. Several researches on *Aloe vera* have indicated its effect on the prevention and healing of skin wounds. Several groups of clinical trials show that aloe can accelerate the re-epithelialization time of STSG patients, accelerate the re-epithelialization and wound healing of II extreme burn patients, and show a better therapeutic effect than SSD. However, aloe had no effect on human skin damage induced by UVB irradiation [7]. *Aloe vera* can relieve postoperative pain after open hemorrhoidectomy and shorten the healing time [8]. It can also improve bleeding and wound healing in patients with chronic anal fissures [9]. The compound ointment of aloe and olive oil also showed a good therapeutic effect on patients with chronic wounds. For example, in the streptozotocin-induced diabetic foot ulcer model, oral aloe gel extract (300mg/kg) or combined with external use for 9 days can evidently improve glucose homeostasis, increase the levels of DNA and glycosaminoglycan (GAG) in granulation tissue, promote ulcer healing and increase tensile strength [10]. In another type 2 diabetic open-wound rat model, *Aloe vera* (30mg) promoted angiogenesis, inflammatory cell infiltration, extracellular matrix deposition and epithelial formation [11]. Furthermore, *Aloe vera* (100μL) shows better therapeutic effect than nigellasativaoil (NSO, 10%) gel in a diabetic ulcer rat model in many aspects, including reducing necrotic tissue, inflammatory reaction, and wound area and increasing epidermal regeneration [12].

Propolis

Bee Products (honey, propolis, *etc.*) have been used as a natural medicine since ancient times. Studies have also indicated that natural bee products can be useful in wound healing. Topical treatment of propolis (5%) can reduce the wound area of patients with diabetic foot ulcers in the first two weeks [13]. Propolis (10 drops of propolis water-soluble ethanol extract in 150 ml water, oral administration) can ameliorate pain and bleeding in patients after tonsillectomy and promote wound healing [14]. Mechanism studies show that propolis 1, 10,100, 250, 500 and 1000 μg/ml can promote the migration of fibroblasts. Brazilian red propolis has the strongest ability to promote the migration of fibroblasts at 10 μg/ml. Malaysian has the strongest ability to promote the proliferation of fibroblasts at 1000 μg/ml. Propolis (0.001%) can significantly increase the wound repair ability of keratinocytes. Cell migration test also shows that propolis can stimulate keratinocytes to seal the wound. Moreover, it is reported that propolis can promote wound contraction, collagen production by increasing hydroxyproline in granulation tissue and levels of hexosamine and uronic acid in wound tissue (both of which are involved in the synthesis of extracellular matrix).

Leonurus

Leonurus is used as a traditional Chinese medicine and is considered to be capable of regulating menstruation and arresting leucorrhoea. The extraction (5-80 μM) of Leonurus can promote the proliferation and migration of HUVECs and enhance the ability of angiogenesis *in vitro* by up-regulating the mTOR/ERK signal pathway. In the rat model of full-thickness skin trauma *in vivo*, Leonurus extraction (20mg/kg/day, injection) can promote the angiogenesis of the wound. Furthermore, Leonurus extraction can promote the process of collagen matrix deposition and remodeling of the wound due to rapid vascularization [15].

Lawsonia Inermis

Lawsonia inermis-extracted oil is famous for its therapeutic application, especially wound healing. In the wound model of skin resection of the back of the neck of rats, *Lawsonia inermis* (50%, topical) promotes the wound contraction rate and the time span of re-epithelialization is shortened. Histological results show that epithelialization, dermal differentiation, collagen fiber orientation, and angiogenesis are all significantly improved by *Lawsonia inermis* treatment [16]. In the rat annular wound resection model, *Lawsonia inermis* (1.5%, 3% and 6%) can shorten the inflammatory period in a dose-dependent manner, accelerate cell proliferation, increase wound contraction, promote angiogenesis, collagen deposition and re-epithelialization, and promote intracellular carbohydrate storage [17]. Another study with the rat wound model indicates that the oil extracted from

Lawsonia inermis (fatty acid methyl ester, 0-1mg/g) can promote wound healing, including increasing wound closure rate, accelerating skin re-epithelialization, reducing epithelial thickness, and making collagen fibers arranged more neatly.

Natural Products In Wound Healing

In addition to traditional natural remedies, natural products also exhibit apparent bioactivities in wound healing. Some typical examples are listed below.

Curcumin

Curcuma longa L. is a medicinal plant and curcumin is a bright yellow compound isolated from its rhizome. Curcumin can improve glucose and lipid metabolism, promote insulin signal transduction, regulate cardiac metabolism, stimulate antioxidant enzymes, and inhibit inflammation, thereby exerting beneficial effects on health. In recent years, the effect of curcumin on promoting skin wound healing has also attracted extensive attention from researchers. For example, in a study, three groups of burn rats received 0.1%, 0.5%, and 2% curcumin ointment, respectively, while the control group received eucerin treatment. After 14 days, mice treated with curcumin ointment had obvious re-epithelialization, and the fibroblasts were arranged in bundles parallel to the epithelial surface with an eosinophilic collagen matrix [18]. Another study has shown that curcumin can promote the healing of burn wounds in mice by up-regulating caveolin-1 in epidermal stem cells. Curcumin can also promote skin wound healing by regulating TNF-α, MMP-9, α-SMA, and collagen. Moreover, the topical application of curcumin can modulate angiogenesis in diabetic-damaged skin wounds. For example, curcumin cream (50mg) applied topically to the diabetic-impaired cutaneous wound twice a day from the day of injury can significantly increase the number of new blood vessels and the expression level of NF-κB in the granulation tissue at the wound after 7 days. Moreover, after 21 days, complete healing and re-epithelialization are found in all animals treated with curcumin [19].

Asperosaponin VI

Asperosaponin VI (ASA VI) is an effective ingredient isolated from the root of the traditional Chinese medicine *Dipsacus asper* Wall, which is used for the treatment of epilepsy, liver disease, waist and knee soreness, rheumatic joint pain, fractures, *etc*. Recent studies also revealed its application in wound healing. ASA VI (20-80 μg/mL) can promote the proliferation and migration of umbilical vein endothelial cells in a dose-dependent manner by regulating the HIF-1α/VEGF pathway and enhancing angiogenesis *in vitro*. In a study using a full-thickness skin wound model of a rat, it is suggested that injection of ASA VI at a dose of

20mg/kg/day can increase the rate of granulation tissue formation, collagen regeneration, and remodeling, and the number of capillaries at the wounds in the ASA VI group is significantly higher than that in the control group. On day 21, wounds in the ASA VI group were completely healed, whereas some of the wounds in the control group remained unhealed, indicating that ASA VI can accelerate the wound healing *in vivo* [20].

Quercetin

Quercetin is a flavanol compound with multiple biological activities. Its powerful antioxidant and anti-inflammatory activities have been fully proven and are believed to play a role in the treatment and prevention of diseases, including diabetes, cancer, neurodegenerative diseases and cardiovascular diseases. In addition, it can increase the proliferation of fibroblasts, reduce immune cell infiltration, and regulate the activity of fibrosis-related signaling pathways, thereby promoting skin wound healing [21]. For example, Osama *et al.* established a full-thickness skin wound model on the back of diabetic rats induced by STZ to investigate the effect of quercetin on skin wound healing. Non-diabetic and diabetic rats with wounds on their backs were orally administered quercetin at a dose of 25mg/kg every other day for two weeks. Compared with the diabetic injury control group, the collagen fibers in the wound of diabetic rats treated with quercetin increased significantly, and the granulation tissue proliferated. Mechanism research results showed that quercetin reduced the levels of serum pro-inflammatory cytokines IL-1β and TNF-α, as well as PGE-2 and LTB-4, and increased serum anti-inflammatory cytokines IL- 10 levels in diabetic trauma rats [22]. Quercetin can also promote skin wound healing by regulating angiogenesis. In a study, three concentrations of quercetin (0.03, 0.1 and 0.3%) were applied to the back wounds of rats every day for 20 days. The wound healing rate was significantly accelerated in the 0.1% and 0.3% quercetin treatment groups. Compared with the control group, the vascular endothelial growth factor and TGF-b1 gene expression of the 0.1% and 0.3% quercetin treatment groups were significantly higher, and the average number of new blood vessels was significantly increased [23].

Moreover, as a natural anti-fibrosis drug, quercetin also plays an extremely important role in reducing scar formation. Karen *et al.* used L929 fibroblasts as an experimental model to conduct scratch experiments *in vitro*. The results showed that after treating the cells with 20 μM quercetins, the B1 integrin on the surface of fibroblasts decreased, and the AV integrin, which is involved in promoting cell migration, significantly increased, which may be the mechanism by which quercetin reduces fibrosis and improves the quality of wound healing in the body [24].

Kirenol

Kirenol is a diterpenoid compound from *Siegesbeckia orientalis*, which plays various roles mainly by regulating inflammation markers. Jia *et al.* investigated the role played by kirenol during the skin wound healing phase. Treatment of L929 cells with different concentrations (5-35 µg) of kirenol for 24 h resulted in significant inhibition of cell migration in the kirenol-treated group. Subsequently, the rat model of diabetes induced by streptozotocin was used to evaluate *in vivo* effect. The results showed that the percentage of wound healing in diabetic rats treated 30% kirenol increased, and the stage of epithelialization was accelerated in kirenol-treated diabetic rats. Compared with the diabetic control group, the expression of NF-κB, COX-2, iNOS, MMP-2 and MMP-9 genes were decreased in the group treated with kirenol, suggesting that kirenol may improve the inflammatory phase of skin wound healing in diabetic rats by regulating the expression of these genes [25].

NEWLY EMERGING THERAPEUTIC TARGETS OF WOUND HEALING FOR NATURAL PRODUCTS

Based on the understanding of the mechanism of wound healing, several conventional therapeutic targets can be proposed corresponding to phases of hemostasis, inflammation, angiogenesis, re-epithelialization, and remodeling. For example, G protein-coupled receptors, integrins, and blood coagulation Factor X are potential therapeutic targets for the hemostasis phase and signals in the Wnt/β-catenin pathway can become potential therapeutic targets for the phase of re-epithelialization. In addition to the conventional target for wound healing, with the growing knowledge of the mechanism of wound healing, an increasing number of factors related to wound healing are unraveled in recent years. In this section, the mechanism and the potential of becoming therapeutic targets for chemokines, connexin 43, the cutaneous microbiome, granzyme B, and non-coding RNAs with respect to wound healing are presented.

Chemokines

Chemokines, which are 8-12 kDa chemotactic cytokines, can be released by a wide array of types of cells, regulating cell migration to the wound. According to the location and the number of cysteine residues of the *N*-terminal, chemokines can be classified into four groups: CC-chemokine group, CXC-chemokine group, CX_3C-chemokine group, and C-chemokine group. Chemokines can exert their effect on all phases of wound healing. For example, chemokines can prevent angiogenesis at the hemostasis phase, and in the remodeling phase, MCP-1, which belongs to the C-C chemokine superfamily, can increase MMP-1 and TIMP-1 expression in dermal fibroblasts to take on the profibrotic and collagen degradative function [26]. However, under most circumstances, they are most significantly differentially expressed and thereby promoting angiogenesis in the phase of inflammation and proliferation, especially during the period of day 3 to day 10 after the wounding, when increased proliferation and migration of various types of cells (endothelial cells, keratinocytes, fibroblasts, *etc.*) occur to facilitate the formation of extracellular matrix, requiring the support of a vast amount of neovessels. And chemokines CXCL1-3, CXCL5-8, and their receptors CXCR1 and CXCR2 are the key factors mediating the angiogenesis of this period [27].

Due to their extensive functions in wound healing, several attempts have been made to promote wound healing through modulating chemokines with the single-target strategy, including CCL2, CCL5, CXCL8, CXCL12, *etc.*, and many intriguing results have been obtained. For example, it has been reported that AMD31000, which is an antagonist of CXCR4, can improve wound healing in diabetic mice, and topical delivery of CXCL12 by lactobacilli vector can promote wound healing in mice [28, 29]. Even so, a few broad-spectrum treatments have also been attempted to avoid the drawbacks of single-target therapy based on chemokine modulation. One typical example is the broad-spectrum chemokine inhibitor 35K, which is a protein produced by the Vaccinia virus, selectively inhibiting chemokines of the CC-chemokine class [30]. It is reported that the 35K can promote wound closure and neovascularization and decrease the collagen deposition that is tightly related to scar formation [31]. Another example is NR58-3.14.3, which is a broad-spectrum inhibitor of CC and CXC chemokines, suppressing CCL2, CCL3, CCL5, CXCL8, and CXCL12 that are related to wound healing. An *in vivo* experiment with a mouse of surgery-induced intraperitoneal adhesions has been carried out, and the result suggests that NR58-3.14.3 can prevent the formation of intraperitoneal adhesion of the model group as well as the number of CD45$^+$ inflammatory cells [32].

Connexin 43

The connexin multigene family encodes protein constituting the intercellular gap junction [33], which functions as an intercellular channel modulating cytoplasmic exchange of small molecules (<1000 Da) among cells. Moreover, intercellular gap junction is also associated with almost all phases of skin wound healing. For example, it can coordinate inflammatory response and is involved in the remodeling phase of wound healing. Among connexin gene family members expressed in the skin, connexin 43 (Cx43) is the most abundant one both in epidermal and dermal cutaneous layers. It is reported that Cx43 is provisionally down-regulated in the epidermis both at and around the wound during the first 24 hours after wound injury but up-regulated in the deep dermis within the same period of time. Subsequently, one week later, the elevated Cx43 level can be observed along with the granulation tissue formation in the remodeling phase [34], suggesting that location-specific manipulation Cx43 expression in a different phase of wound healing might be able to promote skin wound healing. Besides, the role of Cx43 in chronic wounds is also demonstrated. It is indicated that Cx43 is ectopically overexpressed throughout the whole dermis of diabetic wounds [35], which further enhances the potential of Cx43 as a therapeutic target for wound healing. Following this line of thinking, several experiments have used peptides targeting specific functions of Cx43 to promote wound healing. However, so far, only CT1 has proceeded with pivotal Phase III clinical testing (NCT02667327). Meanwhile, natural remedies, including natural products, have not been reported to target Cx43 regarding wound healing. Thus, establishing reliable *in vitro* models to screen Cx43-targeting natural products in future studies would accelerate the discovery of natural therapeutic agents with respect to wound healing.

The Cutaneous Microbiome

The microbiome refers to the ecological community of microorganisms in/on humans. The close association between microbiome and intestinal homeostasis is extensively acknowledged, while the role of the cutaneous microbiome in skin wound healing is thus far much less investigated. Through studies manipulating the microbiome of skin wounds, it can be concluded that balanced organisms are essential for all skin wound healing aspects [36, 37]. Furthermore, the composition of the cutaneous microbiome is not static, varying significantly from acute wounds to those chronic ones. For instance, a clinical study has shown that in the acute burn wound, the abundance of *Aeribacillus*, *Caldalkalibacillus* and *Nesterenkonai* are elevated, and the growth of *Corynebacterium* is repressed [38], whereas another clinical observation has indicated that in the wound caused by blunt or penetrating traumas *Pseudomonas* is the most abundant specie as detected *via* the initial inspection from the emergency department [39]. Therefore, clarifying the detailed function (either positive and/or negative) of the cutaneous microbiome is necessary for further cutaneous microbiome-targeting treatment in wound healing. To date, the specific effect of some commensals on host skin tissues is demonstrated [40], providing a new perspective for the therapeutic strategy of human skin wound healing.

Granzyme B

Granzyme B is one of the most abundant granzymes, inducing cell apoptosis as it functions as a serine protease [41]. Recent studies also show that it can affect wound closure and remodeling. For example, it is reported that granzyme B can suppress the wound healing of HaCaT keratinocytes by interfering with EGFR signaling and mediating vitronectin cleavage to inhibit re-epithelialization [42-44]. As far as we know, there is no endogenous extracellular inhibitor for granzyme B in human bio-fluids, which means the up-regulated granzyme B in the chronic wound is beyond control, and targeting granzyme B may be a novel strategy for wound healing. Supporting this notion, in the ultraviolet light irradiation-induced skin injury model, knockout of granzyme B in mice can significantly improve the healing outcomes [45]. Actually, several granzyme B inhibitors have already elicited promising *in vivo* effects on wound healing in animal experiments. Typical examples of granzyme B inhibitors include VTI-1002, which can enhance the remodeling of impaired burn wound healing, and serpina3n, which can ameliorate delayed wound healing and promote tissue repair of diabetic mice [46, 47].

Non-Coding RNAs

Non-coding RNAs, including microRNAs, long non-coding RNAs, and circular RNAs, can regulate gene expression post-transcriptionally. With advancing knowledge about gene regulation in the past decade, the consensus can be reached that the non-coding RNA-mediated mechanism is linked to the pathogenesis of many diseases [48, 49]. MicroRNAs are the most studied non-coding RNAs due to the relatively high conservative feature among species, and several drugs targeting microRNAs have been subjected to clinical trials, such as RG-101 [50]. However, compared to other diseases like cancers, the role of microRNAs in wound healing is relatively less investigated and explored with *in vivo* experiments [51]. Of note is that recently a few *in vivo* studies have indicated that microRNAs can also modulate skin wound healing through various pathways. For example, it is observed that the level of miR-31 is potently elevated in keratinocytes located at the wound edge, and NF-kB and STAT3 activation can regulate miR-31 expression during the inflammation phase of wound healing. Further investigation in the mouse has shown that through directly targeting *Rasa1*, *Spred1*, *Spred2* and *Spry4* in the RAS/MAPK pathway, miR-31 can promote proliferation and migration of keratinocytes, suggesting that miR-31 is able to promote re-epithelialization of skin wound healing [52]. Both these *in vitro* and *in vivo* results imply that in addition to diseases like cancers, non-coding RNAs, especially microRNAs, are also potential therapeutic targets for wound healing.

THE REMAINING HURDL FOR THE NATURAL PRODUCT-BASED TREATMENT IN WOUND HEALING

Although many researches report the effect of natural remedies on wound healing, there are very few examples of natural molecules becoming clinical drugs for treating wound healing. The hurdles for this low rate of pharmaceutical drug conversion for the bio-active natural molecules with respect to wound healing are complicated, including both technical and intrinsic factors.

Research Model: The Technical Hurdle

The main technical factor preventing natural remedies from being an effective treatment of wound healing is the research model. On the one hand, a large proportion of studies on natural products in the context of skin wound healing using *in vitro* cell models. Although these *in vitro* results are intriguing, the uncertainty of *in vivo* efficacy for the bio-active natural product discovery based on *in vitro* experiments still limits their practical application. On the other hand, even though there are several *in vivo* murine models for skin wound healing, the big discrepancy in mechanism between the human and murine wound healing processes makes the discovery of effective natural products for the treatment of wound healing an intricate task. For example, panniculus carnosus promotes skin contraction and can be found in murine subcutaneous tissue but not in humans [53]. Therefore, more efforts should be made to improve translational studies on wound healing. Actually, attempts have been made to address this critical issue with adapted wound models and genetically modified models. Recently, the humanized mice model carrying functional human genes, cells, or organs rendered a possible way for translational study [54]. For example, the one with human keratinocytes encoding green fluorescent protein enables scientists to observe a wide span of parameters of each phase of wound healing and thereby evaluate the effect of natural products on human skin wound healing [55].

The Intrinsic Factor

Although great nature generates valuable bio-active molecules for humans, we must admit that these natural products are primarily created to be functional for their "hosts", not humans. Therefore, most of the therapeutic effects elicited by natural products are not strong enough for an industrialized drug without structural modification. For wound healing, increasing the rate of skin penetration for a natural product can also strengthen its therapeutic effect to overcome the intrinsic hurdle, for example, the small bi-layered lipid sphere. It has been shown that small bi-layered lipid spheres are able to penetrate the skin barrier and release bio-active encapsulated natural products (either hydrophobic or hydrophilic ones) like curcumin to promote wound healing [56]. Another tactic to increase the effect of natural products on skin wound healing is the combination of "Dressing" and natural products. Wound dressing refers to the sterile compress directly contacting the wound to exert a protective effect; generally, a bandage is used to hold the dressing in place. Among all types of dressings, the one made of fibrous sheets with bioactive agents like natural products is most favorable for wound healing [57]. With the aid of the modern drug delivery system and tools for wound healing, the therapeutic effect of natural products would be significantly promoted to a higher level, making them more likely to meet the demand for modern drugs.

CONCLUSION

Wound healing is a complex mechanism involving injured blood vessels, the immune system, angiogenesis, and remodeling. A fibrotic scar that affects the beauty of the skin is formed during mechanical stress. The wound-healing process in patients with diabetes or vascular diseases is also complicated. This chapter overviews the various aspects of wound healing, the role of natural remedies, and newly emerging therapeutic targets and hurdles involved.

REFERENCES

[1]   Grabowski G, Pacana MJ, Chen E. Keloid and hypertrophic scar formation, prevention, and management. J Am Acad Orthop Surg 2020; 28(10): e408-14.
[http://dx.doi.org/10.5435/JAAOS-D-19-00690] [PMID: 32109921]

[2]   Kaushik K, Das A. Endothelial progenitor cell therapy for chronic wound tissue regeneration. Cytotherapy 2019; 21(11): 1137-50.
[http://dx.doi.org/10.1016/j.jcyt.2019.09.002] [PMID: 31668487]

[3]   Abd Jalil MA, Kasmuri AR, Hadi H. Stingless bee honey, the natural wound healer: a review. Skin Pharmacol Physiol 2017; 30(2): 66-75.
[http://dx.doi.org/10.1159/000458416] [PMID: 28291965]

[4]   Akbik D, Ghadiri M, Chrzanowski W, Rohanizadeh R. Curcumin as a wound healing agent. Life Sci 2014; 116(1): 1-7.
[http://dx.doi.org/10.1016/j.lfs.2014.08.016] [PMID: 25200875]

[5]   Alavi A, French LE, Davis MD, Brassard A, Kirsner RS. Pyoderma gangrenosum: an update on pathophysiology, diagnosis and treatment. Am J Clin Dermatol 2017; 18(3): 355-72.
[http://dx.doi.org/10.1007/s40257-017-0251-7] [PMID: 28224502]

[6]   Desmoulière A, Redard M, Darby I, Gabbiani G. Apoptosis mediates the decrease in cellularity during the transition between granulation tissue and scar. Am J Pathol 1995; 146(1): 56-66.
[PMID: 7856739]

[7]   Burusapat C, Supawan M, Pruksapong C, Pitiseree A, Suwantemee C. Topical *Aloe Vera* gel for accelerated wound healing of split-thickness skin graft donor sites. Plast Reconstr Surg 2018; 142(1): 217-26.
[http://dx.doi.org/10.1097/PRS.0000000000004515] [PMID: 29649056]

[8]   Eshghi F, Hosseinimehr SJ, Rahmani N, Khademloo M, Norozi MS, Hojati O. Effects of *Aloe vera* cream on posthemorrhoidectomy pain and wound healing: results of a randomized, blind, placebo-control study. J Altern Complement Med 2010; 16(6): 647-50.
[http://dx.doi.org/10.1089/acm.2009.0428] [PMID: 20569031]

[9]   Rahmani N, Khademloo M, Vosoughi K, Assadpour S. Effects of *Aloe vera* cream on chronic anal fissure pain, wound healing and hemorrhaging upon defection: a prospective double blind clinical trial. Eur Rev Med Pharmacol Sci 2014; 18(7): 1078-84.
[PMID: 24763890]

[10]   Daburkar M, Lohar V, Rathore A, Bhutada P, Tangadpaliwar S. An *in vivo and in vitro* investigation

of the effect of *Aloe vera* gel ethanolic extract using animal model with diabetic foot ulcer. J Pharm Bioallied Sci 2014; 6(3): 205-12.
[http://dx.doi.org/10.4103/0975-7406.135248] [PMID: 25035641]

[11]   Atiba A, Ueno H, Uzuka Y. The effect of *Aloe vera* oral administration on cutaneous wound healing in type 2 diabetic rats. J Vet Med Sci 2011; 73(5): 583-9.
[http://dx.doi.org/10.1292/jvms.10-0438] [PMID: 21178319]

[12]   Sari Y, Purnawan I. Kurniawan DWSutrisna E. A comparative study of the effects of *Nigella sativa* oil gel and *Aloe vera* gel on wound healing in diabetic rats. J Evid Based Integr Med 2018; 23 2515690x18772804.

[13]   Afkhamizadeh M, Aboutorabi R, Ravari H, *et al.* Topical propolis improves wound healing in patients with diabetic foot ulcer: a randomized controlled trial. Nat Prod Res 2018; 32(17): 2096-9.
[http://dx.doi.org/10.1080/14786419.2017.1363755] [PMID: 28826262]

[14]   Moon JH, Lee MY, Chung YJ, Rhee CK, Lee SJ. Effect of topical propolis on wound healing process after tonsillectomy: randomized controlled study. Clin Exp Otorhinolaryngol 2018; 11(2): 146-50.
[http://dx.doi.org/10.21053/ceo.2017.00647] [PMID: 29665628]

[15]   Wang C, Zhang Z, Xu T, *et al.* Upregulating mTOR/ERK signaling with leonurine for promoting angiogenesis and tissue regeneration in a full-thickness cutaneous wound model. Food Funct 2018; 9(4): 2374-85.
[http://dx.doi.org/10.1039/C7FO01289F] [PMID: 29589609]

[16]   Yassine KA, Houari H, Mokhtar B, Karim A, Hadjer S, Imane B. A topical ointment formulation containing leaves' powder of *Lawsonia inermis* accelerate excision wound healing in Wistar rats. Vet World 2020; 13(7): 1280-7.
[http://dx.doi.org/10.14202/vetworld.2020.1280-1287] [PMID: 32848301]

[17]   Daemi A, Farahpour MR, Oryan A, Karimzadeh S, Tajer E. Topical administration of hydroethanolic extract of *Lawsonia inermis* (henna) accelerates excisional wound healing process by reducing tissue inflammation and amplifying glucose uptake. Kaohsiung J Med Sci 2019; 35(1): 24-32.
[http://dx.doi.org/10.1002/kjm2.12005] [PMID: 30844141]

[18]   Mehrabani D, Farjam M, Geramizadeh B, Tanideh N, Amini M, Panjehshahin MR. The healing effect of curcumin on burn wounds in rat. World J Plast Surg 2015; 4(1): 29-35.
[PMID: 25606474]

[19]   Dehghani S, Dalirfardouei R, Jafari Najaf Abadi MH, Ebrahimi Nik M, Jaafari MR, Mahdipour E. Topical application of curcumin regulates the angiogenesis in diabetic - impaired cutaneous wound. Cell Biochem Funct 2020; 38(5): 558-66.
[http://dx.doi.org/10.1002/cbf.3500] [PMID: 32030812]

[20]   Wang C, Lou Y, Tong M, *et al.* Asperosaponin VI promotes angiogenesis and accelerates wound healing in rats *via* up-regulating HIF-1α/VEGF signaling. Acta Pharmacol Sin 2018; 39(3): 393-404.
[http://dx.doi.org/10.1038/aps.2017.161] [PMID: 29219948]

[21]   Hatahet T, Morille M, Hommoss A, *et al.* Quercetin topical application, from conventional dosage forms to nanodosage formsEur J Pharm Biopharm 2016; 108: 41-53.

[22]   Ahmed OM, Mohamed T, Moustafa H, *et al.* Quercetin and low level laser therapy promote wound healing process in diabetic rats *via* structural reorganization and modulatory effects on inflammation and oxidative stress. Biomed Pharmacother 2018; 101: 58-73.

[23]   Kant V, Jangir BL, Kumar V, Nigam A, Sharma V. Quercetin accelerated cutaneous wound healing in rats by modulation of different cytokines and growth factors. Growth Factors 2020; 38(2): 105-19.
[http://dx.doi.org/10.1080/08977194.2020.1822830] [PMID: 32957814]

[24]   Doersch KM, Newell-Rogers MK. The impact of quercetin on wound healing relates to changes in αV and β1 integrin expression. Exp Biol Med (Maywood) 2017; 242(14): 1424-31.
[http://dx.doi.org/10.1177/1535370217712961] [PMID: 28549404]

[25]   Ren J, Yang M, Chen J. Ma SWang N. Anti-inflammatory and wound healing potential of kirenol in diabetic rats through the suppression of inflammatory markers and matrix metalloproteinase expressions. Biomed Pharmacother 2020; 129: 110475.

[26]   Yamamoto T, Eckes B, Mauch C, Hartmann K, Krieg T. Monocyte chemoattractant protein-1 enhances gene expression and synthesis of matrix metalloproteinase-1 in human fibroblasts by an autocrine IL-1 alpha loop. J Immunol 2000; 164(12): 6174-9.
        [http://dx.doi.org/10.4049/jimmunol.164.12.6174] [PMID: 10843667]

[27]   Zaja-Milatovic S, Richmond A. CXC chemokines and their receptors: a case for a significant biological role in cutaneous wound healing. Histol Histopathol 2008; 23(11): 1399-407.
        [PMID: 18785122]

[28]   Nishimura Y, Ii M, Qin G, *et al.* CXCR4 antagonist AMD3100 accelerates impaired wound healing in diabetic mice. J Invest Dermatol 2012; 132(3): 711-20.
        [http://dx.doi.org/10.1038/jid.2011.356] [PMID: 22048734]

[29]   Vågesjö E, Öhnstedt E, Mortier A, *et al.* Accelerated wound healing in mice by on-site production and delivery of CXCL12 by transformed lactic acid bacteria. Proc Natl Acad Sci USA 2018; 115(8): 1895-900.
        [http://dx.doi.org/10.1073/pnas.1716580115] [PMID: 29432190]

[30]   Zhang L, DeRider M, McCornack MA, *et al.* Solution structure of the complex between poxvirus-encoded CC chemokine inhibitor vCCI and human MIP-1β. Proc Natl Acad Sci USA 2006; 103(38): 13985-90.
        [http://dx.doi.org/10.1073/pnas.0602142103] [PMID: 16963564]

[31]   Ridiandries A, Bursill C, Tan J. Broad-spectrum inhibition of the cc-chemokine class improves wound healing and wound angiogenesis. Int J Mol Sci 2017; 18(1): 155.
        [http://dx.doi.org/10.3390/ijms18010155] [PMID: 28098795]

[32]   Berkkanoglu M, Zhang L, Ulukus M, *et al.* Inhibition of chemokines prevents intraperitoneal adhesions in mice. Hum Reprod 2005; 20(11): 3047-52.
        [http://dx.doi.org/10.1093/humrep/dei182] [PMID: 16006464]

[33]   Söhl G, Willecke K. Gap junctions and the connexin protein family. Cardiovasc Res 2004; 62(2): 228-32.
        [http://dx.doi.org/10.1016/j.cardiores.2003.11.013] [PMID: 15094343]

[34]   Goliger JA, Paul DL. Wounding alters epidermal connexin expression and gap junction-mediated intercellular communication. Mol Biol Cell 1995; 6(11): 1491-501.
        [http://dx.doi.org/10.1091/mbc.6.11.1491] [PMID: 8589451]

[35]   Mendoza-Naranjo A, Cormie P, Serrano AE, *et al.* Targeting Cx43 and *N*-cadherin, which are abnormally upregulated in venous leg ulcers, influences migration, adhesion and activation of Rho GTPases. PLoS One 2012; 7(5): e37374.
        [http://dx.doi.org/10.1371/journal.pone.0037374] [PMID: 22615994]

[36]   Canesso MCC, Vieira AT, Castro TBR, *et al.* Skin wound healing is accelerated and scarless in the absence of commensal microbiota. J Immunol 2014; 193(10): 5171-80.
        [http://dx.doi.org/10.4049/jimmunol.1400625] [PMID: 25326026]

[37]   Zhang M, Jiang Z, Li D, *et al.* Oral antibiotic treatment induces skin microbiota dysbiosis and influences wound healing. Microb Ecol 2015; 69(2): 415-21.
        [http://dx.doi.org/10.1007/s00248-014-0504-4] [PMID: 25301498]

[38]   Plichta JK, Gao X, Lin H, *et al.* Cutaneous burn injury promotes shifts in the bacterial microbiome in autologous donor skin. Shock 2017; 48(4): 441-8.
        [http://dx.doi.org/10.1097/SHK.0000000000000874] [PMID: 28368977]

[39]   Bartow-McKenney C, Hannigan GD, Horwinski J, *et al.* The microbiota of traumatic, open fracture wounds is associated with mechanism of injury. Wound Repair Regen 2018; 26(2): 127-35.

[http://dx.doi.org/10.1111/wrr.12642] [PMID: 29802752]

[40]   Johnson T, Gómez B, McIntyre M, *et al.* The cutaneous microbiome and wounds: new molecular targets to promote wound healing. Int J Mol Sci 2018; 19(9): 2699.
[http://dx.doi.org/10.3390/ijms19092699] [PMID: 30208569]

[41]   Shi L, Kam CM, Powers JC, Aebersold R, Greenberg AH. Purification of three cytotoxic lymphocyte granule serine proteases that induce apoptosis through distinct substrate and target cell interactions. J Exp Med 1992; 176(6): 1521-9.
[http://dx.doi.org/10.1084/jem.176.6.1521] [PMID: 1460416]

[42]   Merkulova Y, Shen Y, Parkinson LG, *et al.* Granzyme B inhibits keratinocyte migration by disrupting epidermal growth factor receptor (EGFR)-mediated signaling. Biol Chem 2016; 397(9): 883-95.
[http://dx.doi.org/10.1515/hsz-2016-0129] [PMID: 27060743]

[43]   Hiebert PR, Wu D, Granville DJ. Granzyme B degrades extracellular matrix and contributes to delayed wound closure in apolipoprotein E knockout mice. Cell Death Differ 2013; 20(10): 1404-14.
[http://dx.doi.org/10.1038/cdd.2013.96] [PMID: 23912712]

[44]   Buzza MS, Zamurs L, Sun J, *et al.* Extracellular matrix remodeling by human granzyme B *via* cleavage of vitronectin, fibronectin, and laminin. J Biol Chem 2005; 280(25): 23549-58.
[http://dx.doi.org/10.1074/jbc.M412001200] [PMID: 15843372]

[45]   Hiebert PR, Boivin WA, Abraham T, Pazooki S, Zhao H, Granville DJ. Granzyme B contributes to extracellular matrix remodeling and skin aging in apolipoprotein E knockout mice. Exp Gerontol 2011; 46(6): 489-99.
[http://dx.doi.org/10.1016/j.exger.2011.02.004] [PMID: 21316440]

[46]   Shen Y, Zeglinski MR, Turner CT, *et al.* Topical small molecule granzyme B inhibitor improves remodeling in a murine model of impaired burn wound healing. Exp Mol Med 2018; 50(5): 1-11.
[http://dx.doi.org/10.1038/s12276-018-0095-0] [PMID: 29849046]

[47]   Hsu I, Parkinson LG, Shen Y, *et al.* Serpina3n accelerates tissue repair in a diabetic mouse model of delayed wound healing. Cell Death Dis 2014; 5(10): e1458.
[http://dx.doi.org/10.1038/cddis.2014.423] [PMID: 25299783]

[48]   Chen G, Han Y, Feng Y, *et al.* Extract of Ilex rotunda Thunb alleviates experimental colitis-associated cancer *via* suppressing inflammation-induced miR-31-5p/YAP overexpression. Phytomedicine 2019; 62: 152941.

[49]   Li B, Zhou D, Li S, *et al.* Licochalcone A reverses NNK-induced ectopic miRNA expression to elicit *in vitro* and *in vivo* chemopreventive effects. Phytomedicine 2020; 76: 153245.

[50]   van der Ree MH, de Vree JM, Stelma F, *et al.* Safety, tolerability, and antiviral effect of RG-101 in patients with chronic hepatitis C: a phase 1B, double-blind, randomised controlled trial. Lancet 2017; 389(10070): 709-17.
[http://dx.doi.org/10.1016/S0140-6736(16)31715-9] [PMID: 28087069]

[51]   Wu P, Cao Y, Zhao R, Wang Y. miR-96-5p regulates wound healing by targeting BNIP3/FAK pathway. J Cell Biochem 2019; 120(8): 12904-11.
[http://dx.doi.org/10.1002/jcb.28561] [PMID: 30883918]

[52]   Shi J, Ma X, Su Y, *et al.* MiR-31 Mediates inflammatory signaling to promote re-epithelialization during skin wound healing. J Invest Dermatol 2018; 138(10): 2253-63.
[http://dx.doi.org/10.1016/j.jid.2018.03.1521] [PMID: 29605672]

[53]   Gerber PA, Buhren BA, Schrumpf H, Homey B, Zlotnik A, Hevezi P. The top skin-associated genes: a comparative analysis of human and mouse skin transcriptomes. Biol Chem 2014; 395(6): 577-91.
[http://dx.doi.org/10.1515/hsz-2013-0279] [PMID: 24497224]

[54]   Walsh NC, Kenney LL, Jangalwe S, *et al.* Humanized mouse models of clinical disease. Annu Rev Pathol 2017; 12: 187-215.

[55] Escámez MJ, García M, Larcher F, *et al.* An *in vivo* model of wound healing in genetically modified skin-humanized mice. J Invest Dermatol 2004; 123(6): 1182-91.
[http://dx.doi.org/10.1111/j.0022-202X.2004.23473.x] [PMID: 15610532]

[56] Gong C, Wu Q, Wang Y, *et al.* A biodegradable hydrogel system containing curcumin encapsulated in micelles for cutaneous wound healing. Biomaterials 2013; 34(27): 6377-87.
[http://dx.doi.org/10.1016/j.biomaterials.2013.05.005] [PMID: 23726229]

[57] Chaudhari A, Vig K, Baganizi D, *et al.* Future prospects for scaffolding methods and biomaterials in skin tissue engineering: a review. Int J Mol Sci 2016; 17(12): 1974.
[http://dx.doi.org/10.3390/ijms17121974] [PMID: 27898014]

CHAPTER 4

The Role of Natural Products in the Management of Skin Pigmentary Anomalies

Luis Alfonso Jiménez Ortega[1], **Manuel Adrián Picos Salas**[1], **Erick Paul Gutiérrez Grijalva**[2] and **José Basilio Heredia**[1,*]

[1] *Centro de Investigación en Alimentación y Desarrollo, A.C., Culiacán, Sinaloa, México*

[2] *Catedras Conacyt-Centro de Investigación en Alimentación y Desarrollo, A.C., Culiacán, Sinaloa, México*

Abstract: The skin is one of the most important organs of the human body. Dermatological ailments and pathologies are important for public health because they cause physical damage and emotional and psychological repercussions that sometimes present high healthcare expenses. Some of the most common pathologies are eczema, psoriasis, acne, rosacea, pyoderma, scabies, tinea capitis, dermatitis, reactions of poisonous insect or reptile bites hives, pigmentary anomalies such as vitiligo, albinism, tinea versicolor, melasma, acanthosis nigricans, and café au Lait spots, such others, can cause serious damage to health, for which extensive pharmacological treatments have been proposed; however, they have serious side effects such as steroid treatments, so in certain regions of the world, medicinal plants are used to treat dermatological complications, where ethnopharmacological records date to treat or aid skin conditions, mainly burns and scars. These effects are due to their anti-inflammatory, healing, antimicrobial, and antioxidant properties, where the compounds most studied have been phenolic (flavonoids such as phloretin), vitamins, and essential oils (terpenes). Some species that stand out are the genera *Dendrobium, Aloe, Acalypha, Acanthus, Achillea, Actinidia, Calendula, Bulbine, Heparinum, Sanguisorba*, and *Buddleja*, among others. This chapter summarizes the most recent information regarding the potential of natural products as biopharmaceutical agents against some of the most evaluated skin pigmentary anomalies.

Keywords: Alkaloids, Antioxidant, Botanicals, Cosmetic, Cosmeceuticals, Dermatology, Ethnopharmacology, Flavonoids, Melanogenesis, Natural Products, Phototherapeutic, Phytochemistry, Phytomedicine, Pigmentary Anomalies, Secondary Metabolites, Skin Care, Skin Diseases, Terpenes, Topical.

* **Corresponding author José Basilio Heredia:** Centro de Investigación en Alimentación y Desarrollo, AC. Carretera a Eldorado Km 5.5, Campo el Diez, 80110 Culiacán, Sinaloa, México; Tel: +52(667)4806950; E-mail: jbheredia@ciad.mx

Heba Abd El-Sattar El-Nashar, Mohamed El-Shazly & Nouran Mohammed Fahmy (Eds.)

INTRODUCTION

The skin is one of the most important organs of the human body; it protects from damage and covers the internal organs, muscles, and bones. It is made up of several layers, such as the epidermis, dermis, and subcutaneous tissue. In turn, these are made up of numerous glands and strata, where the *Stratum corneum* stands out, responsible for receiving the first contact with irritants, organisms, and toxic products [1]. Pigmentation is due to the mixture of melanin (quantity and distribution), oxyhemoglobin, and carotene [2, 3].

The skin can suffer pathologies and alterations, causing serious damage to health; these can be due to genetic defects, chronic degenerative pathologies, inflammation, infections, reactions to medications, exposure to toxic products, poisonous animal bites, and light UV. Some of the most frequent conditions in clinical practice are vitiligo, ichthyosis, psoriasis, impetigo, atopic dermatitis, freckle, contact dermatitis, pityriasis alba, tinea versicolor, melasma, cutaneous lupus erythematosus, urticaria, granuloma annulare, hematomas, cold panniculitis, and acne. In addition, pigmentation-related conditions are divided into hyperpigmentation which is the increase in melanin production and the number of melanocytes; and hypopigmentation, related to the reduction in skin pigmentation and mixed conditions [1, 3 - 5]. The most common conditions/disorders are shown in Table **1**.

Table 1. Pigmentation disorders and conditions [1, 2, 4, 6].

Disorder/Condition	Pathogenesis/Causes	Characteristics	Pharmacological Treatment and Therapy
Melasma	Pregnancy (stimulates melanocytes), use birth control pills, phenytonin, hepatic disease, endocrine disorders	Acquired condition, characterized by changes in the pigmentation of the face and arms, mainly in pregnant women, with well-demarcated patches.	Bleaching cream with a hydroquinone, tretinoin, azelic acid, kogic acid, licorice extract, pulsed light, sunscreens (SPF< 30).
Vitiligo	Selective destruction of melanocytes	Vitiligo is acquired during a person's life, making it a psychologically depleting condition. This is characterized by completely losing skin pigmentation, the lesions are characterized by well-demarcated depigmented macules and patches, which occur mainly around the feet, hands, elbows, eyes, and genitals.	Psoralens, UVA-UVB light, monobenzone, camouflage cosmetics, sunscreens, potent steroids.

Disorder/Condition	Pathogenesis/Causes	Characteristics	Pharmacological Treatment and Therapy
Albinism/piebaldism	Autosomal recessive condition in which reduced melanization and number of melanosomes	It is a congenital disorder of the hypopigmentation type, which manifests in the hair, skin, and eyes. On the other hand, piebaldism is partial albinism characterized by presenting a white forelock and a circumscribed congenital leukoderma. The lesions appear as a triangular patch of depigmentation and white hair on the frontal scalp, they can manifest other macular ones on the extremities, flanks, face, and neck.	Sunscreens use, and strict sun avoidance from childhood.
Acanthosis nigricans	Related to obesity and endocrine disorders	Hyperpigmentation disorder manifests as marked lines on the skin's surface, with a leathery and warty appearance. Four forms of manifestation have been identified, the benign one that is related to hyperinsulinemia or insulin resistance, the hereditary, endocrine-associated acanthosis nigrans, and the malignancy-related one.	Hypoglycemic drugs, contraceptives, glucocorticoids.
Café-au-lait	Unclear, associated with neurofibromatosis	It manifests in the form of macules, which can be related to neurofibromatosis type 1, McCune-Albright syndrome, polyostotic fibrous dysplasia, endocrinopathy, hyperthyroidism, and precocious puberty.	Copper vapor laser, frequency-doubled 1064-nm neodymium-doped yttrium aluminum garnet, Q-switched ruby laser, Q-switched alexandrite laser, erbium-doped YAG, and pulsed-dye laser.

These conditions are normally characterized by presenting skin lesions, changes in tonality, and hyper or hypopigmentation, and may or may not be accompanied by the presence of other chronic degenerative pathologies, such as diabetes in the case of acanthosis nigricans, which represents greater harm to the patient, also represents emotional damage, lowering self-esteem [5]. In Table **1**, we summarize the most common skin pigmentary anomalies and their conventional pharmaceutical treatment.

Although pharmacological treatments are effective, natural and phytochemical products can contribute to the treatment of certain ailments. In different regions of the world, it is used as first-line medicine to treat pathologies and ailments. These products come from roots, leaves, stems, and flowers of certain botanical species and are usually consumed/applied through decoctions, tinctures and extracts [7]. The effectiveness of these products will depend on the concentration, amount of secondary metabolites present, dose, conservation, method of obtaining, the region from where the plant is obtained, as well as metabolic and genetic factors of who consumes them, as well as the types of phytochemicals present as phenolic compounds (phenolic acids/flavonoids), alkaloids, terpenes, triterpenes, saponins, among others.

NATURAL PRODUCTS AND PHYTOCHEMICALS FOR SKIN PIGMENTARY ANOMALIES

Phenolic compounds are one of the most studied regarding pigmentary anomalies; *p*-coumaric acid and kojic acid can reduce pigmentation [8, 9], while flavonoids like naringenin and galangin promote melanogenesis [10, 11]; meanwhile, terpenes from different plants also inhibit melanogenesis, mostly by tyrosinase inhibition [12, 13]; contrary, alkaloids like piperine and capsaicin are more related to the promotion of melanogenesis [14, 15]; and glucosinolates, not so studied according to recent literature, can suppress melanogenesis [16].

Some traditional formulations have been developed to treat pigmentation disorders (hyper or hypo), such as the product called ubtan, which is commonly used in India, is prepared is composed of rhizome powder of *Curcuma longa*, the heartwood of *Santalum album*, and *Cicer arietum* seeds. This product is used as a tyrosinase inhibitor, momentarily providing a better appearance of the skin. Another product used is "Kumkumadi Tailan", where the compound is mainly *Crocous sativus*, responsible for the inhibitory activity of tyrosinase [17]. Likewise, natural products have been evaluated to help treat periorbital hyperpigmentation, where phytochemicals and other compounds such as hyaluronic acid, lactic acid, lycopene, retinol, niacinamide, pycnogenol, arabinoxylans, beta-carotene, glucuronic acid, among others [18]. In addition, compounds with anti-pigment activity have been isolated from various natural sources, in addition to highlighting plants, marine organisms, bacteria, and fungi [19].

In Vitro and *In Vivo* Studies

Multiple phytochemicals have shown benefits against skin pigmentary anomalies, especially promoting or decreasing melanogenesis (Fig. **1**), including phenolic compounds, alkaloids, terpenes, and glucosinolates. Assessing the different effects of phytochemicals against skin pigmentary anomalies is usually done by a variety of studies.

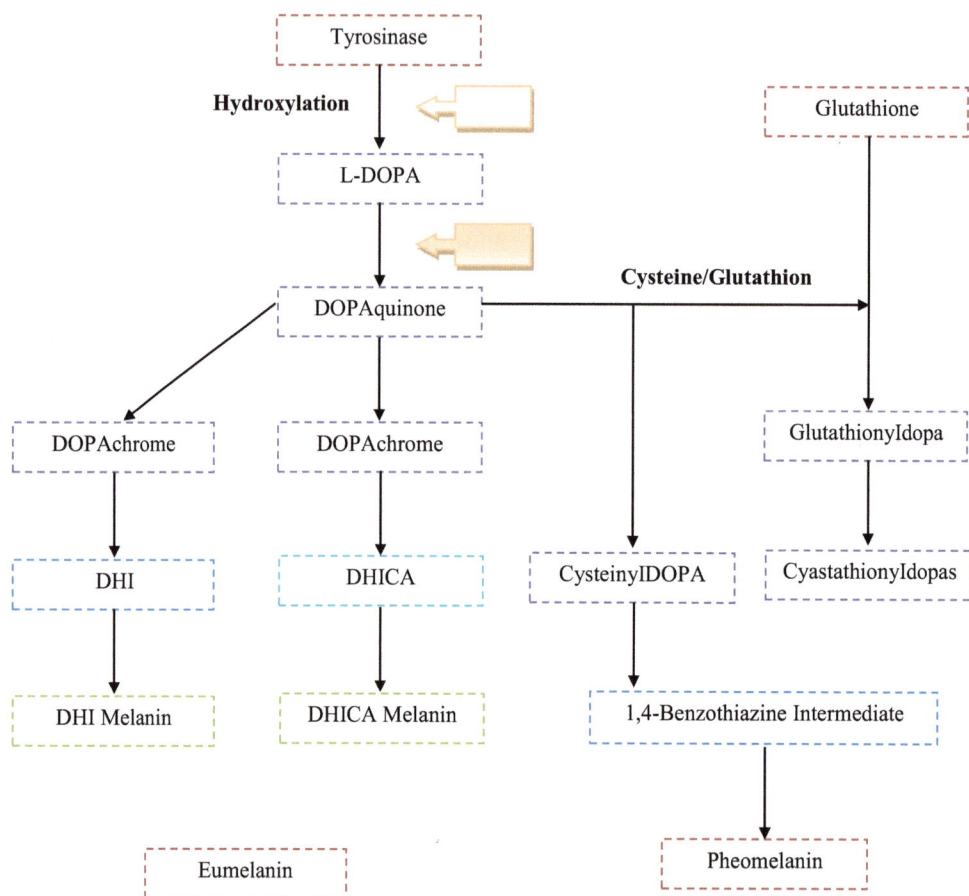

Fig. (1). Melanogenesis pathway (*Abbreviations:* TYR: Tyrosinase; LDopa: Levo Dopa; TYRP-1: Tyrosinase related protein-1; TYRP-2: Tyrosinase related protein-2; DHICA: 5,6-dihydroxyindole-2-carboxylic acid; DHI: 5,6-dihydroxyindole; GST: Glutathione-S-transferase; DCT: DOPAchrome tautomerase).

In vitro studies using murine melanomas cells are the most employed, although human cells are also used. Two important proteins related to melanin modulation are tyrosinase, a key enzyme produced in melanocytes, associated with the production of melanin [20], and microphthalmia-associated transcription factor (MITF), which is important for melanocytes development and melanogenesis regulation [21]; for this reason, the modulation of these proteins by phytochemicals is a popular topic of research. A summary of recent literature regarding *in vitro* and *in vivo* studies is shown in Table **2**.

Table 2. *In vitro* **and** *in vivo* **studies of phytochemicals against skin pigmentary anomalies.**

Plant Part/Standard	Extraction Method	Compound(s)	Identification	Model	Effect	Refs.
Phenolics compounds						
Argania spinosa leaves	70% ethanol	Gallic acid, gallocatechin, epigallocatechin, catechin, epicatechin, quercetin-3-*O*-glucuronide, myricetin-3-*O*-galactoside, myricitrin, quercitrin, quercetin 7-*O*-rhamnoside, myricetin, rutin, quercetin	UPLC-ESI-HRMS	B16 cells	Increased expression of tyrosinase, dopachrome tautomerase, and tyrosinase-related protein-1	[22]
Gentiana veitchiorum Hemsl. Flowers.	Milli-Q water	Isoorientin	HPLC	B16F10 cells	Inhibitory effect on melanogenesis in a dose-dependent manner. Suppressed expression of tyrosinase, TRP1, and DOPA-chrome tautomerase	[23]
Vaccinium dunalianum buds	H₂O-acetone 4:6 v/v	6'-*O*-caffeoyl arbutin	IR, TLC, ¹H and ¹³C NMR MS	Zebrafish embryos	Anti-melanin activity in a dose-dependent manner, through competitive inhibition	[24]
Pistacia vera hulls	80% methanol	Gallic acid, pyrogallol, catechin, myricetin, naringenin, quercetin, rutin	RP-HPLC	Tyrosinase enzyme/ B16F10	Anti-melanogenic activity, inhibition the tyrosinase enzyme. Modulation of melanin biosynthesis genes in B16F10 melanoma cells	[25]
Mistletoe from oak tree	70% ethanol	Vetulin (aglycone)	HPLC, ¹H and ¹³C NMR	Mushroom tyrosinase /Zebrafish embryos	Inhibited melanocyte development and melanin synthesis in a dose-dependent manner	[26]
Mixture of seeds of *A. graveolens, P. anisum, F. campestreis*	Methanol	Umbelliprenin	HPLC	Melan-a-cells. Non-tumoral murine melanocytes	Modulate melanogenesis due to the mixture of phytochemicals presents	[27]
Malpighia emarginata juice fruits	-	Dehydroascorbic acid	HPLC-ECD	SMP30/GNL KO hairless mice	Suppressing UVB-induced skin pigmentation through inhibiting melanogenesis-related genes	[28]
Pinus densiflora leafs	80% ethanol	*Trans*-communic acid	-	Human melanoma cells line MNT1	Decreased melanin levels in melanocytes through activation of gene FoxO3a	[29]
Arthrophytum scoparium stems	70% ethanol	Coumaric acid, cinnamic acid, chrysoeriol, cyanidin, catechol, caffeoylquinic acid	HPLC-ESI-TOF-MS	B16 cells	Inhibition of Tyr and Trp1 gene expressions by downregulation of MITF and Mc1R expressions	[30]

(Table 2) cont.....

Plant Part/Standard	Extraction Method	Compound(s)	Identification	Model	Effect	Refs.
Bamboo Stems (*Phyllostachys nigra* variety *henosis*)	80% ethanol extraction, partitioned with ethyl acetate	Catechin, chlorogenic acid, caffeic acid, *p*-coumaric acid, ferulic acid, rutin, luteolin	HPLC-qTOF-MS	B16F10 cells	Decrease in mRNA levels of tyrosinase-related protein 1, and MITF. Downregulation of PKA/CREB mediated by MITF downregulation	[31]
Citrus sinensis, Citrus aurantium, and *Citrus Reticulata* material grade extracts	Hydrolyzed with HCl, ethyl acetate	Hesperetin	HPLC-UV	B16F10 cells	Upregulation of tyrosinase activity, activation of CREB and MAPKs in Wnt/β-catenin pathway	[32]
Juniperus communis fruits	Methanolic extraction, subsequent fractionation	Hypolaetin 7-*O*-β-xylopyranoside	^{1}H NMR, ^{13}C NMR, COSY, HMQC, HMBC, NOESY	B16F10 cells	Inhibition of tyrosinase activity	[33]
Pomegranate concentrate powder	Juice	Ellagic acid, punicalagin A and B	HPLC-PAD	B16F10 cells	Inhibition of tyrosinase activity and melanin production by inactivation of p38 and PKA/CREB pathways	[34]
Black, green, white tea	Water	Catechin, theaflavins	HPLC-PAD	Melan-A cells	Decrease in tyrosinase activity and protein levels	[35]
Citrus depressa peel	Methanolic extraction, subsequent fractionation	Nobiletin	^{1}H NMR, ^{13}C NMR	Normal human melanocyte	Reduction in tyrosinase activity, downregulation of MITF, and tyrosinase expression *via reduction of Raf-1 phosphorylation*	[36]
Scutellaria baicalensis root	70% ethanolic extraction, subsequent fractionation	Wogonide, wogonoside	HPLC-DAD-MS	B16F10 cells	Inhibition of melanogenesis, suppression of melanosome transportation by MLPH downregulation	[37]
Panax ginseng root	Water extraction, subsequent fractionation	Vanillic acid	HPLC-MS	B16F10 cells	Decrease in melanin levels and tyrosinase activity, suppression of melanogenesis *via* inhibition of NO/PKG pathways	[38]
Ziziphus jujuba seeds	70% ethanolic	Spinosin	HPLC-DAD-MS	B16F10 cells, human skin	Suppression of melanogenesis, *via* possible competitive inhibition of tyrosinase	[39]
Ziziphora taurica subsp. *Cleonioides* aerial parts	Methanolic, ethyl acetate, and water extraction	Rosmarinic acid, chlorogenic acid, luteolin, apigenin-7-glucoside, protocatechuic acid, caffeic acid, hyperoside, hesperidin, among others	LC–ESI–MS/MS	Tyrosinase	Inhibition of tyrosinase activity	[40]

(Table 2) cont.....

Plant Part/Standard	Extraction Method	Compound(s)	Identification	Model	Effect	Refs.
Alnus cordata stem bark	80% methanolic	Gallic acid, vanillic acid, caffeic acid, *p*-coumaric acid, *m*-coumaric acid, epicatechin, orientin, isovitexin, oregonin, naringenin-7-*O*-glucoside, eriodictyol, naringenin, hyperoside, isoquercetin, rutin, isorhamnetin-3-*O*-glucoside, isorhamnetin-3-*O*-rutinoside	RP-LC-DAD	Tyrosinase, zebrafish embryos	Inhibition of tyrosinase activity, whitening of zebrafish embryos	[41]
Vernonia anthelmintica seeds	80% ethanolic	4-*O*-caffeoylquinate, 3-*O*-caffeoylquinate, 5,7,3′,4′-tetrahydroxy-flavanone-3-*O*-glucoside, 3′-methoxy-5,7,4′-trihydroxy-dihydrochalcone-3-*O*-rutinoside, 3,4-di-*O*-caffeoylisoquinic acid, 3,4-di-*O*-caffeoylquinic acid, liquiritigenin, luteolin, apigenin, methoxyisorhamnetin, kaempferide,	HPLC-qTOF-ESI-MS/MS	B16 cells	Increase in tyrosinase activity; and expression of tyrosinase, tyrosinase-related protein 1 and 2 through MITF	[42]
Juniperus chinensis fruits	95% ethanolic extraction, subsequent fractionation	Quercetin-7-*O*-α-L-rhamnoside	RP-HPLC-UV, ^{1}H NMR, ^{13}C-NMR, HR-MS, IR	B16F10 cells	Downregulation of tyrosinase activity	[43]
Hibiscus sabdariffa anthocyanins	-	-	-	A375 cells	Downregulation of tyrosinase activity, inhibition of tyrosinase, and MITF protein expression	[44]
Diosmetin, acacetin, kaempferide, luteolin, apigenin, kaempferol	-	-	-	B16F10 cells	Upregulation of tyrosinase activity through activation of the CREB pathway	[45]
Naringenin	-	-	-	B16F10 cells	Upregulation of tyrosinase activity and Induction of melanogenesis through activation of PI3K/Akt or Wnt/β-catenin pathways	[10]
Galangin	-	-	-	C57BL/6 mice with induced vitiligo	Increase in melanocytes, melanin-containing epidermal cells, tyrosinase in serum, tyrosinase expression	[11]
Afzelin	-	-	-	Normal human epidermal melanocyte	Activation of the Nrf2-ARE pathway through inhibition of GSK-3β	[46]

(Table 2) cont.....

Plant Part/Standard	Extraction Method	Compound(s)	Identification	Model	Effect	Refs.
Gallic acid	-	-	-	B16F10 cells	Inhibition of tyrosinase, tyrosinase-related protein 1, dopachrome tautomerase, and MITF genes; inhibition of cAMP/PKA/CREB and MITF pathways *via* blocking the MCR-1 receptor system; induction of proteasomal degradation through activation of ERK and AKT kinases	[47]
Gallic acid	-	-	-	Zebrafish embryos	Inhibition of pigmentation	[47]
Gallic acid	-	-	-	C57B/6 mice with UVB-induced melanogenesis, zebrafish	Inhibition of melanin production, decrease in tyrosinase and MITF expression	[47]
Swertiajaponin	-	-	-	B16F10 cells, human skin model	Inhibition of melanogenesis in both models, possible competitive bind with tyrosinase, inhibition of MAPK/MITF signaling in B16F10 cells	[48]
Chlorogenic acid	-	-	-	B16 cells	Suppression of tyrosinase activity	[49]
Isoliquiritigenin	-	-	-	Human skin culture; SK-MEL-2 cells and HaCaT cells	Inhibition of melanogenesis, melanocyte dendricity, and melanosome transport through activation of the ERK pathways; causing MITF degradation and suppressing the expression of tyrosinase, dopachrome tautomerase, and tyrosinase related protein-1, Rab27a and Cdc42	[50]
Baicalein	-	-	-	PIG3V cells	Upregulation of the Nrf2 pathway, enhance the expression of HO-1	[51]
Triacylresveratrol, tetraacetyl oxyresveratrol	-	-	-	HEK293 cells reconstituted human skin model MEL-300-B	Inhibition of melanogenesis	[52]

(Table 2) cont.....

Plant Part/Standard	Extraction Method	Compound(s)	Identification	Model	Effect	Refs.
Paeonol and salidroside	-	-	-	Brown guinea pigs with UVB-induced melanogenesis	Anti-melanogenic effect	[53]
Hesperidin	-	-	-	B16F10 cells, HEMa cells	Increase of melanin synthesis in both cell lines, and tyrosinase activity in HEMa cells	[54]
Ellagic acid	-	-	-	B16F10 cells, HaCaT cells, zebrafish embryos	Inhibition of tyrosinase activity and melanogenesis, tyrosinase-related protein 1 and 2 through downregulation of CREB/MITF expression *via* JNK, ERK, and AKT pathways in B16F10 cells. Activation of autophagy *via* an increase of LC3-II accumulation, AVO formation, AGT4B downregulation p62/SQSTM1 activation, PI3K/AKT/mTOR inhibition, Beclin-1/Bcl-2 dysregulation in B16F10 cells. Suppression of ROS-mediated POMC/ α-MSH generation; and activation of the Nrf2 pathway, and suppression of the UVA-activated α-MSH pathways in HaCaT cells. Inhibition of endogenous pigmentation and tyrosinase activity in zebrafish embryos.	[55]
Sulfuretin	-	-	-	B16 cells, normal primary human melanocytes PCS-200-012, tyrosinase	Inhibition of melanogenesis, inhibition of tyrosinase, a decrease of MITF expression	[56]
Terpenes						
Metasequoia glyptostroboides cones	Ethyl acetate	Sugiol	^{1}H NMR, ^{13}C-NMR	Tyrosinase	Inhibition of tyrosinase	[57]

(Table 2) cont.....

Plant Part/Standard	Extraction Method	Compound(s)	Identification	Model	Effect	Refs.
Inula britannica flowers	Methanolic extraction, subsequent fractionation	1-O-acetyl-britannilactone	^{1}H NMR, ^{13}C-NMR, EI-MS	B16F10 cells	Inhibition of melanogenesis and tyrosinase activity and expression, reduction of tyrosinase-related protein 1 and 2 levels; through suppression of CREB and activation of ERK and AKT pathways	[12]
Eucalyptus camaldulensis flowers	Hydodistillation	1,8-Cineole, γ-terpinene, α-eudesmol, γ-eudesmol, terpinen-4-ol, α-terpineol, elemol, τ-cadinol, among others	GC/MS	B16F10 cells	Inhibition of tyrosinase activity, downregulation of MAPK and PKA pathways	[13]
Pogostemon plectranthoides leaves	Hydrodistillation	Cyclosativene, α-guaiene, spathulenol, caryophyllene oxide, humulene epoxide II, 1,10-di-*epi*-cubenol, among others	GC-FID, GC-MS	Tyrosinase	Inhibition of tyrosinase	[58]
Citrus grandis leaves	Hydrodistillation	Citronellal, citronellol	GC–MS	Tyrosinase	Inhibition of tyrosinase	[59]
Copaifera guianensis, Copaifera langsdorffi, Copaifera multijuga, unidentified *Copaifera* species	Previously obtained oleoresin	3-hydroxy-copalic acid	^{1}H NMR, ^{13}C NMR, IR, ESI-MS, ^{13}C-^{1}H COSY, HSQC, HMBC	Tyrosinase	Inhibition of tyrosinase	[60]
Carvacrol	-	-	-	B16F10 cells	Inhibition of tyrosinase activity, expression of tyrosinase, tyrosinase and related protein 1; inhibition of CREB phosphorylation; inhibition of MITF expression *via* ERK phosphorylation	[61]
Loliolide	-	-	-	B16F10 cells, HaCaT cells	Decrease in melanin content and expression of MITF, *p*-CREB, and tyrosinase in B16F10 cells; increase in expression of Nrf2 and HO-1 in HaCaT cells	[62]
Bilobalide	-	-	-	Normal human melanocytes	Reduction in H_2O_2-induced apoptosis, intracellular ROS increase, and Hsp70 release; increase in catalase and glutathione peroxidase mRNA levels	[63]

(Table 2) cont.....

Plant Part/Standard	Extraction Method	Compound(s)	Identification	Model	Effect	Refs.
Ginkgolide B	-	-	-	B16F1 cells	Reduction in ROS production, inhibition of tyrosinase activity; decrease in melanin content through a reduction in protein expression of tyrosinase-related protein 1 and 2, and MITF	[64]
Peel of *Citrus x aurantium*; whole flowering plant of *Salvia officinalis* and *Origanum vulgare*; buds of *Cupressus sempervirens*; flowers and herbs of *Salvia sclarea*; whole plant of *Thymus vulgaris*; leaves of *Rosmarinus officinalis*, flowers of *Syzgium aromaticum*	Stem distillation	Linalyl acetate, bornyl acetate, thymol, carvacrol, eugenol, β-caryophyllene	GC-MS, GC-FID	Mushroom tyrosinase/ murine B16 melanoma	Several essential oils show activity in a dose-dependent manner inhibition of mushroom tyrosinase. Almost two compounds inhibited the tyrosinase from murine B16 melanoma cells	[65]
Alkaloids						
Germinated barley (*Hordeum vulgare*)	Ultrasonication in water extraction	Hordenine	HPLC-DAD	Human epidermal melanocytes	Inhibition of melanin content *via* suppression of cAMP pathway, inhibition of CREB phosphorylation, and MITF expression, along with tyrosinase and tyrosinase-related protein 1 and 2	[66]
Berberis aristata stem bark and wood	Methanolic extraction, subsequent fractionation	Berberine	HPLC-UV/Vis	Tyrosinase	Inhibition of tyrosinase	[67]
Berberis vulgaris root bark	Ultrasound-assisted extraction with water/glycerol	Berberine	HPLC-DAD	Tyrosinase	Inhibition of tyrosinase	[68]
Piper caninum aerial parts, *Piper magnibaccum* leaves, and stems	Hexane extraction, subsequent fractionation	Cepharadione A	^{1}H NMR, ^{13}C NMR, IR, HRMS, UV	Tyrosinase	Inhibition of tyrosinase	[69]
Piperine	-	-	-	B16F10 cells	Increase in melanin content and expression of tyrosinase and MITF	[14]
Capsaicin	-	-	-	B16 cells	Increase of tyrosinase expression	[15]
Berberine	-	-	-	PIG1 cells	Decrease in H_2O_2-induced apoptosis; increase in Nrf2 expression, MITF, tyrosinase, tyrosinase-related protein 1, and L-dopachrome Delta-isomerase	[70]

(Table 2) cont.....

Plant Part/Standard	Extraction Method	Compound(s)	Identification	Model	Effect	Refs.
Berberine	-	-	-	B16F10 cells	Decrease in melanin synthesis and tyrosinase activity through a decrease in MITF and tyrosinase expression; induction of PI3K/AKT, ERK, and GSK3β phosphorylation	[71]
Glucosinolates						
7-methylsulfinylheptyl isothiocyanate	-	-	-	B16F1	Suppression of melanogenesis *via* reduction of MITF, tyrosinase, and tyrosinase-related protein 1 levels; probably by activation of the ERK pathway	[16]

Abbreviations: MITF: microphthalmia-associated transcription factor, CREB: cAMP response element-binding protein, PKA: protein kinase A, MLPH: melanophilin; PKG: protein kinase G, PI3K: phosphoinositide 3-kinases, AKT: protein kinase B, Nrf2: nuclear factor erythroid 2-related factor 2, ARE: antioxidant response element, GSK-3β: glycogen synthase kinase-3β, MCR-1: melanocortin receptor 1, ERK: extracellular signal-regulated protein kinase, HO-1: heme oxygenase 1, JNK: c-Jun N-terminal kinase, LC3-II: microtubule-associated protein light chain-3, AVO: acidic vesicular organelle, SQSTM1: sequestosome 1, mTOR: mechanistic target of rapamycin, ROS: reactive oxygen species, α-MSH: α-melanocyte- stimulating hormone.

Phenolic compounds are commonly extracted from plants using polar solvents like methanol, ethanol, or water. Tyrosinase, generally from mushrooms, is usually evaluated as a first step to determine if a compound can modulate melanogenesis; for instance, the *Ziziphora taurica* aerial parts extract rich in rosmarinic acid, *Alnus cordata* stem bark methanolic extract rich in hydroxycinnamic acids, and sulfuretin inhibits the activity of this enzyme [40, 41, 56]. Concerning studies using mouse melanoma cells, hypolaetin 7-*O*-β-xylopyranoside from *Juniperus communis* fruits methanolic extract can inhibit tyrosinase activity [33]; the ethanolic extract of *Argania spinosa* leaves can upregulate the expression of important protein related to melanin synthesis, including tyrosinase, dopachrome tautomerase (DCT), and tyrosinase-related protein 1 (TRP-1) and 2 (TRP-2) [22]. At the same time, hesperetin from *Citrus* species upregulates the activity of tyrosinase through activation of the Wnt/ β-catenin signaling pathway [32], although the flavonoid naringenin may also induce melanogenesis by activation of this pathway, but also can be attributed to activation of the PI3K/Akt pathway [10]; furthermore, the flavonoids diosmetin, acacetin, kaempferide, luteolin, apigenin, and kaempferol upregulate the activity of tyrosinase *via* activation of the CREB pathway [45].

On the other hand, anti-melanogenic properties of phenolic compounds are more studied, and MITF modulation is greatly affected by these compounds; downregulation of this transcription factor is accompanied by a decrease in the gene expression of important enzymes related to melanogenesis like tyrosinase and TRP-1, as seen in ethanolic extracts of *Arthrophytum scoparium* stems and bamboo stems [30, 31]; similarly, sulfuretin and swertiajaponin also can inhibit the expression of MITF and inhibit tyrosinase activity, the former probably by competitive inhibition [56]. Moreover, quercetin-7-*O*-α-L-rhamnoside and spinosin from ethanolic extracts of *Ziziphus jujuba* seeds and *Juniperus chinensis* fruits, respectively, downregulate the activity of tyrosinase [43]; similarly, vanillic acid from *Panax ginseng* root water extract inhibits this enzyme and inhibits the NO/PKG signaling pathway [38]; furthermore, wogonide and wogonoside extracted from *Scutellaria baicalensis* roots suppress melanosome transportation due to the mono-*O*-methyl group in the A ring of the flavone *via* melanophilin [MLPH] downregulation [37]. In contrast, some compounds from ethanolic extract of *Vernonia anthelmintica* seeds upregulate the expression of tyrosinase, TRP-1, and TRP2 *via* MITF expression upregulation [42].

More detailed studies of modulation of signaling pathways by phenolic compounds in murine cells include p38 and PKA/CREB as seen by ellagic acid and punicalagin A and B from pomegranate [34]; cAMP/PKA/CREB *via* blocking the MCR-1 receptor, and activation of ERK and AKT kinases causing proteasomal degradation, by gallic acid [47]. Particularly, ellagic acid also can downregulate CREB/MITF expression *via* JNK, ERK, and AKT signaling pathways; activate autophagy *via* an increase of LC3-II accumulation, AVO formation, AGT4B downregulation p62/SQSTM1 activation, PI3K/AKT/mTOR inhibition, and Beclin-1/Bcl-2 dysregulation [54].

In addition to murine cells, human cells have also been used to study the modulation of phenolic compounds in melanogenesis. For instance, nobiletin from *Citrus depressa* peel reduces tyrosinase activity and downregulates MITF and tyrosinase expression, *via* Raf-1 phosphorylation in normal human melanocytes [36]; while catechins and theaflavins from tea reduce protein levels of tyrosinase and inhibit it activity in Melan-A cells. Similarly, MITF expression and tyrosinase activity are reduced by *Hibiscus sabdariffa* anthocyanins in A375 cells [44], and by sulfuretin in normal human melanocytes [56]. Moreover, in a human skin model, swertiajaponin and resveratrol derivatives can inhibit melanogenesis [48, 52]; spinosin from *Ziziphus jujuba* seeds inhibits tyrosinase activity [39]; while isoliquiritigenin can inhibit melanocyte dendricity and melanosome transport, this *via* activation of the ERK signaling pathway, causing degradation of MITF, tyrosinase, tyrosinase-related protein 1, dopachrome tautomerase, Rab27a and Cdc42 [50].

The health benefit effect of phenolic compounds is usually associated with their ability to induce an antioxidant response in cells; for instance, baicalein upregulates the Nrf2 pathway and enhances HO-1 expression, protecting vitiligo PIG3V cells from antioxidant damage [51]; while a similar effect in activating the Nrf2-ARE pathway is promoted by afzelin in normal human melanocytes [46]. On the other hand, *in vivo* studies have shown similar results; the methanolic extract of *Alnus cordata* stem bark whitened zebrafish embryos; moreover, gallic acid can inhibit its pigmentation [47]; and tyrosinase activity is inhibited by ellagic acid [55]. Other models include mice, in which gallic acid exhibited a decrease in tyrosinase and MITF expression [47]; contrary, galangin increases melanocytes, melanin-containing epidermal cells, and an increase of tyrosinase expression and tyrosinase in serum [11]; while in guinea pigs, an anti-melanogenic effect was exhibited by hesperitin [53].

Different organs of the persimmon fruit (*Diospyros kaki*) contain a large number of phytochemicals, including phenolic acids such as gallic, *p*-coumaric, vanillic, cinnamic, caffeic, chlorogenic, ferulic, tannic acid, flavonoids like anthocyanidins (cyanidin), flavan-3-ols (catechin, catechin-gallate, gallocatechin-gallate, ellagitannins), flavonols (kaempferol, quercetin), carotenoids mainly xanthophylls and carotenes (lutein, zeaxanthin, β-cryptoxanthin, and β-carotene), terpenes such as ursolic acid, rosolic acid, lupeol, betulinic acid, pomolic acid, which thanks to their antioxidant capacity, contribute to the maintenance of skin cells and the treatment of hypopigmentation due to inhibiting melanin biosynthesis, tyrosinase activity, reducing the expression of melanogenic proteins, and have shown anti-inflammatory, photoprotective, anti-aging capacity. Glycosylated quercetin, isoquercitrin, and hyperin inhibit metallogenesis and tyrosinase activity *in vitro* models [72].

The apolar extract of twigs of *Broussonetia papyrifera* contains flavonols with tyrosinase inhibitory activity; also, the polar extracts of stem bark of *Sideroxylon inerme*, *Hyaenanche globose*, and *Myrsine africana* inhibit *in vitro* the activity of the monophenolase and diphenolase (a form of tyrosinase). *Garcinia livingstonei*, on the other hand, has a depigmenting effect and is less toxic than hydroquinone [7]. *Hyptis mociniana* aerial parts present rutin, isoquercitroside, boehmerin, hyprhombins, glucopyranosyl rosmarinic acid, which due to their wavelength, can act as photochemoprotectors; this is due to the presence of antioxidants. For that reason, it did not present cytotoxicity in HaCaT keratinocytes. It also presented photoprotective effects, preserving cell *viability* up to 113.5%. Finally, the extract is protected from photocarcinogenesis, reducing the incidence of skin carcinomas in SKH-1 mice [73].

The methanolic extracts of *Hypericum perforatum* L., *H. calycinum* L., and *H. confertum*, showed chlorogenic acid, quinic acid, gallic acid, rutin, quercitrin, isoquercitrin, which acted as tyrosinase inhibitors, highlighting *H. calycinum* with inhibition of 54.30% [74]. The ethanolic extract of *Eucalyptus camaldulensis,* for its content of rutin, ellagic acid, ferulic acid, quercetin, presented tyrosinase inhibitory activity with 51%, with an IC_{50} of 555.55µg/mL [75]. Bioactive flavonoids were identified from methanolic extracts and their fractions with solvents of increasing polarities from *Juniperus communis* fruits, where hypolaetin 7-*O*-β-xylopyranoside stood out, which inhibited mushroom tyrosinase activity with an IC_{50} value of 45.15 µM; this may be due to the inhibited α-MSH-stimulated melanin synthesis dose-dependently [76]. Apolar stems extracts of *J. curcas*, identified by NMR scoparone, scopoletin, glaberide I, pinoresinol, medioresinol, syringaresinol, matairesinol, secoisolariciresinol showed anti-melanogenic activity *in vitro* with an IC_{50} of 22.7µg/mL, likewise, their bioactive fractions inhibited the expression of the gene *Tyr* [77].

4-hexyl-1,3-phenylenediol showed effectiveness both *in vitro* and in a clinical study reducing melanogenesis, due to the inhibition of tyrosinase; in addition, the treatment did not present cytotoxicity [78]. Abolangelone identified from *Angelica koreana* Maxim roots dose-dependently inhibited melanin production in B16 melanoma cells, with an IC_{50} of 9-17µM [79]. The aqueous extract of *Azadirachta indica* var siamensis valeton (neem), reduced melanin levels in a dose-dependent manner, up to 69%, and also reduced the intracellular activity of tyrosinase in B16F10 melanoma cells, up to 180% compared to the control, without presenting toxicity, this due to its high flavonoid contents [80].

Although less studied, terpenes also have properties against melanogenesis; they can inhibit tyrosinase activity, compounds like sugiol from *Metasequoia glyptostroboides* cones [57], the cyclosativene from *Pogostemon plectranthoides* leaves [58], citronellal and citronellol from *Citrus grandis* leaves [59], and 3-hydroxy-copalic acid from *Copaifera* species [60], exhibit this property. In murine cells, terpenes modulate signaling pathways. For instance, suppression of CREB and activation of ERK and AKT pathways are produced by 1-*O*-acetylbritannilactone, causing a reduction of the expression of tyrosinase, TRP-1, and TRP-2 [12]; MITF expression is reduced by ginkgolide B, accompanied by a reduction in the expression of tyrosinase, TRP-1, and TRP-2 [64]. Carvacrol inhibits CREB phosphorylation, and MITF expression *via* ERK phosphorylation [61], and loliolide decrease the expression of *p*-CREB and MITF [62].

On the other hand, terpenes like cyclosativene, α-guaiene and spathulenol from *Eucalyptus camaldulensis* flowers downregulate the MAPK and PKA pathways [13]. Furthermore, terpenes can induce an antioxidant response in human cells.

Loliolide increases the expression of Nrf2 and HO-1 [62], whereas bilobalide reduces intracellular ROS, reduces the H_2O_2-induced apoptosis, increases Hsp70 release and the mRNA levels of the antioxidant enzymes catalase and glutathione peroxidase [63]. However, a similar effect can also be observed in murine cells [64]. Diterpene extracts from aerial parts of *Euphorbia antiquorum* L. showed antivitiligo activity, which was related to melanogenesis stimulation in B16 cells [81].

Among the recently studied alkaloid compounds, berberine has been widely analyzed. This compound can be obtained from *Berberis aristata* stem bark and wood and *Berberis vulgaris* root bark and can inhibit the activity of mushroom tyrosinase [67, 68]. In murine cells, it can also activate the PI3K/AKT, ERK, and GSK3β signaling pathways, therefore decreasing MITF and tyrosinase expression [71]. While in human cells, it has been observed protection against oxidative stress by increasing Nrf2 expression and reducing H_2O_2-induced apoptosis, with MITF activation [70]. Other alkaloids promote melanogenesis in murine cells; for instance, piperine increases the expression of MITF and tyrosinase, causing an increase in melanin content [14], whereas capsaicin has improved the expression of this enzyme [15]; on the other hand, cepharadione A from *Piper* species inhibits mushroom tyrosinase [69]. In addition, a study of the glucosinolate 7-methylsulfinylheptyl isothiocyanate in murine cells showed a probable activation of the ERK signaling pathway, causing a reduction in levels of MITF, tyrosinase, and TRP-1 [16].

Other compounds, like withaferin A, isolated from *Whitania somnifera,* showed depigmenting potential in EDN1 cells, with doses of 10µg/mL. This was attributed to the suppression of melanocyte's mRNAs and proteins [82]. Aqueous extracts of seaweed such as *Schizymenia dubyi, Ecklonia cava, Sargassum silquastrum,* and *Endarachne binghamiae* have also shown the inhibitory potential of mushroom tyrosinase, showing inhibitory effects of up to 50%, with IC_{50} of 9.08, 18.00, 19.85, and 27µg/mL, respectively [83].

Clinical Studies

Usually, the population is small, and the subjects are adult women; a summary of various studies of this kind is shown in Table **3**. In this regard, ingestion of phenolic compounds from apple (procyanidins, flavan-3-ols, hydroxycinnamic acids, phloretin glucosides) help to prevent skin pigmentation caused by UV light [84]; while *p*-coumaric acid from *Asplenium australasicum* topical application can decrease skin melanization [85]; also, the combination of phenolic compounds and ginsenoside of Korean red ginseng not only reduce melasma and erythema levels but also improve their score in a melasma quality of life scale [86];

moreover, decrease in melanin index is observed after consumption of Oligometric proanthocyanidins from *Pinus maritima* bark and gallic acid, flavones, anthocyanins, punicalagin and other hydrolyzable tannins from *Polypodium leucotomos* with pomegranate; finally, topical application of piperine after narrowband UVB phototherapy, caused repigmentation in the patients treated [87].

Table 3. Clinical and observational studies of phytochemicals against skin pigmentary anomalies.

Plant/Fruit	Subjects	Treatment	Attributed Compound(s)	Effect	References
Malus domestica	59 healthy women. Mean age: 34.09 ± 4.41 years	300 or 600 mg/day, for 12 weeks	Procyanidins, flavan-3-ols, hydroxycinnamic acids, phloretin glucosides	Prevention of UV-induced skin pigmentation and inhibition of erythema formation	[84]
Asplenium australasicum water and ethanolic extract	46 healthy women. Age 18-40 years	Application of emulsion in forearm skin 2 times per day, for 4 weeks	*p*-coumaric acid	Decrease in skin melanization	[85]
Korean red ginseng powder	23 healthy women. Mean age: 43.2 years	3 g/day, for 24 weeks	Phenolic compounds, ginsenoside	Decrease in melasma and severity index, erythema levels, and level of pigmentation; improvement in melasma quality of life scale	[86]
Pinus maritima bark	112 healthy women with photodamaged skin. Age: <60 years	100 or 40 mg/day; for 18 months	Oligometric proanthocyanidins	Decrease in melanin index	[91]
Polypodium leucotomos with pomegranate	40 healthy subjects. Mean age: 37.2 ± 5.5 years	480 mg/day, for 3 months	Gallic acid, flavones, anthocyanins, punicalagin, and other hydrolyzable tannins	Decrease in melanin index	[92]
Piperine	63 subjects with facial vitiligo. Mean age: 35.8 ± 10.9 years	Application of treatment after phototherapy, for 3 months	-	Topical piperine with narrowband UVB caused re-pigmentation	[87]

(Table 3) cont.....

Plant/Fruit	Subjects	Treatment	Attributed Compound(s)	Effect	References
Zingiber officinale	31 healthy subjects. Mean age 44 ± 7 years.	Application of a cream twice per day, for 8 weeks.	Acetyl zingerone	Decrease in wrinkle severity. Improves photodamage, dyspigmentation and redness intensity	[93]
Prunus dulcis	91 postmenopausal females witch Fitzpatrick skin types I or II. Mean age 61.72 ± 8.76 years	Consumption of almond snack for 16-24 weeks.	Tocopherols, Vit. E,	Decrease the wrinkle severity, facial pigment was decreased 20%.	[94]

Topical treatment of *Nigella sativa* in which thymoquinone, saponins, and alkaloids have been identified, demonstrated in a clinical study repigmentation in 10 treated patients (p=.001), after 6 months of treatment [88]. Natural products such as a mixture of herbs from China, grape seeds, green tea extracts, coffee, mulberry, *Glycine max*, have shown in clinical trials significant improvements in terms of the degree of pigmentation, greater moisturization, and reduction in the diameter of the spots. Most of the compounds responsible for this activity are polyphenols, such as flavanols, flavan-3-ols, catechins, and phenolic acids, mainly due to their antioxidant and reactive oxygen species scavenging activity, can exert bioactivity, as well as some inhibit the tyrosinase [89].

A randomized, double-blind, during 12 weeks with 44 patients evaluated the topical application of a cream with bakuchiol 0.5% twice a day, obtaining favorable results in terms of the reduction of the area of the spots, being better tolerated than retinol [90].

CONCLUDING REMARKS

Natural products play an important role in both traditional medicine and pharmacology. Phenolic compounds are a large group of phytochemicals that can inhibit melanogenesis through different mechanisms, but the most common is by enzymatic inhibition, as the inhibition of tyrosinase activity. Also, natural products from plants have shown low toxicity, placing them as potential candidates for melanogenesis inhibitors. Thus, we encourage further studies on the pharmaceutical applications and safe use of natural products as biopharmaceutical treatments for skin pigmentary anomalies.

REFERENCES

[1]   Gehris RP. Dermatology. In: Za D, Ed. Zitelli and Davis' Atlas of Pediatric Physical Diagnosis. 7th ed. Elsevier 2018; p. 1032.

[2]   David J. Gawkrodger MRA-J Pigmentation Dermatology. 7th ed. Elsevier 2021; p. 184.

[3]   Lakhan MK, Lynch M. Skin pigmentation. Medicine (Abingdon) 2021; 49(7): 447-52.
[http://dx.doi.org/10.1016/j.mpmed.2021.04.010]

[4]   Patterson JW. Disorders of pigmentation Weedson's Skin Pathology. 5th ed. Elsevier 2021; p. 1320.

[5]   Rose PT. Pigmentary disorders. Med Clin North Am 2009; 93(6): 1225-39.
[http://dx.doi.org/10.1016/j.mcna.2009.08.005] [PMID: 19932328]

[6]   Rebat M. Halder ARH-M Pigmentary Disorders Conn's Current Therapy 2021. 1st ed. Elsevier 2020; p. 1536.

[7]   Dlova NC, Ollengo MA. Traditional and ethnobotanical dermatology practices in Africa. Clin Dermatol 2018; 36(3): 353-62.
[http://dx.doi.org/10.1016/j.clindermatol.2018.03.009] [PMID: 29908577]

[8]   Boo YC. *p*-coumaric acid as an active ingredient in cosmetics: a review focusing on its antimelanogenic effects. Antioxidants 2019; 8(8): 275.
[http://dx.doi.org/10.3390/antiox8080275] [PMID: 31382682]

[9]   Saeedi M, Eslamifar M, Khezri K. Kojic acid applications in cosmetic and pharmaceutical preparations. Biomed Pharmacother 2019; 110: 582-93.
[http://dx.doi.org/10.1016/j.biopha.2018.12.006] [PMID: 30537675]

[10]   Huang YC, Yang CH, Chiou YL. Citrus flavanone naringenin enhances melanogenesis through the activation of Wnt/β-catenin signalling in mouse melanoma cells. Phytomedicine 2011; 18(14): 1244-9.
[http://dx.doi.org/10.1016/j.phymed.2011.06.028] [PMID: 21802267]

[11]   Huo SX, Liu XM, Ge CH, *et al.* The effects of galangin on a mouse model of vitiligo induced by hydroquinone. Phytother Res 2014; 28(10): 1533-8.
[http://dx.doi.org/10.1002/ptr.5161] [PMID: 24820380]

[12]   Choo SJ, Ryoo IJ, Kim KC, *et al.* Hypo-pigmenting effect of sesquiterpenes from *Inula britannica* in B16 melanoma cells. Arch Pharm Res 2014; 37(5): 567-74.
[http://dx.doi.org/10.1007/s12272-013-0302-4] [PMID: 24346861]

[13]   Huang HC, Ho YC, Lim JM, Chang TY, Ho CL, Chang TM. Investigation of the anti-melanogenic and antioxidant characteristics of *Eucalyptus camaldulensis* flower essential oil and determination of its chemical composition. Int J Mol Sci 2015; 16(12): 10470-90.
[http://dx.doi.org/10.3390/ijms160510470] [PMID: 25961954]

[14]   Heriniaina RM, Dong J, Kalavagunta PK, Wu HL, Yan DS, Shang J. Effects of six compounds with different chemical structures on melanogenesis. Chin J Nat Med 2018; 16(10): 766-73.
[http://dx.doi.org/10.1016/S1875-5364(18)30116-X] [PMID: 30322610]

[15]   Liu Q, Hong J-H, Chen H-J, *et al.* Capsaicin reverses the inhibitory effect of licochalcone A/β-Arbutin on tyrosinase expression in b16 mouse melanoma cells. Pharmacogn Mag 2018; 14(53): 110-5.
[http://dx.doi.org/10.4103/pm.pm_103_17] [PMID: 29576710]

[16]   Kim AJ, Park JE, Cho YH, Lim DS, Lee JS. Effect of 7-Methylsulfinylheptyl Isothiocyanate on the Inhibition of Melanogenesis in B16-F1 Cells. Life (Basel) 2021; 11(2): 162.
[http://dx.doi.org/10.3390/life11020162] [PMID: 33672463]

[17]   Mukherjee PK, Biswas R, Sharma A, Banerjee S, Biswas S, Katiyar CK. Validation of medicinal herbs for anti-tyrosinase potential. J Herb Med 2018; 14: 1-16.
[http://dx.doi.org/10.1016/j.hermed.2018.09.002]

[18]   Sawant O, Khan T. Management of periorbital hyperpigmentation: an overview of nature-based agents

and alternative approaches. Dermatol Ther 2020; 33(4): e13717.
[http://dx.doi.org/10.1111/dth.13717] [PMID: 32472659]

[19]   Kim K, Huh Y, Lim KM. Anti-pigmentary natural compounds and their mode of action. Int J Mol Sci 2021; 22(12): 6206.
[http://dx.doi.org/10.3390/ijms22126206] [PMID: 34201391]

[20]   Pillaiyar T, Manickam M, Namasivayam V. Skin whitening agents: medicinal chemistry perspective of tyrosinase inhibitors. J Enzyme Inhib Med Chem 2017; 32(1): 403-25.
[http://dx.doi.org/10.1080/14756366.2016.1256882] [PMID: 28097901]

[21]   Wan P, Hu Y, He L. Regulation of melanocyte pivotal transcription factor MITF by some other transcription factors. Mol Cell Biochem 2011; 354(1-2): 241-6.
[http://dx.doi.org/10.1007/s11010-011-0823-4] [PMID: 21519923]

[22]   Bourhim T, Villareal MO, Couderc F, Hafidi A, Isoda H, Gadhi C. Melanogenesis promoting effect, antioxidant activity, and UPLC-ESI-HRMS characterization of phenolic compounds of *Argan* leaves extract. Molecules 2021; 26(2): 371.
[http://dx.doi.org/10.3390/molecules26020371] [PMID: 33445748]

[23]   Wu QY, Wong ZCF, Wang C, *et al.* Isoorientin derived from *Gentiana veitchiorum* Hemsl. flowers inhibits melanogenesis by down-regulating MITF-induced tyrosinase expression. Phytomedicine 2019; 57: 129-36.
[http://dx.doi.org/10.1016/j.phymed.2018.12.006] [PMID: 30668315]

[24]   Xu M, Lao QC, Zhao P, *et al.* 6′-*O*-Caffeoylarbutin inhibits melanogenesis in zebrafish. Nat Prod Res 2014; 28(12): 932-4.
[http://dx.doi.org/10.1080/14786419.2014.883395] [PMID: 24498931]

[25]   Oskoueian E, Karimi E, Noura R, Ebrahimi M, Shafaei N, Karimi E. Nanoliposomes encapsulation of enriched phenolic fraction from pistachio hulls and its antioxidant, anti-inflammatory, and anti-melanogenic activities. J Microencapsul 2020; 37(1): 1-13.
[http://dx.doi.org/10.1080/02652048.2019.1692941] [PMID: 31714165]

[26]   Jung SH, Kim J, Eum J, *et al.* Velutin, an aglycone extracted from korean mistletoe, with improved inhibitory activity against melanin biosynthesis. Molecules 2019; 24(14): 2549.
[http://dx.doi.org/10.3390/molecules24142549] [PMID: 31336931]

[27]   Taddeo V, Epifano F, Preziuso F, *et al.* HPLC analysis and skin whitening effects of umbelliprenin-containing extracts of *Anethum graveolens*, *Pimpinella anisum*, and *Ferulago campestris*. Molecules 2019; 24(3): 501.
[http://dx.doi.org/10.3390/molecules24030501] [PMID: 30704124]

[28]   Sato Y, Uchida E, Aoki H, *et al.* Acerola (*Malpighia emarginata* DC.) juice intake suppresses UVB-induced skin pigmentation in SMP30/GNL knockout hairless mice. PLoS One 2017; 12(1): e0170438.
[http://dx.doi.org/10.1371/journal.pone.0170438] [PMID: 28114343]

[29]   Kim J, Kang YG, Choi D, *et al.* The natural phytochemical trans-communic acid inhibits cellular senescence and pigmentation through FoxO3a activation. Exp Dermatol 2019; 28(11): 1270-8.
[http://dx.doi.org/10.1111/exd.14025] [PMID: 31461579]

[30]   Chao HC, Najjaa H, Villareal MO, *et al.* *Arthrophytum scoparium* inhibits melanogenesis through the down-regulation of tyrosinase and melanogenic gene expressions in B16 melanoma cells. Exp Dermatol 2013; 22(2): 131-6.
[http://dx.doi.org/10.1111/exd.12089] [PMID: 23362872]

[31]   Choi MH, Jo HG, Yang J, Ki S, Shin HJ. Antioxidative and Anti-Melanogenic Activities of Bamboo Stems (*Phyllostachys nigra* variety *henosis*) *via* PKA/CREB-Mediated MITF Downregulation in B16F10 Melanoma Cells. Int J Mol Sci 2018; 19(2): 409.
[http://dx.doi.org/10.3390/ijms19020409] [PMID: 29385729]

[32]   Huang YC, Liu KC, Chiou YL. Melanogenesis of murine melanoma cells induced by hesperetin, a

Citrus hydrolysate-derived flavonoid. Food Chem Toxicol 2012; 50(3-4): 653-9.
[http://dx.doi.org/10.1016/j.fct.2012.01.012] [PMID: 22266363]

[33]   Jegal J, Park S, Chung K, *et al.* Tyrosinase inhibitory flavonoid from *Juniperus communis* fruits. Biosci Biotechnol Biochem 2016; 80(12): 2311-7.
[http://dx.doi.org/10.1080/09168451.2016.1217146] [PMID: 27492585]

[34]   Kang S, Choi B, Lee E, *et al.* Inhibitory Effect of Dried Pomegranate Concentration Powder on Melanogenesis in B16F10 Melanoma Cells; Involvement of p38 and PKA Signaling Pathways. Int J Mol Sci 2015; 16(10): 24219-42.
[http://dx.doi.org/10.3390/ijms161024219] [PMID: 26473849]

[35]   Kim M, Shin S, Lee JA, Park D, Lee J, Jung E. Inhibition of melanogenesis by *Gaillardia aristata* flower extract. BMC Complement Altern Med 2015; 15(1): 449.
[http://dx.doi.org/10.1186/s12906-015-0972-1] [PMID: 26702819]

[36]   Kim HJ, Yonezawa T, Teruya T, Woo JT, Cha BY. Nobiletin, a polymethoxy flavonoid, reduced endothelin-1 plus SCF-induced pigmentation in human melanocytes. Photochem Photobiol 2015; 91(2): 379-86.
[http://dx.doi.org/10.1111/php.12400] [PMID: 25488359]

[37]   Kudo M, Kobayashi-Nakamura K, Tsuji-Naito K. Bifunctional effects of O-methylated flavones from *Scutellaria baicalensis* Georgi on melanocytes: Inhibition of melanin production and intracellular melanosome transport. PLoS One 2017; 12(2): e0171513.
[http://dx.doi.org/10.1371/journal.pone.0171513] [PMID: 28182699]

[38]   Liu J, Xu X, Jiang R, Sun L, Zhao D. Vanillic acid in *Panax ginseng* root extract inhibits melanogenesis in B16F10 cells *via* inhibition of the NO/PKG signaling pathway. Biosci Biotechnol Biochem 2019; 83(7): 1205-15.
[http://dx.doi.org/10.1080/09168451.2019.1606694] [PMID: 30999826]

[39]   Moon KM, Hwang YH, Yang JH, Ma JY, Lee B. Spinosin is a flavonoid in the seed of *Ziziphus jujuba* that prevents skin pigmentation in a human skin model. J Funct Foods 2019; 54: 449-56.
[http://dx.doi.org/10.1016/j.jff.2019.01.044]

[40]   Sarikurkcu C, Kakouri E, Sarikurkcu RT, Tarantilis PA. Study on the chemical composition, enzyme inhibition and antioxidant activity of *Ziziphora taurica* subsp. *cleonioides.* Appl Sci (Basel) 2019; 9(24): 5515.
[http://dx.doi.org/10.3390/app9245515]

[41]   Smeriglio A, D'Angelo V, Denaro M, Trombetta D, Raimondo FM, Germanò MP. Polyphenol characterization, antioxidant and skin whitening properties of *Alnus cordata* stem bark. Chem Biodivers 2019; 16(9): e1900314.
[http://dx.doi.org/10.1002/cbdv.201900314] [PMID: 31397975]

[42]   Tuerxuntayi A, Liu Y, Tulake A, Kabas M, Eblimit A, Aisa HA. Kaliziri extract upregulates tyrosinase, TRP-1, TRP-2 and MITF expression in murine B16 melanoma cells. BMC Complement Altern Med 2014; 14(1): 166.
[http://dx.doi.org/10.1186/1472-6882-14-166] [PMID: 24884952]

[43]   Park S, Jegal J, Chung KW, *et al.* Isolation of tyrosinase and melanogenesis inhibitory flavonoids from *Juniperus chinensis* fruits. Biosci Biotechnol Biochem 2018; 82(12): 2041-8.
[http://dx.doi.org/10.1080/09168451.2018.1511367] [PMID: 30130471]

[44]   Hwang JM, Kuo HC, Lin CT, Kao ES. Inhibitory effect of liposome-encapsulated anthocyanin on melanogenesis in human melanocytes. Pharm Biol 2013; 51(8): 941-7.
[http://dx.doi.org/10.3109/13880209.2013.771376] [PMID: 23570521]

[45]   Horibe I, Satoh Y, Shiota Y, *et al.* Induction of melanogenesis by 4'-O-methylated flavonoids in B16F10 melanoma cells. J Nat Med 2013; 67(4): 705-10.
[http://dx.doi.org/10.1007/s11418-012-0727-y] [PMID: 23208771]

[46]   Jung E, Kim JH, Kim MO, Lee SY, Lee J. Melanocyte-protective effect of afzelin is mediated by the Nrf2-ARE signalling pathway *via* GSK-3β inactivation. Exp Dermatol 2017; 26(9): 764-70.
        [http://dx.doi.org/10.1111/exd.13277] [PMID: 27992083]

[47]   Kumar KJS, Vani MG, Wang SY, *et al*. *In vitro* and *in vivo* studies disclosed the depigmenting effects of gallic acid: A novel skin lightening agent for hyperpigmentary skin diseases. Biofactors 2013; 39(3): 259-70.
        [http://dx.doi.org/10.1002/biof.1064] [PMID: 23322673]

[48]   Lee B, Moon KM, Lee BS, *et al*. Swertiajaponin inhibits skin pigmentation by dual mechanisms to suppress tyrosinase. Oncotarget 2017; 8(56): 95530-41.
        [http://dx.doi.org/10.18632/oncotarget.20913] [PMID: 29221146]

[49]   Li HR, Habasi M, Xie LZ, Aisa H. Effect of chlorogenic acid on melanogenesis of B16 melanoma cells. Molecules 2014; 19(9): 12940-8.
        [http://dx.doi.org/10.3390/molecules190912940] [PMID: 25157464]

[50]   Lv J, Fu Y, Cao Y, *et al*. Isoliquiritigenin inhibits melanogenesis, melanocyte dendricity and melanosome transport by regulating ERK-mediated MITF degradation. Exp Dermatol 2020; 29(2): 149-57.
        [http://dx.doi.org/10.1111/exd.14066] [PMID: 31785162]

[51]   Ma J, Li S, Zhu L, *et al*. Baicalein protects human vitiligo melanocytes from oxidative stress through activation of NF-E2-related factor2 (Nrf2) signaling pathway. Free Radic Biol Med 2018; 129: 492-503.
        [http://dx.doi.org/10.1016/j.freeradbiomed.2018.10.421] [PMID: 30342186]

[52]   Park J, Park JH, Suh HJ, Lee IC, Koh J, Boo YC. Effects of resveratrol, oxyresveratrol, and their acetylated derivatives on cellular melanogenesis. Arch Dermatol Res 2014; 306(5): 475-87.
        [http://dx.doi.org/10.1007/s00403-014-1440-3] [PMID: 24414332]

[53]   Peng LH, Xu SY, Shan YH, *et al*. Sequential release of salidroside and paeonol from a nanosphere-hydrogel system inhibits ultraviolet B-induced melanogenesis in guinea pig skin. Int J Nanomedicine 2014; 9: 1897-908.
        [http://dx.doi.org/10.2147/IJN.S59290] [PMID: 24790432]

[54]   Usach I, Taléns-Visconti R, Magraner-Pardo L, Peris JE. Hesperetin induces melanin production in adult human epidermal melanocytes. Food Chem Toxicol 2015; 80: 80-4.
        [http://dx.doi.org/10.1016/j.fct.2015.02.017] [PMID: 25765751]

[55]   Yang HL, Lin CP, Vudhya Gowrisankar Y, *et al*. The anti-melanogenic effects of ellagic acid through induction of autophagy in melanocytes and suppression of UVA-activated α-MSH pathways *via* Nrf2 activation in keratinocytes. Biochem Pharmacol 2021; 185: 114454.
        [http://dx.doi.org/10.1016/j.bcp.2021.114454] [PMID: 33545118]

[56]   Zhou Z, Hou J, Xiong J, Li M. Characterization of sulfuretin as a depigmenting agent. Fundam Clin Pharmacol 2019; 33(2): 208-15.
        [http://dx.doi.org/10.1111/fcp.12414] [PMID: 30216535]

[57]   Bajpai VK, Kang SC. A diterpenoid sugiol from *Metasequoia glyptostroboides* with α-glucosidase and tyrosinase inhibitory potential. Bangladesh J Pharmacol 2014; 9(3)
        [http://dx.doi.org/10.3329/bjp.v9i3.19026]

[58]   Suganya P, Jeyaprakash K, Mallavarapu GR, Murugan R. Comparison of the chemical composition, tyrosinase inhibitory and anti-inflammatory activities of the essential oils of *Pogostemon plectranthoides* from India. Ind Crops Prod 2015; 69: 300-7.
        [http://dx.doi.org/10.1016/j.indcrop.2015.02.045]

[59]   Tsai ML, Lin CD, Khoo K, *et al*. Composition and bioactivity of essential oil from *Citrus grandis* (L.) Osbeck 'mato peiyu' leaf. Molecules 2017; 22(12): 2154.
        [http://dx.doi.org/10.3390/molecules22122154] [PMID: 29206180]

[60] de S Vargas F, D O de Almeida P, Aranha ES, *et al.* Biological activities and cytotoxicity of diterpenes from *Copaifera* spp. Oleoresins. Molecules 2015; 20(4): 6194-210.
[http://dx.doi.org/10.3390/molecules20046194] [PMID: 25859778]

[61] Jeon NJ, Kim YS, Kim EK, *et al.* Inhibitory effect of carvacrol on melanin synthesis *via* suppression of tyrosinase expression. J Funct Foods 2018; 45: 199-205.
[http://dx.doi.org/10.1016/j.jff.2018.03.043]

[62] Park S, Choi E, Kim S, *et al.* Oxidative stress-protective and anti-melanogenic effects of loliolide and ethanol extract from fresh water green algae, *Prasiola japonica.* Int J Mol Sci 2018; 19(9): 2825.
[http://dx.doi.org/10.3390/ijms19092825] [PMID: 30231594]

[63] Lu L, Wang S, Fu L, Liu D, Zhu Y, Xu A. Bilobalide protection of normal human melanocytes from hydrogen peroxide-induced oxidative damage *via* promotion of antioxidase expression and inhibition of endoplasmic reticulum stress. Clin Exp Dermatol 2016; 41(1): 64-73.
[http://dx.doi.org/10.1111/ced.12664] [PMID: 26178968]

[64] Zhao Z, Ma S, Dong X. Anti-melanogenesis efficacy of ginkgolide B is favored by attenuating oxidative stress and melanin synthesis in B16F1 melanoma cell model. Int J Pharmacol 2019; 15(5): 560-6.
[http://dx.doi.org/10.3923/ijp.2019.560.566]

[65] Fiocco D, Arciuli M, Arena MP, Benvenuti S, Gallone A. Chemical composition and the anti-melanogenic potential of different essential oils. Flavour Fragrance J 2016; 31(3): 255-61.
[http://dx.doi.org/10.1002/ffj.3315]

[66] Kim SC, Lee JH, Kim MH, *et al.* Hordenine, a single compound produced during barley germination, inhibits melanogenesis in human melanocytes. Food Chem 2013; 141(1): 174-81.
[http://dx.doi.org/10.1016/j.foodchem.2013.03.017] [PMID: 23768344]

[67] Biswas R, Mukherjee PK, Chaudhary SK. Tyrosinase inhibition kinetic studies of standardized extract of *Berberis aristata.* Nat Prod Res 2016; 30(12): 1451-4.
[http://dx.doi.org/10.1080/14786419.2015.1062376] [PMID: 26212353]

[68] Dulić M, Ciganović P, Vujić L, Zovko Končić M. Antidiabetic and cosmeceutical potential of common barbery *(Berberis vulgaris L.)* root bark extracts obtained by optimization of 'green' ultrasound-assisted extraction. Molecules 2019; 24(19): 3613.
[http://dx.doi.org/10.3390/molecules24193613] [PMID: 31597237]

[69] Hashim NA, Ahmad F, Salleh WMNHW, Khamis S. Phytochemicals and tyrosinase inhibitory activity from *Piper caninum* and *Piper magnibaccum.* Ulum-i Daruyi 2019; 25(4): 358-63.
[http://dx.doi.org/10.15171/PS.2019.47]

[70] Jiang W, Li S, Chen X, *et al.* Berberine protects immortalized line of human melanocytes from H_2O_2-induced oxidative stress *via* activation of Nrf2 and Mitf signaling pathway. J Dermatol Sci 2019; 94(1): 236-43.
[http://dx.doi.org/10.1016/j.jdermsci.2019.03.007] [PMID: 30987854]

[71] Song YC, Lee Y, Kim HM, *et al.* Berberine regulates melanin synthesis by activating PI3K/AKT, ERK and GSK3β in B16F10 melanoma cells. Int J Mol Med 2015; 35(4): 1011-6.
[http://dx.doi.org/10.3892/ijmm.2015.2113] [PMID: 25716948]

[72] Kashif M, Akhtar N, Mustafa R. An overview of dermatological and cosmeceutical benefits of *Diospyros kaki* and its phytoconstituents. Rev Bras Farmacogn 2017; 27(5): 650-62.
[http://dx.doi.org/10.1016/j.bjp.2017.06.004]

[73] Espinosa-González AM, Estrella-Parra EA, Nolasco-Ontiveros E, *et al. Hyptis mociniana*: phytochemical fingerprint and photochemoprotective effect against UV-B radiation-induced erythema and skin carcinogenesis. Food Chem Toxicol 2021; 151: 112095.
[http://dx.doi.org/10.1016/j.fct.2021.112095] [PMID: 33689855]

[74] Ersoy E, Eroglu Ozkan E, Boga M, Yilmaz MA, Mat A. Anti-aging potential and anti-tyrosinase

activity of three *Hypericum* species with focus on phytochemical composition by LC–MS/MS. Ind Crops Prod 2019; 141: 111735.
[http://dx.doi.org/10.1016/j.indcrop.2019.111735]

[75]   Radwan RA, El-Sherif YA, Salama MM. A novel biochemical study of anti-ageing potential of eucalyptus camaldulensis bark waste standardized extract and silver nanoparticles. Colloids Surf B Biointerfaces 2020; 191: 111004.
[http://dx.doi.org/10.1016/j.colsurfb.2020.111004] [PMID: 32335357]

[76]   Jegal J, Park NJ, Park S, *et al.* Juniperus chinensis fruits attenuate oxazolone- and 2, 4-dinitrochlorobenzene-induced atopic dermatitis symptoms in mice. Biol Pharm Bull 2018; 41(2): 259-65.
[http://dx.doi.org/10.1248/bpb.b17-00818] [PMID: 29386485]

[77]   Woo SY, Wong CP, Win NN, *et al.* Anti-melanin deposition activity and active constituents of *Jatropha multifida* stems. J Nat Med 2019; 73(4): 805-13.
[http://dx.doi.org/10.1007/s11418-019-01314-7] [PMID: 31055728]

[78]   Won YK, Loy CJ, Randhawa M, Southall MD. Clinical efficacy and safety of 4-hexyl-1-3-phenylenediol for improving skin hyperpigmentation. Arch Dermatol Res 2014; 306(5): 455-65.
[http://dx.doi.org/10.1007/s00403-014-1439-9] [PMID: 24402285]

[79]   Roh E, Yun CY, Lee J, *et al.* Hypopigmenting activity of bisabolangelone isolated from *Angelica koreana* Maxim. in α-melanocyte stimulating hormone-activated B16 or melan-a cells. Planta Med 2011; 77(3): 248-51.
[http://dx.doi.org/10.1055/s-0030-1250285] [PMID: 20814852]

[80]   Thanitsara S, Benjamart P, Warachin G, Jarinyaporn N. *Azadirachta indica* (Neem) water leaf extract inhibits melanin production and tyrosinase activity in B16F10 melanoma cells. Pharmacogn J 2021; 13(4)

[81]   Yuan WJ, Gao WF, Zhao JY, *et al.* Diterpenes with potential treatment of vitiligo from the aerials parts of *Euphorbia antiquorum* L. Fitoterapia 2020; 144: 104583.
[http://dx.doi.org/10.1016/j.fitote.2020.104583] [PMID: 32234374]

[82]   Bungau S, Vesa CM, Abid A, *et al.* Withaferin a—a promising phytochemical compound with multiple results in dermatological diseases. Molecules 2021; 26(9): 2407.
[http://dx.doi.org/10.3390/molecules26092407] [PMID: 33919088]

[83]   Kanlayavattanakul M, Lourith N. Skin hyperpigmentation treatment using herbs: A review of clinical evidences. J Cosmet Laser Ther 2018; 20(2): 123-31.
[http://dx.doi.org/10.1080/14764172.2017.1368666] [PMID: 28853960]

[84]   Shoji T, Masumoto S, Moriichi N, Ohtake Y, Kanda T. Administration of apple polyphenol supplements for skin conditions in healthy women: a randomized, double-blind, placebo-controlled clinical trial. Nutrients 2020; 12(4): 1071.
[http://dx.doi.org/10.3390/nu12041071] [PMID: 32294883]

[85]   Zeng WW, Lai LS. Anti-melanization effects and inhibitory kinetics of tyrosinase of bird's nest fern (*Asplenium australasicum*) frond extracts on melanoma and human skin. J Biosci Bioeng 2019; 127(6): 738-43.
[http://dx.doi.org/10.1016/j.jbiosc.2018.11.005] [PMID: 30639118]

[86]   Song M, Mun JH, Ko HC, Kim BS, Kim MB. Korean red ginseng powder in the treatment of melasma: an uncontrolled observational study. J Ginseng Res 2011; 35(2): 170-5.
[http://dx.doi.org/10.5142/jgr.2011.35.2.170] [PMID: 23717059]

[87]   Shafiee A, Hoormand M, Shahidi-Dadras M, Abadi A. The effect of topical piperine combined with narrowband UVB on vitiligo treatment: A clinical trial study. Phytother Res 2018; 32(9): 1812-7.
[http://dx.doi.org/10.1002/ptr.6116] [PMID: 29781089]

[88]   Sarac G, Kapicioglu Y, Sener S, *et al.* Effectiveness of topical *Nigella sativa* for vitiligo treatment.

Dermatol Ther 2019; 32(4): e12949.
[http://dx.doi.org/10.1111/dth.12949] [PMID: 31025474]

[89]   Fisk WA, Agbai O, Lev-Tov HA, Sivamani RK. The use of botanically derived agents for hyperpigmentation: A systematic review. J Am Acad Dermatol 2014; 70(2): 352-65.
[http://dx.doi.org/10.1016/j.jaad.2013.09.048] [PMID: 24280646]

[90]   Dhaliwal S, Rybak I, Ellis SR, *et al.* Prospective, randomized, double-blind assessment of topical bakuchiol and retinol for facial photoageing. Br J Dermatol 2019; 180(2): 289-96.
[http://dx.doi.org/10.1111/bjd.16918] [PMID: 29947134]

[91]   Furumura M, Sato N, Kusaba N, Takagaki K, Nakayama J. Oral administration of French maritime pine bark extract (Flavangenol®) improves clinical symptoms in photoaged facial skin. Clin Interv Aging 2012; 7: 275-86.
[http://dx.doi.org/10.2147/CIA.S33165] [PMID: 22956863]

[92]   Emanuele E, Bertona M, Biagi M. Comparative effects of a fixed *Polypodium leucotomos*/Pomegranate combination *versus* Polypodium leucotomos alone on skin biophysical parameters. Neuroendocrinol Lett 2017; 38(1): 38-42.
[PMID: 28456146]

[93]   Dhaliwal S, Rybak I, Pourang A, *et al.* Randomized double-blind vehicle controlled study of the effects of topical acetyl zingerone on photoaging. J Cosmet Dermatol 2021; 20(1): 166-73.
[http://dx.doi.org/10.1111/jocd.13464] [PMID: 32369655]

[94]   Rybak I, Carrington AE, Dhaliwal S, *et al.* Prospective randomized controlled trial on the effects of almonds on facial wrinkles and pigmentation. Nutrients 2021; 13(3): 785.
[http://dx.doi.org/10.3390/nu13030785] [PMID: 33673587]

CHAPTER 5

Treatment of Scabies with Herbal Medicines

Om Prakash[1,*], **Priyanka Bajpai**[1], **Shazia Usmani**[2], **Ruchi Singh**[3], **Amita Pandey**[2], **Rajesh Kumar**[4] and **Nadeem Rais**[5]

[1] *Goel Institute of Pharmacy and Sciences, Ayodhya (Faizabad) Road, Lucknow, Uttar Pradesh, 226 028, India*

[2] *Herbal Bioactive Research Lab Faculty of Pharmacy, Integral University, Dasauli, Kursi Road, Lucknow, Uttar Pradesh, 226 026, India*

[3] *Goel Institute of Pharmaceutical and Sciences, Ayodhya (Faizabad) Road, Lucknow, Uttar Pradesh, 226 028, India*

[4] *Narayan Institute of Pharmacy, Gopal Narayan Singh University, Jamuhar, Sasaram, Bihar, 821 305, India*

[5] *Department of Pharmacy, Bhagwant University, Ajmer, Rajasthan, 305 004, India*

Abstract: Scabies is a chronic and serious community disorder caused by a parasite commonly known as a mite *(Sarcoptes scabiei var hominis)*. The long-term infection may lead to chronic complications such as septicemia, acute post-streptococcal glomerulonephritis, heart disease, and secondary infections. The majority of novel medicinal agents from various plant sources are responsible for the management and treatment of several types of chronic disorders. The safe and cost-effective alternative treatment strategy is the use of medicinal plants that plays a potential role against a variety of diseases due to the presence of numerous types of active phytochemicals with no or negligible adverse effect. This study gives a unique summary, including a correlation between traditional medicinal plants and their derived active phytochemicals for the significant treatment of scabies. The literature search was carried out *via* search engines through different databases, including Google Scholar, PubMed, Medline, ScienceDirect, *etc.* A large number of medicinal plants and their active medicinal agents have been reviewed with remarkable therapeutic effects against scabies. There are some limitations due to insufficient data related to limited pre-clinical and clinical trials in this particular area. This review provides a baseline to explore the therapeutic potential of these medicinal plants against skin diseases, especially scabies. However, extensive studies are required to identify, authenticate, and characterize the bioactive compounds present in these plants, which may lead to value addition in pharmaceutical industries by providing a cost-effective way of treatment with minimal side effects.

* **Corresponding author Om Prakash:** Goel Institute of Pharmacy and Sciences Ayodhya (Faizabad) Road, Lucknow, Uttar Pradesh, India; Tel: +91-9412573776; E-mail: opverma2007@gmail.com

Heba Abd El-Sattar El-Nashar, Mohamed El-Shazly & Nouran Mohammed Fahmy (Eds.)
All rights reserved-© 2023 Bentham Science Publishers

Keywords: Burrows, Clinical Study, Epidemiology, Future Prospective, Herbal Medicines, Mites, Natural Products, Skin diseases, Scabies, *Sarcoptes scabiei var hominis*, Therapeutic Agents, Transmission, World Health Organization.

INTRODUCTION

Human scabies (also known as seven-year itch) is a highly contagious and itchy ectoparasitic skin infestation caused by microscopic scabies mites - *Sarcoptes scabiei var. hominis* and it is a public health concern in all countries, regardless of socioeconomic class [1, 2]. The scabies mite tunnels into the epidermis and lays eggs, provoking an immunological reaction in the host that results in severe itching and a rash. Scabies mites can live for up to two months on a human. Scabies mites rarely live longer than 48-72 hours outside a human. If scabies mites are exposed to a temperature of 50°C (122°F) for 10 minutes, they will die. Scabies infestation can be worsened by bacterial infection, resulting in skin sores that can lead to more serious complications such as septicemia, cardiovascular disease, and chronic renal disease. With respect to the Individual Countries' requests and the Council's suggestions, by the World Health Organization (WHO)- Strategic and Technical Advisory Group (STAG), scabies and other ectoparasites were added to the list of Neglected Tropical Diseases (NTDs) in 2017. In March 2018, the WHO NTDs Worldwide Working Group on Monitoring and Evaluation suggested that a global scabies burden be determined, diagnostic criteria are developed and, interim guidelines for public health interventions be issued (Table **1**) [3, 4].

Table 1. What exactly is scabies?

• Scabies is a skin rash caused by tiny bugs called mites.
• *Sarcoptes scabiei var. hominis* is the parasitic mite that causes human scabies.
• To lay eggs and the mite penetrates the skin.
• Scabies burrows beneath the skin and causes itching & tiny red lumps.
• Physical contact is an easy way for the mites to spread to other people.
• Scabies can also be contracted by touching scabies-infected towels, beds, or clothing.
• The rash is quite itchy to the point of being infuriating.

Scabies Epidemiology

Scabies is among the most frequent dermatological disorders, popular for a large percentage of skin illnesses in underdeveloped nations. It is appraised that it affects greater than 200 million individuals worldwide at any given moment, while additional research is required to quantify the current burden. In current scabies-associated work, prevalence estimates covered from 0.2 percent to 71 percent. Throughout many tropical regions with insufficient resources, scabies is prevalent, with a 5–10% proportion among youngsters. Scabies infestation and its possible consequences put a significant financial burden on healthcare systems [5]. Cases are infrequent in high-income economies, but outbreaks in health facilities and vulnerable groups cost national health services a lot of money. Scabies is found all over the world. Little youngsters in places with limited resources are among the most exposed to scabies and their related issues. Infestation rates are much higher in hot, tropical countries, especially where there is a high prevalence of overpopulation and poverty and when access to treatment is constrained (Table **2**) [6].

Table 2. Scabies epidemiology.

• At every given time, 2 billion people globally are thought to be affected by scabies.
• Scabies affects 5-10 percent of youngsters in resource-limited regions.
• Scabies can affect people of all ages and socioeconomic backgrounds.
• Scabies is present throughout the world, but it is much more prevalent in warm, tropical nations and densely populated locations.
• Scabies outbreaks are common in places like nursing homes, extended-care facilities, and jails.

Symptoms

The mature female of the scabies mite burrows into the epidermis' top layer, where it lays eggs. In 3–4 days, the eggs hatch, and in 1–2 weeks, the adult mites emerge. After 4–6 weeks, the patient develops an allergic reaction to mite proteins and feces found in the scabies burrow, resulting in severe itching and redness. The majority of people are afflicted with 10–15 mites (Table **3**). Mostly in finger webs, wrists, upper and lower limbs, and waistline region, there is frequently intense itching, linear burrows, as well as vesicles [7, 8].

Table 3. How can you know if you have scabies?

• The itching gets progressively worse over time, especially at night.
• A rash of tiny red lumps that occasionally appear in a line.
• The lumps are most commonly found on the fingers, wrists, and arms, but they can appear anywhere on the body (except on the face of an adult).
• The rash can also appear on the cheeks, scalp (particularly behind the ears), palms of the hands, and soles of the feet in babies.
• The rash may be extremely minor in older people, making it difficult to see.
• Scabies can spread all over a person's body if he or she has HIV.

In infants and young children, a much more widespread rash may cover the palms, soles of the feet, ankles, and occasionally the scalp. Inflammatory scabies nodules can be found on adult males' penis and scrotums, as well as around females' breasts. Burrows could be seen in close contacts who still haven't displayed itching due to the time lag between infection and onset of symptoms. People with crusted scabies have thick, peeling crusts that can be found all over the body, including the face. Symptoms may take 4-8 weeks to appear if a person has never had scabies previously. It's crucial to note that even if one doesn't have symptoms, an infected individual might spread scabies during this period. Symptoms normally occur significantly sooner (1-4 days) in a person who has previously had scabies [9].

Burrows

Female scabies mites could be seen digging just below the skin's surface, causing microscopic tunnels to be seen on the body. Burrows seems on the skin surface as arched and curved (serpiginous) grayish-white or skin-colored threads. These burrows can be difficult to discover because mites are usually small in number (about 10-15 per individual). The penis, breast, or upper arms are the most typical places to find them, along with the folds of skin on the forearm, elbow, or knee, as well as between fingers. The burrow is a scabies diagnostic indication. The egg-laying female produces an intraepidermal path that is usually less than a centimeter long. The burrow's opening may have a modest scale, while the female is confined in the blind end. Most adult humans have burrows on their hands or wrists, while children frequently have burrows on their feet [10]. Burrows can be found in a variety of places (Fig. **1**).

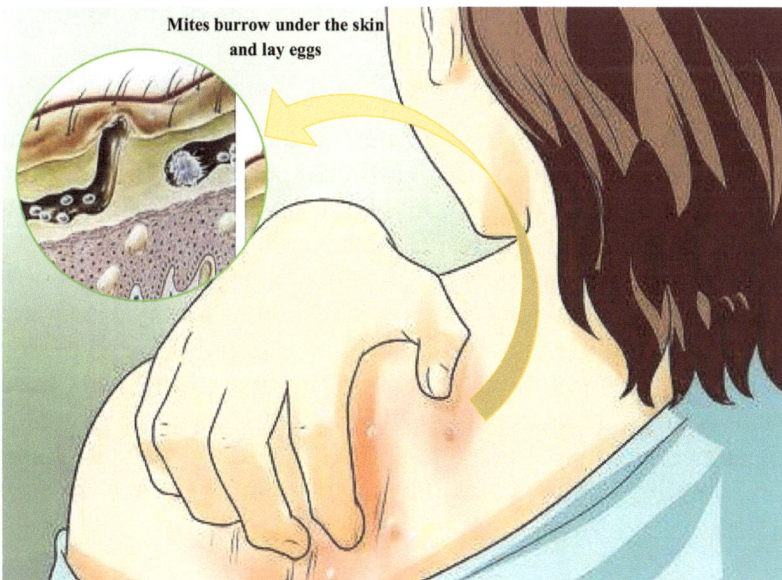

Fig. (1). Mites burrow under the skin and lay eggs.

Anatomy of the Scabies Mite

The scabies mite is an ectoparasitic arthropod with eight legs that is hardly visible to the human eye. The adult female mite is between 0.3 and 0.5 mm in length. The female mite has an oblong body with two pairs of anterior and posterior legs, which are fat on the under-side and convex on the upper side, respectively. The anterior legs end in long, unjointed stalks called 'suckers,' whereas the posterior legs end in long bristles. The eggs are laid through the tocostome, which is a slit in the middle of the female mite's ventral surface. Male mites are smaller and have a genital apparatus on the outside [11].

Biology of the Scabies Mite

A mite's life cycle is divided into three stages: egg, nymph, and larva. Larvae hatch two to four days after the eggs are laid, and the full development life cycle takes around 15 days from egg to adult mite. Adult female mites use their front legs and mouth to burrow into the epidermis of human skin, which takes around 15–30 minutes. Adult females survive for four to six weeks and lay four eggs every day in the burrowed cave. She leaves behind empty shells, as well as mite excretory and secretory materials, in addition to her eggs. When the larvae hatch from the eggs, they emerge from their burrow, reach the skin's surface, and seek food and shelter in hair follicles. Experiments on mite reproduction revealed that the largest numbers of mites in an infected host were discovered between 80 and 115 days after infestation, with a maximum parasite rate of 50 to 380 mites [9].

Transmission

Scabies is mainly transmitted person-to-person through close skin contact (*e.g.*, residing in the same household) with an afflicted person. The risk of transmission increases with the degree of infestations, with the highest risk owing to contact with individuals with crusted scabies. Contact with infested personal goods (*e.g.*, clothes and bed linens) is unlikely to transmit common scabies, but it may be significant for those with crusted scabies. Since there is an asymptomatic phase of infestation, the transmission may occur before the initial infested person exhibits symptoms. As a scabies mite takes 15 to 20 minutes to infect its host, holding hands, sexual contact, breastfeeding, and nursing newborns are all high-risk behaviors if someone comes into touch with an infected person. As a result of these factors, family members are the most common source of transmission (Table **4**) [10].

Human scabies is not spread by animals. An epidermal barrier breach brought on by scratching and the body's reaction to it can result in secondary bacterial skin infections , which are most frequently brought on by *Streptococcus pyogenes* as well as *Staphylococcus aureus*. A kind of surface bacterial skin disease known as impetigo has the potential to worsen and cause immune-mediated issues with vital organs, including the kidney and heart. A distinct type of scabies mite can infect pets, one that does not live or reproduce in people but produces "mange" in animals. If a person comes into close contact with an animal that has "mange," the animal mite can enter under the person's skin and produce brief itching and irritation [11].

Table 4. How can scabies be prevented from spreading?

Mites can quickly travel from person to person, and in some cases, to everyone in your home. To prevent the spread of scabies: • Consult a doctor as soon as any symptoms are noticed.   • Scabies can only be kept at bay by avoiding lengthy, close, and skin-to-skin contact with an infected person.   • Also, until infected patients have completed treatment, avoid touching or sharing clothes, mattresses, or towels with them.   • It's advised to hold off on having sex until the affected partner has finished treatment.   *Also, if someone has mites on clothing, towels, or bedding, use one of the following methods to kill them:*   • All clothing should be washed in hot, soapy water and then dried on high heat.   • Items that cannot be washed at home should be dry cleaned professionally.   • Stowaway non-washable things, such as stuffed animals and upholstery, in a sealed plastic bag for at least 72 hours so that the mites die.   • Throw away the vacuum cleaner bag after cleaning and vacuuming each room in the house.

Crusted (Norwegian) Scabies

Crusted, or Norwegian, scabies is one of the chronic types of scabies that affects immunocompromised, old, crippled, or debilitated people. Itching and redness are classic indications and indicators of scabies that may not appear in people with crusted scabies (pruritus). These patients have thick skin crusts that are packed with scabies mites and eggs. Crusted scabies mites are not more virulent than non-crusted scabies mites, although they are far more numerous (up to 2 million per patient). People with crusted scabies are extremely contagious to others because they are afflicted with so many mites. Persons with crusted scabies can transmit scabies indirectly by shedding mites that contaminate items such as their clothing, bedding, and furniture, in addition to direct skin-to-skin contact. To avoid scabies epidemics, those with crusted scabies should undergo prompt and aggressive medical treatment for their infestation. If left untreated, this illness has a high death rate due to secondary sepsis [12].

Diagnosis

There are still no standardized scientific assays known for the detection of scabies. There have been several candidate antigens and antibody immunoassays studied, but their performance has been unsatisfactory, and none have been widely accepted. Formerly, scabies infestations were detected using traditional PCR targeting on *Sarcoptes scabiei* mitochondrial cytochrome c oxidase subunit 1 (cox1) genome; nevertheless, the confirmed identification frequency was too low to provide reliable results [13]. In most cases, healthcare providers diagnose scabies in their clinics. The diagnosis can sometimes, but not always, be confirmed by looking at skin scrapings under a microscope, although this takes time and can be traumatic for youngsters. The use of a dermatoscope, a hand-held magnifier, may be beneficial; however, dermatoscopes are expensive and not widely available in resource-poor places. Other diagnostic aids in development include low-cost magnification and a quick antigen detection testing procedure [14]. Identifying the mite, mite eggs, or feces (scybala) should be done whenever possible to confirm the diagnosis of scabies. This can be done by carefully removing the mites first from the end of the burrow with the top of a syringe, or by getting a skin scrape to look at under a microscope for mites, larvae, or mite faces. Even if no mites, eggs, or feces are observed, a person can still be infested; less than 10-15 mites may be present in an otherwise healthy infected person (Table **5**) [15].

Table 5. How can doctors tell if someone has scabies?

• Rash symptoms are generally enough for doctors to figure it out.
• One or two lumps may be scraped open by doctors.
• Under a microscope, doctors examine the scrapings for mites.
Major diagnostic criteria (one required to validate the diagnosis)
• Burrows that can be identified have an itchy rash.
• Positive scrapings of the epidermis containing eggs or mites or feces.
Minor diagnostic criteria (two required for a probable diagnosis)
• Typical irritating rash.
• Sudden start of unexplained itchy rash.
• In contact with a person with scabies.
• Penis papules.

TREATMENT

There is little research on new scabies medications. Probably the two most often utilized scabies therapy at the moment are oral ivermectin as well as topical permethrin. Furthermore, only a small number of nations worldwide have access to these medications, and they are both pricey [16]. For the first line of protection, infected individuals are treated with a topical scabicide, including 5 percent permethrin, 0.5 percent malathion in an aqueous base, 10–25 percent benzyl benzoate emulsion, or 5–10 percent Sulphur ointment. Ivermectin used orally, is also extremely effective and is legal in many nations. The safety of ivermectin in kids under 15 kg or pregnant women has not been proven; hence it should not be used in these populations until additional safety information becomes available. Itching usually worsens for 1-2 weeks after effective treatment, and those who have been treated should be aware of this. Existing scabicides have several drawbacks, including toxicity, side effects, poor safety evidence in critical populations, resistance development, and treatment failures [17, 18].

Plants have been utilized to cure skin problems throughout human history, and this technique is still used today. This is because most of these herbals are readily available, and inexpensive, and the extracted compounds have few or no adverse effects when compared to drugs created in a laboratory. Plants' therapeutic properties are attributed to phytochemicals, which are organic molecules that have a specific physiological function on the human body. They are plant-derived chemicals, and the term is frequently used to refer to the enormous number of secondary metabolic products found in plants. Novel medicinal agents like Polyphenols, resins, alkaloids, flavonoids, coumarin derivatives, vitamins, and tannins provide medicinal plants their therapeutic potential (Table 6) [19].

Table 6. Advantages of herbal medicines for scabies treatment.

• Safety of the patient with no or few negative impacts.
• Cost-effectiveness.
• Patient acceptability, adaptability, and compliance.
• Multiple biologically active compounds reduce the potential for resistance.
• Herbal medicines' antipruritic, anti-inflammatory, and antibacterial properties can also assist to decrease scabies complications.

TRADITIONAL MEDICINAL PLANTS USED FOR THE TREATMENT OF SCABIES

Globally the use of herbal medicine and Phytochemicals has expanded tremendously over the past three decades; there are more than four billion people (about 80% of the global population) who utilize medicinal plants and their products as a primary source of healthcare and traditional medical practice which involves the use of herbs is viewed as an integral part of the culture in those communities [20 - 22]. Traditional medicine (TCM) is an important example of how ancient and accumulated knowledge is applied in a holistic approach in present-day health care [23]. Compared to existing medications, traditional herbal treatments are said to be cheap, effective, and have few to no adverse effects [24]. Active biometabolites such as glycosides, alkaloids, flavonoids, coumarin compounds, vitamins, and tannins are what give significant therapeutic potential [25, 26]. Although they have little or no negative impacts, biopharmaceutical businesses, and medical practices now rely on medicines made from plants [27, 28]. Different cultures around the world have their native medicinal plants, and some of these distinct varieties of herbs have various therapeutic benefits [29, 30]. Indigenous knowledge is useful for conducting biomedical investigations [31]. The cultural heritage of the medical applications of plants is extremely important for understanding the pharmacological importance of herbal medicines (Fig. **2**) [32, 33].

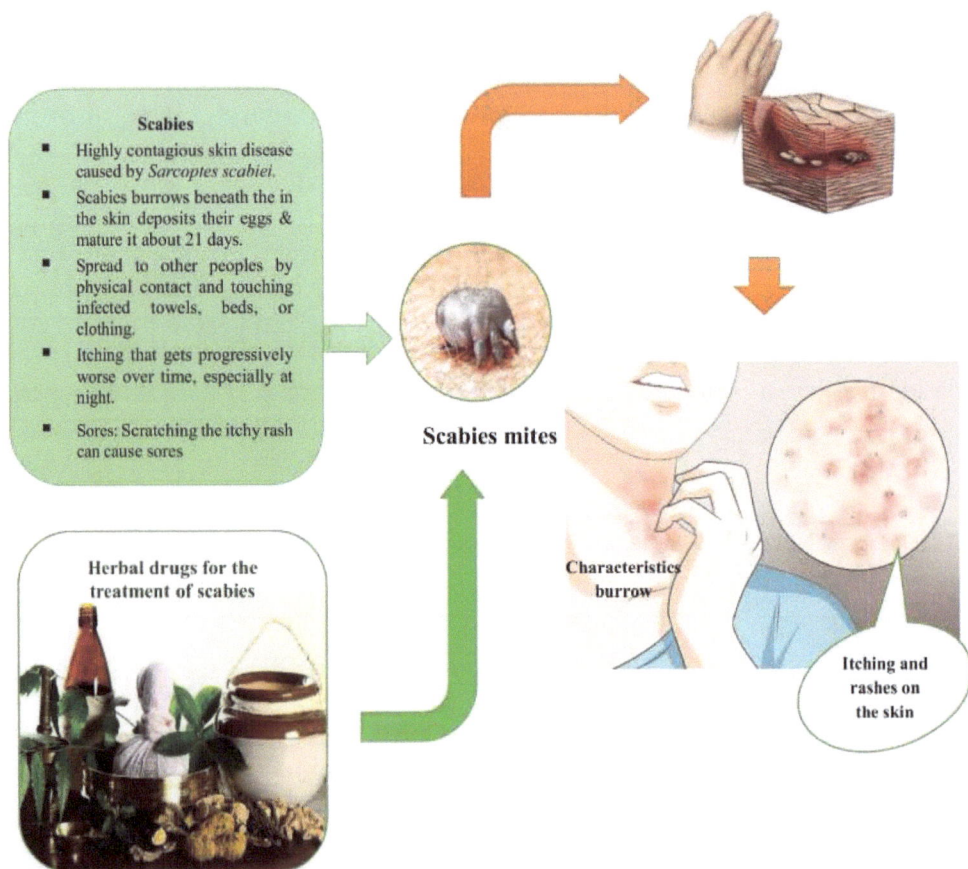

Scabies
- Highly contagious skin disease caused by *Sarcoptes scabiei.*
- Scabies burrows beneath the in the skin deposits their eggs & mature it about 21 days.
- Spread to other peoples by physical contact and touching infected towels, beds, or clothing.
- Itching that gets progressively worse over time, especially at night.
- Sores: Scratching the itchy rash can cause sores

Scabies mites

Herbal drugs for the treatment of scabies

Characteristics burrow

Itching and rashes on the skin

Fig. (2). Graphical representation of scabies and their treatment with traditional medicinal plants.

Chrysanthemum Cinerariifolium

Insecticides called pyrethrins are frequently found in chrysanthemum blossoms. They are a combination of six poisonous compounds for insects. Permethrin is emphasized as a phototoxic insecticide with low cytotoxic effects and almost no allergic side effects that are particularly efficient against a wide range of insects and mites. Permethrin (1 percent cream rinse or 0.5 percent in ethanol) demonstrated safety, dependability, and cosmetic acceptability in the treatment of head lice infestations and the prevention of reinfestations, as well as in failures with lindane leading to the advancements of sensitivity in the lice. These results were seen only 10–20 minutes after implementation. The permethrin cream used to treat scabies had a 5 percent concentration (2.5 percent for children under 5 years old). Small amounts of permethrin are absorbed through the skin, where it is quickly digested and eliminated in the urine. For eradication campaigns, a single "head to toe" administration is appropriate since it allows lice to be targeted and reduces the occurrence of microbial infection at around the same time. The outcomes of treating 48 children as well as 56 adults with scabies provide evidence for this. Permethrin is suggested in the management of scabies in premature babies, young children, patients with epilepsy and neurological issues, patients who have failed lindane medication and require further medication, pregnant women, breastfeeding mothers, and patients suffering *scabies crustose* [34].

Melaleuca Alternifolia

Scabies mites were isolated from 20-year-old women who were admitted to the Royal Darwin Hospital with crusted scabies to correlate the acaricidal action of tea tree oil, specifically *M. alternifolia,* and its bioactive constituents on *Sarcoptes scabiei* itch mite varhominis. After three hours of the collection, which governs the use of acaricides, scabies mites were usually placed with the tea tree oil preparations and inspected at defined intervals. Through constant interaction with acaricides and tea tree oil products, the percentage of dead mites is monitored at regular intervals. The active constituents in tea tree oil (5%) and terpinen-4-ol were very efficient in decreasing mite survival. Administering 5% tea tree oil, 100 g/g ivermectin (Emulsifying Ointment), 2.1% terpinen-4-ol, as well as 5% permethrin allowed researchers to identify mite viability. *M. alternifolia*, a surface biocide, is the source of tea tree oil. According to the studies, acaricide is a highly effective topical medication. Tea tree oil is a helpful natural and conventional remedy for skin disorders, bruising, and insect bites [35, 36].

Aloe Barbadensis Miller

Aloe vera's scientific name is *Aloe barbadensis* Miller. It is a pea-green, perennial, xerophytic plant belonging to the family Liliaceae that is succulent, with small shrubs, or arborescent in shape. The drier parts of Africa, Asia, Europe, and North America are where it is most frequently found. It can be cultivated in the Indian states of Rajasthan, Andhra Pradesh, Gujarat, Maharashtra, and Tamil Nadu, among others. Amino acids, enzymes, vitamins, minerals, lignin, saponins, salicylic acids, and saponins are some of the other *Aloe vera's* 75 theoretically active components. *Aloe vera*, a medical plant, has been known and utilized for its health, beauty, therapeutic, and skincare characteristics for generations. *Aloe vera* is mostly constituted of water and polysaccharides (pectin, cellulose, hemicellulose, glucomannan, acemannan, and mannose derivatives), with a long chain of acetylated mannose [37].

In an open, non-comparative study carried out between August and December 2002 at the Obafemi Awolowo University Teaching Hospitals Complex, Ile-Ife, Nigeria, 5 patients with scabies were successfully treated with crude gel of *Aloe vera*; thereafter, the efficacy of the extract was compared with that of benzoate lotion among 30 patients. Sixteen patients were treated with *Aloe vera* and 14 patients had benzyl benzoate lotion. The itching was still present in 3 patients in the benzyl benzoate group and 2 patients in the *Aloe vera* group after 2 courses of treatment. The scabietic lesions virtually disappeared in all of them. None of these patients had any noticeable side effects. It is concluded that *Aloe vera* gel is as effective as benzyl benzoate in the treatment of scabies [38].

Azadirachta Indica

Herbal shampoo made with *A. indica* seed extract effectively eliminates pathogens. *A. indica* has been tested in Egypt towards *S. scabiei*-affected canines. Ten naturally infected canines from various regions of the Nile delta were gathered. Skin irritation, lesions, and hair loss were noted as indicators of infiltration, and their prevalence was confirmed by the discovery of mature parasites and their growth stages in infected areas. For 14 days straight, appropriate shampoo was given externally to the affected areas. To complete the healing process, evaluations of scraping were also used. On the seventh day after application, four canines were mite-free, and it was also demonstrated that the mites' developmental stages had vanished. The six remaining dogs showed a significant decrease in the number of mites. Eight dogs were treated after 14 days of treatment, as evidenced by lower mite counts and improved clinical symptoms; just a small proportion of mites were identified in two dogs [39].

Neem oil contains an anti-parasite component called azadirachtin. The triterpene azadirachtin is responsible for the majority of the pesticide activity. This substance disrupts parasites' hormonal cycles, inhibits mite growth and development, turns eggs sterile, and has an antifeedant effect. Neem oil does not kill scabies mites directly, but it does stop them from reproducing and multiplying, resulting in a decrease in the parasite population over time. This is why; the cream should be applied daily. Neem oil at a concentration of 5 percent was said to be effective against scabies, with a 20–21 day recovery period [40].

Sarcoptes scabiei var. cuniculi were highly susceptible to the powerful acaricidal effects of Octadecanoic acid-3,4-tetrahydrofuran diester, isolated from neem

(*Azadirachta indica*) oil. Depending on histopathological and enzyme functions, the acaricidal strategy of octadecanoic acid-3,4-tetrahydrofuran diester towards Sarcoptes scabiei var. cuniculi has been assessed in this article. The outcomes demonstrated that mite lesions were noticeable under transmission electron microscopy following compound therapy for 24 hours at a dose of 20 mg/mL. The lesions included spinal problems that had disappeared, lysis of dermal cellular membrane as well as nuclear membranes, aberrant mitochondrial morphology, and vacuolization of the mitochondria. Octadecanoic acid-3,4-tetrahydrofuran diester treatment significantly altered the activities of superoxide dismutase (SOD), peroxidase (POD), glutathione-s-transferases (GSTs), as well as Ca (2+)-ATPase in mites compared to a control group. SOD, POD, and Ca (2+)-ATPase functions were all reduced significantly, but GST activity was enhanced. These findings suggested that the mechanism of octadecanoic acid-3,4-tetrahydrofuran diester's acaricidal activity was mostly achieved by interfering with mites' mitochondrial respiration, leading to insect mortality [41, 42].

Another study suggests that the acaricidal activity of *Azadirachta indica* (neem) aqueous fruit extracts was evaluated against *Sarcoptes scabiei* var. suis (mange mites) in an on-farm trial using grower pigs. Aqueous neem fruit extracts of three concentrations of 5%, 10%, and 25% w/v, and a commercial acaricide, 12.5% amitraz-based Triatix spray (positive control), were compared with pigs that received no treatment (negative control). Thirty grower pigs of the Dalland breed were allocated to the five treatments in a completely randomized experiment. Each experimental animal was sprayed on day 0 and again on day 7. Counts of mange mites, scoring of lesion index, and calculation of rubbing index were done weekly. The topical application of 25% aqueous neem fruit extract had a higher efficacy ratio ($p < 0.05$) than the other fruit extract concentrations, and performed similarly to an amitraz-based acaricide, suggesting a dose-dependent response. Amitraz (positive control) cured clinical mange on grower pigs after 5 weeks and 25% aqueous neem fruit extract 6 weeks post-treatment. The results indicated that aqueous neem fruit extracts have acaricidal effects against mange mites and can provide a cheaper, safer, and more eco-friendly alternative for the control of Sarcoptes mange in pigs [43].

Rosmarinus Officinalis

Globally, *R. officinalis* was utilized as a therapeutic herb. That plant includes significant active ingredients like camphor and 8-cineole. It possesses astringent, antibacterial, and anti-inflammatory properties that aid in the treatment of scabies illness. While rosemary oil helps to dry out wounds and quickly heal bruises, it is not recommended for internal usage [44, 45]. Rosemary oil also kills mites.

Capsicum Annuum

Capsaicin, a molecule that lessens pain perception when employed correctly, is a component of cayenne [46]. Capsaicin can help reduce itching because it makes skin neurons less sensitive. However, according to one study, 30% of patients who apply capsaicin topically experience burning [47]. Studies have also demonstrated that rubbing *C. annuum* into the skin will kill scabies mites. In a boiling water bath with cayenne administered, the patient waits until the water cools before washing their bodies. Cayenne burns the eyes, so be able to keep yours away from any contact with it. One or two drops of water can also be used to create the cayenne paste. The paste is rubbed onto visible warrens under the top layer of the skin [48].

Cinnamomum Camphor

For several years, that tree has been used successfully to treat scabies. C. camphor is an analgesic and aromatic herb with a pleasant scent. This tree's insecticidal properties may have therapeutic benefits. For the management of muscular discomfort, it works well. This tree's oil will completely cure the scabies infection if used consistently for ten days. In the repellent assay, the highest repellent rate was found in the seed essential oil at the concentration of 20 µL/mL after 24 h of treatment. Linalool was found to be a significant contributor to insecticidal and repellent activities [49].

Eupatorium Adenophorum

The possible acaricidal activity of *Eupatorium adenophorum* was analyzed using extracts created by water decocting, ethanol thermal circumfluence, and steam distillation. The toxic effect of each extract was tested against Psoroptes cuniculi and *Sarcoptes scabiei in vitro*. Ethanol, thermal circumfluence extract, had strong toxicity against mites, killing all *Sarcoptes scabiei* at 0.5 and 1.0 g/ml (w/v) concentration, while 1g/ml extract was also found to kill all P. cuniculi within a 4-h period. Similarly, 0.25, 0.5 and 1.0 g/ml concentrations of extract had strong toxicity against *S. scabiei*, with median lethal time (LT (50)) values at 0.866, 0.785 and 0.517 h, respectively. 0.5 g/ml and 1g/ml showed strong acaricidal action against P. cuniculi; the LT (50) values were 0.93 h and 1.29 h, respectively. The median lethal concentration (LC (50) values were 0.22 g/ml for Scabies mite and 0.64 g/ml for *P. cuniculi* in 1h. The results indicated that *E. adenophorum* contains potent acaricidal ingredients; as a first step in the potential development of novel drugs, it may provide new acaricidal compounds for the effective control of animal acariasis [50].

Ailanthus Altissima

Psoroptes cuniculi and *Sarcoptes scabiei* var. *cuniculi*, the two most common taxa of animal ectoparasitic mites, are being used as *in-vitro* test subjects to determine the possible acaricidal effects of an *Ailanthus altissima* stem bark. *A. altissima* bark extract was made using ethanol thermal circumfluence and evaluated against rabbit mites at four different concentrations (1.0, 0.5, 0.25, and 0.125 g/ml). The bark of *A. altissima* displayed considerable acaricidal capabilities for both mite species treated in comparison to the fenvalerate-treated group. Only 1.0 and 0.5 g/ml of extract killed all treated *P. cuniculi*, although doses of 1.0, 0.5, and 0.25 g/ml killed all tested *Sarcoptes scabiei* in 7 hours. *Sarcoptes scabiei* median lethal time (LT_{50}) values at 1, 0.5, and 0.25 g/ml were 0.60, 0.78, and 1.48 h and *P. cuniculi* were 0.74, 1.29, and 3.33 h. At 4 hours, *P. cuniculi* median lethal concentration (LC_{50}) was almost 1.6 times higher than that of *Sarcoptes scabiei* var. *cuniculi*. *Sarcoptes scabiei* was more sensitive to the extract's toxicity than *P. cuniculi*. The acaricidal effect of *A. altissima* crude extracts is time- and dose-dependent, as evidenced by the fact that mortality rates rose with increasing extract concentration supplied, even with increasing time post-treatment. The acaricidal activity of *A. altissima* against *P. cuniculi* and *Sarcoptes scabiei* var. *cuniculi* has never been documented before. It suggests that *A. altissima* may contain substances that have acaricidal properties. The development of possibly novel chemicals from *A. altissima* for the efficient control of mites in livestock is underway with the help of our investigation [51].

Cymbopogon Citratus

Tropical and subtropical areas frequently cultivate the plant *Cymbopogon citratus*. Lemongrass oil is an essential oil derived from the *C. citratus* genus, with citral as the main component. The essential oil of Cymbopogon species is in high demand around the world. Lemongrass essential oil is derived from dried or fresh leaves using steam distillation. Essential oils, as well as hydrosols or aromatic fluids, are produced by steam distillation and are frequently used to treat inflammatory illnesses and microbiological infections. Lemongrass oil has a number of pharmacological characteristics, including antiparasitic, antioxidant, antibacterial, and anti-inflammatory qualities. Lemongrass oil has been shown to have a miticidal impact on a plant pathogen (*Tetranycchus urticae*) as well as domestic dust mites [52].

Essential oils may represent an alternative strategy for controlling scabies, a neglected tropical disease caused by the infestation of mites from the species *Sarcoptes scabiei*. Lemongrass (*Cymbopogen citratus*) oil is reported to possess pharmacological properties, including antiparasitic, antioxidant, antimicrobial, and anti-inflammatory. The present study aimed to assess the potential efficacy of lemongrass oil against the mites and eggs of *Sarcoptes scabiei*. Mass spectrometry analysis confirmed that the main component presented in lemongrass oil was citral. Lemongrass oil at concentrations of 10% and 5% killed all Sarcoptes mites within 10 and 25 min, respectively. The median lethal concentration value was 1.37%, 1.08%, 0.91%, 0.64%, and 0.48% at 1, 3, 6, 12, and 24 h, respectively. Lemongrass oil at all concentrations (10%, 5%, 1%, 0.5%, 0.1%) was able to significantly decrease the hatching rate of Sarcoptes eggs. Lemongrass oil should be considered a promising miticidal and ovicidal agent for scabies control [53].

Eucalyptus Globulus

In Egypt, *Scarcoptes scabiei* is the most prevalent mites of medical importance infesting man. This is true in overcrowded and poorly hygienic areas. Many effective acaridical regimens are available, but being compounds used as insecticides. With the success of camphor oil in treating human demodicidosis, it was applied to treating human scabies. Camphor oil with or without glycerol dilutions gave a complete cure, with concentrations (100%, 75%, and 50%) within five to ten days [54].

Curcuma Longa

In the Ayurvedha and Sidha systems of medicine (Indian system of medicine), *Azadirachta indica* ADR ('Neem') and *Curcuma longa* ('Turmeric') have been used for healing chronic ulcers and scabies. 'Neem' and 'Turmeric' were used as a paste for the treatment of scabies in 814 people. In 97% of cases, a cure was obtained within 3 to 15 days of treatment. We find that this is a very cheap, easily available, effective, and acceptable mode of treatment for villagers in developing countries. We have noticed no toxic or adverse reactions so far. However, further research is needed [55].

Syzygium Aromaticum Oil

Syzygium aromaticum, commonly known as clove oil, is a traditional spice that has been used for food preservation and possesses various pharmacological activities. *S. aromaticum* is rich in many phytochemicals, as follows: sesquiterpenes, monoterpenes, hydrocarbon, and phenolic compounds. Eugenyl acetate, eugenol, and β-caryophyllene are the most significant phytochemicals in clove oil. Anti-microbial, anti-oxidant, and anaesthetic activities, can boost the inclination to heal. Pests can also be killed by it. Numerous other oils, including lavender, thyme, lemongrass, orange, and mint, are also used to treat scabies [56].

Additionally, it works well when combined with coconut oil. It seems to have narcotic effects. Rashes and blisters can also be treated with it [57].

Melaleuca Alternifolia (Tea Tree) Oil

Scabies affects approximately more than 130 million individuals worldwide. In the industrialised world, outbreaks in healthcare facilities and vulnerable areas have a substantial financial impact. In addition to its successful usage as a topical adjuvant agent for the treatment of crusted scabies, particularly in instances that did not answer to traditional treatments, tea tree oil has also shown potential acaricidal actions against scabies mites *in vitro*. The effectiveness of the currently prescribed gold standard treatments for scabies (oral ivermectin and topical permethrin) in the prospective is threatened by the emergence of acaricide resistance. It's unlikely that any new chemical entities will emerge anytime soon. Tea tree oil's combined acaricidal, antibacterial, antipruritic, anti-inflammatory, and wound-healing properties may have the power to significantly lessen the incidence of scabies infection and the bacterial problems that go along with it. This review provides an overview of the most recent research on the use of tea tree oil in the treatment of scabies. Larger-scale, randomised controlled clinical investigations are called for depending on the merits of the available findings for tea tree oil [58, 59].

The 5% *Melaleuca alternifolia* oil and active component terpinen-4-ol were highly effective in reducing mite survival times. Statistically significant differences in mite survival curves were observed for 5% Tea tree oil, 2.1% terpinen-4-ol, 5% permethrin, and ivermectin (100 micro/g of Emulsifying Ointment British Pharmacopoeia 88). Tea tree oil is a membrane-active biocide extracted from the tree *M alternifolia*. It is a principal antimicrobial in a wide range of pharmaceuticals sold in Australia, with the main active component being oxygenated terpenoids. The results suggest that *Melaleuca alternifolia* oil has a potential role as a new topical acaricide and confirms terpinen-4-ol as the primary active component [60, 61].

Heliotropium Indicum

An assessment of Siddha herbal preparation *Thelkodukku Chooranam* (*Heliotropium indicum*), a total number of 50 patients with scabies were treated with *Thelkodukku Chooranam* orally at the dose of 500 mg twice a day with milk after food and for external use; the fresh leaf paste was applied over the affected area twice a day for one month. Clinical assessment of scabies lesions based on clinical grading score; itching intensity was assessed at weekly intervals for four weeks. From the result, it was observed that oral and topical administration of *Thelkodukku Chooranam* significantly reduced all the signs and symptoms after one month of treatment. As compared to baseline, *Thelkodukku Chooranam* treatment significantly reduced clinical grading score and itching grading score from 3.02 ± 0.08 and 2.04 ± 0.099 to 0.08 ± 0.03 and 0.04 ± 0.03 respectively ($P < 0.001$). The complete disappearance of scabies lesions was observed in all patients. No adverse effect has been noticed during the study period. Hence it is concluded that *Thelkodukku Chooranam* exhibits scabicidal activity and is a promising Siddha herbal preparation that has an effective and safe anti-scabies agent [62].

Crinum Asiaticum

Scabies is an enervating parasitic infestation of the skin caused by *Sarcoptes scabiei*, affecting 130 million people at any time. Globally, this neglected tropical disease is amenable to 0.07% of the total burden of disease. *Crinum asiaticum* Linn. (Amaryllidaceae) plant parts are used in traditional medicines used for the treatment and management of various ailments, including insecticidal properties. Studies evaluate the anti-scabies and mosquito-repellent activity of ethanol and aqueous extracts of *Crinum asiaticum* leaves. Ethanol extract of *C. asiaticum* showed 100.00 ± 0.00% mortality of *Sarcoptes scabiei* at 10% concentration within 80 min. of contact and also at its 10% concentration; it provided 97.00 ± 0.42% protection effect and 78.25 ± 0.53% after 6 h treatment comparable to DEET. This present study revealed that the ethanol extract of *C. asiaticum* exhibited excellent scabicidal activity against adult *Sarcoptes scabiei* mites and mosquito-repellent activity against mosquito vector *A. stephensi* [63].

Lippia Multiflora Moldenke

Lippia multiflora Moldenke, a perennial aromatic plant found primarily in tropical West Africa, yields lippia oil. Bush tea, Gambian tea bush, and healer herb are all names for it. Several studies have shown that the components of this plant have antihypertensive, anti-inflammatory, anti-analgesic, anti-pyretic, anti-malaria, anti-oxidant, anti-microbial, muscle relaxant, pedicucidal, and scabicidal qualities. Linalool, α-pinene, β-pinene, geraniol, limonene, β-cymene, thymol, terpineol, and citronellyl acetate are among the essential oils extracted from leaves. Body and head lice are known to be resistant to terpineol with α-pinene, while β-pinene with α-pinene is an efficient insecticide [64]. A 20 percent v/v dilution of lippia oil in mild liquid paraffin BP (British Pharmacopoeia) preparation of lippia oil applied to scabietic patients for 5 consecutive days resulted in 100% cure, compared to 87.5 percent cure for the same concentration of benzyl benzoate preparation. Lippia oil had fewer side effects and was more tolerable. Researchers and producers may be able to replace crude ingredients with lippia oil because it is an economically underutilised resource [65]. Another study found that *L.*

multiflora oil is a better and more efficient scabicidal than benzyl benzoate. In a randomised, double-blind, and group parallel investigation, the researchers compared two topical emulsion formulations (Lippia oil emulsions A and B), each containing 20 percent weight-for-weight essential oil of Lippia multiflora (Lippia oil), to benzyl benzoate emulsion BP. On application for 3, 5, and 7 days, the percentage cure attained for the Lippia oil emulsions (A and B) was around 50 percent, 80 percent, and 80 percent, respectively, compared to 30 percent, 60 percent, and 70% for much the same therapy using the benzyl benzoate emulsion BP at a time [66].

Nicotiana Tobacum

Sarcoptic scabies-infested rabbits were treated with *Nicotiana tabacum* decoctions ad-lib at weekly intervals on 3, 2, and 1 occasions required for severely, moderately, and mildly infested rabbits, respectively, for complete healing of lesions and disappearance of different stages of *Sarcoptic scabiei*. Both macroscopic and microscopic examination of lesions was done throughout the period. Reinfestation was not observed even after 1 and a half months of treatment. Thus, tobacco decoction was highly effective in controlling *Sarcoptes scabiei* infestation in rabbits with no side effects. In addition, the decoction is convenient and simple to prepare, economical, costing only 1/10th of the cost involved in using acaricide [67].

Tinospora Cordifolia

The current study evaluated the clinical efficacy and safety of *Tinospora cordifolia* lotion, including its cure rate and clearance time compared with permethrin lotion. A single-blind, randomized, controlled, pilot clinical study was performed in three government institutions to investigate the clinical efficacy of *T. cordifolia* lotion in sixty-six clinically diagnosed scabies-infected patients. The patients were treated with *T. cordifolia* or permethrin lotions for three consecutive days for two weeks and a clinical assessment of each patient was performed for five weeks. *T. cordifolia* lotion and permethrin significantly reduced the mean global evaluation score after four weeks of treatment. The two lotions showed comparable effects as an anti-scabies agent. Moreover, the clearance time (days) and cure rate using the two lotions did not differ. Clinical improvement, mean clearance time and cure rate of *T. cordifolia* lotion are comparable with permethrin. *Tinospora cordifolia* lotion exhibits anti-scabies activity comparable with permethrin. Its incorporation as a therapeutic reagent in *Sarcoptes scabiei* infections is highly recommended [68].

Denis Elliptica

Rotenone was originally extracted from derris root (*Denis elliptica*) of which it constitutes 5-9 percent, and now from *Lonchocarpus nicou* (South American cuberoot), which has a content of about 7 percent. It is widely used in veterinary medicine for demodectic mange and as a constituent of flea powders. It is colorless, crystalline, and insoluble in water but readily soluble in alcohol, ether, acetone, chloroform, benzene, or carbon tetrachloride. Though toxic by mouth, it is not absorbed by the skin. For the trial in scabies cases, 1 gm of rotenone was dissolved in 3 cc. chloroform, and added, with vigorous shaking, to a mucilage of quince seed and Irish moss to make a 1-2 percent, lotion; 0.1 percent, sodium benzoate is added as a preservative [69].

Allium Sativum

Garlic is an alternative therapy for various parasites, therefore, the assumption that it might help with scabies infestations is convincing [70]. Garlic has a long history of use as a preventive and therapeutic medicinal plant in various cultures. Throughout antiquity, garlic has played important dietary and therapeutic roles. Garlic possesses hundreds of phytochemicals, including sulfur-containing compounds such as ajoenes (E & Z), allicin, sulphides (diallyl disulfide - DADS, diallyl trisulfide - DATS), and others, which make up 82% sulfur content. Enzymes like alliinase, sulfur-containing substances like alliin, and enzymatically generated compounds like allicin are among their constituents. The four garlic formulations are aged garlic extract (AGE), dried garlic powder (DGP), heated garlic juice (HGJ), and raw garlic juice (RGJ). Different types of garlic formulations have different pharmacological characteristics, and among the four garlic preparations, AGE is the most efficacious preparation. S-allyl cysteine, Allin, S-methyl-L-cysteine, cycloalliin, S-ethylcysteine, S-1-proponyl-L-cysteine, S-allylmercapto-L-cysteine, fructosyl-arginine, and beta-chlorogenin are some of the components of AGE [71]. Some of the medicinal plants and their active metabolites with significant scabicidal activities are described in (Table 7) [72 - 93].

CLINICAL AND PRECLINICAL STUDIES

Herbal products have become an important and indispensable part of public healthcare around the world [94]. Plant-based agents have been used in indigenous medicine for several years and are now entering clinical trials. However, to further widen their forum of acceptance, clinical trials of these herbal products should be encouraged. To prove the efficacy of clinical trials, it is advised to use single and consistent batches of formulations [95]. Direct and network meta-analyses were applied to 13 antiscabietic agents on 3 outcomes (cure, persistent itching, and adverse events). Their probability of having the highest efficacy and safety was estimated and ranked. A network meta-analysis of 52 trials, including 9917 patients, indicated that permethrin (the reference treatment) had a significantly higher cure rate than sulfur, malathion, lindane, crotamiton, and benzyl benzoate. Combination permethrin plus oral ivermectin had a nonsignificantly higher cure rate than permethrin. Combination permethrin plus oral ivermectin was ranked highest in terms of cure, topical ivermectin in terms of persistent itching, and synergized pyrethrins in terms of adverse events. Based on clustered ranking, permethrin, oral ivermectin, and synergized pyrethrins seemed to retain a balance between cure and adverse events [96, 97].

Table 7. Common traditional medicinal plants for the treatment and management of scabies.

Vernacular Name	Botanical Name	Family	Parts Used	Active Metabolites	Pharmacological Significance	Refs.
Arrow-poison-tree	*Acokanthera schimperi*	Apocynaceae	Leaves	Triterpenoids, including lupeol, ursolic aldehyde	It is used to treat convulsion, oedema, warts, wounds, amnesia, syphilis, rheumatic pain, scabies, leprosy, elephantiasis, headaches, and amnesia.	[72]
Falling stars	*Calamagrostis aurea*	Fabaceae	Leaves	Not Known	Is used for elephantiasis, syphilis, scabies, intestinal parasites, tinea capitis, diarrhoea, leishmaniasis, as well as respiratory disease.	[72, 73]
Lippia	*Lippia adoensis*	Verbenaceae	Leaves	1,8-cineole, camphor and *para*-cymene, carvacrol	Used for eczema and cutaneous fungal infections.	[74]
Amargna	*Olinia rochetiana*	Oliniaceae	Leaves	-	In eczema, scabies, and acne.	[72]
Black cohosh	*Actaea racemosa*	Euphorbiaceae	Roots and leaves	Triterpene glycosides, Actein, 27-deoxyactein, cimicifugoside M and cimicifugoside	It is used for scabies.	[75]
Small taro	*Canna esculenta*	Araceae	Leaves and rhizome	Γ-eudesmol, δ-cadinol, γ- selinene, luciferin	It is used for skin diseases.	[76]

(Table 7) cont.....

Vernacular Name	Botanical Name	Family	Parts Used	Active Metabolites	Pharmacological Significance	Refs.
Smooth crotalaria	*Crotalaria pallida*	Fabaceae	Leaves, roots, and bark	Cyclopentyliene, crotolidene, octacosane hydroxydihydrobovolide,	It is used for skin diseases.	[77]
Caesar weed or Congo jute	*Urena lobata*	Malvaceae	Leaves	Alkaloids, cardiac glycoside, tannins, terpenoid	It is used in itching and scabies.	[78]
Tall pine barren milkwort	*Polygala cymosa*	Urticaseae	Leaves	Apigenin, quercetin	In skin disorders.	[79]
Rough Mexican clover	*Richardia scabra*	Rubiaceae	Leaves	Isopsoralen, Oleic acid	In skin disorders, pruritis, and scabies.	[80]
Hard pear tree	*Graptopetalum pentandrum*	Santalaceae	Bark	Not known	In itching as well as eczema.	[81]
Sannale gida	*Euphorbia heyneana*	Euphorbiaceae	Leaves and bark	Flavonoids, naringenin, quercetin	In skin Disorders.	[82]
Spiny pigwee	*Amaranthus spinosus*	Amaranthaceae	Whole plant	Diglycoside flavonoids hesperidin, rutin, phenolic acid (E)-ferulic acid	In gonorrhea, piles, dermatitis and STD.	[80, 83]
Licorice weed	*Scoparia dulcis*	Plantaginaceae	Leaves and flower	Benzoxazinone, phenylethanoid, flavone, and lignan	It is used for toothache and itching.	[80]
Jersey cudweed	*Gnaphalium luteoalbum*	Asteraceae	Whole plant	5, 7, 3, 4 tetrahydroxy flavone; 5, 3, 4 trihydroxy flavonol	Use It is applied against dermatitis, arthritis, and tumours.	[80]
Papaya	*Carica papaya*	Caricaceae	Whole plant	Tannins, alkaloids, flavonoids, terpenes, anthraquinone, saponins, phenolics	It treats hyperglycemia, dermatitis, hepatitis, constipation, scabies, rheumatoid arthritis.	[84]
Wild cabbage	*Brassica oleracea*	Cruciferae	Leaves and fruits	Indole-3-carbinole (^{13}C), sulforaphane and indoles	It treats a variety of skin conditions, including eczema, cancer, and gynaecological issues.	[85]

(Table 7) cont.....

Vernacular Name	Botanical Name	Family	Parts Used	Active Metabolites	Pharmacological Significance	Refs.
Himalayan cedar	*Cedrus deodara*	Pinaceae	Leaves and bark	Wikstromal, matairesinol, dibenzylbutyrolactol	It is used for psoriasis, gastritis, hemorrhoids, and sexual difficulties.	[86]
Zebra cactus	*Haworthia aristata*	Asphodelaceae	Whole plant	Berberine, oxyberberine, berbamine, aromoline	It treats coughs and scabies.	[83, 72]
Common vervain	*Verbena officinalis*	Verbenaceae	Whole plant	Iridoids, phenylpropanoids, flavonoids, luteolin and terpenoids	It treats eczema, leukemia, TB, and helminthiasis.	[77]
Dwarf bulrush	*Typha minima*	Typhaceae	Whole plant	Trianthemine	It helps treat dermatitis, wounds, and other disorders that cause cutaneous itching.	[76]
African senna	*Senna didymobotrya*	Fabaceae	Whole plant	Alkaloids, flavonoids, saponins, steroids, tannins, terpenoids	It helps treat dermatitis, sores, and other conditions that cause skin irritation.	[87]
Fig-mulberry	*Ficus sycomorus*	Moraceae	Fruit juice	Tannins, flavonoids, saponins, glycosides and alkaloids	It treats scabies as well as boils.	[88]
Vernonia	*Vernonia lasiopus*	Asteraceae	Leaves	Alkaloids, *phenols and flavonoids*	It treats scabies, acne, and dermatitis.	[88]
Arrowhead	*Sagittaria secundifoli*	Aloaceae	Leaves	Tannin, saponins	It is applied to injuries, tumors, rashes, dermatitis, and acne.	[88]
Siam weed	*Chromolaena odorata*	*Compositeae*	Leaf	Essential oil, flavonoids, oxalates, tannins, Antibiotic	Skin sepsis, scabies. Wound dressing.	[89]
Thorny pigweed	*Amaranthus spinosus*	*amaranthaceae*	Whole plant	Tannins, saponins, hydrocyanic Acid anti-prostaglandin synthesis	Scabies, Eczema, Psoriasis, Burns & Sunburn, Insect bites, Scorpion stings, Cobra bites.	[90, 91]

(Table 7) cont.....

Vernacular Name	Botanical Name	Family	Parts Used	Active Metabolites	Pharmacological Significance	Refs.
Mango	*Mangifera indica*	*Anacardineae*	leaf, stem bark, root, sap	Tannins, resins, volatile oil, cyanogenic Glycoside methylsalicylate quercetin	Burns, Scabies, Eczema recipe.	[91]
Botuje red, Botuje white	*Jatropha curcas*	*euphorbiaceae*	Fresh latex, Ash of leaves	A-epi-cadinol, α-Cadinol	It treats yaws, wounds, sores, ringworm, eczema, scabies, and alopecia caused by guinea parasites.	[92, 93]

FUTURE PROSPECTIVE

Natural products and their structural analogs have historically made a major contribution to pharmacotherapy, especially for cancer and infectious diseases [98, 99]. Nevertheless, natural products also present challenges for drug discovery, such as technical barriers to screening, isolation, characterization, and optimization, which contributed to a decline in their pursuit by the pharmaceutical industry from the 1990s onwards. In recent years, several technological and scientific developments, including improved analytical tools, genome mining, and engineering strategies, and microbial culturing advances, are addressing such challenges and opening up new opportunities against several types of chronic disorders, including scabies. Consequently, interest in natural products as drug leads is being revitalized, particularly for the treatment and mitigation of scabies and other communicable diseases [100].

DISCUSSION

One of the most prevalent dermatological disorders, scabies, contributes significantly to skin disorders in emerging economies. More work is needed to determine the burden, although it is expected to affect more than 200 million individuals worldwide at any given moment. In the most recent scabies-related studies, prevalence estimates ranged from 0.2 percent to 71 percent [101]. In the developed world, outbreaks in health institutions and vulnerable communities result in a significant economic burden [102]. It is caused by infection with the female mite *Sarcoptes scabiei var. hominis*, an ectoparasite. The most common symptoms are severe itchiness and a pimple-like rash [103]. Several medications are available to treat those infected, including permethrin, crotamiton, and lindane creams, and ivermectin pills [104]. Healing with medicinal plants is as old as mankind itself. Plants are used for various ailments and have been an age-old practice since time immemorial [105, 106]. About 80% of people worldwide rely on herbal medicines for some aspects of their primary health care [107]. The documentation of medicinal plants is gaining recognition in recent times to preserve the knowledge for the next generation and also make effective use of the resources. In this connection majority of medicinal plants and their parts utilized for scabies treatments were documented. Globally, huge numbers of traditional healers are practicing from generation to generation by obtaining knowledge from their elders and also through learning. From the collected and documented medicinal plants, *Melaleuca alternifolia* (Tea tree oil), *Aloe barbadensis* mill (*Aloe vera*), *Azadirachta indica* (Neem oil), *Curcuma longa* (Turmeric), *Chrysanthemum cinerariifolium* (Pyrethrins), *etc.* was the most popular medicinal plant used for the treatment of scabies.

CONCLUSION

According to reports, medicinal plants contain potent therapeutic compounds that are readily available, reasonably priced, and utilised to treat a wide range of illnesses. In this review paper, medicinal plants having therapeutic potential against the scabies condition are investigated, and their beneficial impacts are thoroughly discussed. Many herbs efficiently become anti-scabies with various content that is potential as an alternative medicine due to drug resistance anti-scabies synthesis. This compound provides resistance to *Sarcoptes scabiei* mites by inhibiting the life cycle of the mite metamorphosis. Due to a dearth of literature studies indicating the scabicidal action of the medicinal herbs under review based on pre-clinical trials, the study had limitations. The present review paper serves as a starting point for investigating the effectiveness of medicinal herbs in treating scabies disease. Exploring additional medicinal plants that can be employed as a therapeutic therapy for the treatment of scabies as well as other skin conditions will demand more investigation. To isolate, identify, authenticate, and describe the bioactive phytochemicals contained in these plants with scabicidal actions, that will ultimately lead to contributing its role in improvement through pharmaceutical research and development, more thorough research at the theoretical level are necessary. Modern methodologies will be employed to characterise and identify the bioactive phytochemical constituents of these plants, which will aid in the exploration of the therapeutic potential of scabies-treating plants.

AUTHOR'S CONTRIBUTIONS

Om Prakash and Shazia Usmani generated an idea, wrote, and revised the manuscript. Nadeem Rais and Rajesh Kumar conducted a literature survey through Science Direct, PubMed, Research Gate, Google Scholar, and various

Textbooks. Ruchi Singh and Amita Pandey modified the language, such as grammar mistakes and spelling checking, rectifying the similarity content. Amresh Gupta and Priyanka Bajpai drafted all references per the author's instructions and online verified all the cited references from various journals.

AVAILABILITY OF DATA AND MATERIAL

All data generated during this study are included.

ACKNOWLEDGEMENTS

The authors are thankful to vice-chancellor Dr. A.P.J. Technical University, Lucknow, Uttar Pradesh, India, for his sustained encouragement, meticulous supervision, and valuable suggestions at all stages of completion of this manuscript. The authors are also thankful to Er. Mahesh Goel, Managing Director, Goel Institute of Pharmacy & Sciences, Lucknow, Uttar Pradesh, India, for providing the library facilities for the compilation of the current review.

REFERENCES

[1]   Welch E, Romani L, Whitfeld MJ. Recent advances in understanding and treating scabies. Fac Rev 2021; 10: 28.
[http://dx.doi.org/10.12703/r/10-28] [PMID: 33817697]

[2]   Thomas C, Coates SJ, Engelman D, Chosidow O, Chang AY. Ectoparasites. J Am Acad Dermatol 2020; 82(3): 533-48.
[http://dx.doi.org/10.1016/j.jaad.2019.05.109] [PMID: 31310840]

[3]   Scabies and other ectoparasites 2020.www.who.int/news-room/fact-sheets/detail/scabies

[4]   Leung AKC, Lam JM, Leong KF. Scabies: a neglected global disease. Curr Pediatr Rev 2020; 16(1): 33-42.
[http://dx.doi.org/10.2174/1875633660Tk3jMjEcTcVY] [PMID: 31544694]

[5]   Anderson KL, Strowd LC. Epidemiology, diagnosis, and treatment of scabies in a dermatology office. J Am Board Fam Med 2017; 30(1): 78-84.
[http://dx.doi.org/10.3122/jabfm.2017.01.160190] [PMID: 28062820]

[6]   Turan Ç, Metin N, Utlu Z. Epidemiological evaluation of scabies cases encountered in the last three years as a tertiary health center. Turkiye Parazitol Derg 2020; 44(2): 77-82.
[http://dx.doi.org/10.4274/tpd.galenos.2020.6796] [PMID: 32482039]

[7]   Chandler DJ, Fuller LC. A review of scabies: an infestation more than skin deep. Dermotology 2019; 235(2): 79-90.
[http://dx.doi.org/10.1159/000495290]

[8]   Cox V, Fuller LC, Engelman D, Steer A, Hay RJ. Estimating the global burden of scabies: what else do we need? Br J Dermatol 2021; 184(2): 237-42.
[http://dx.doi.org/10.1111/bjd.19170] [PMID: 32358799]

[9]   Siddig EE, Hay R. Laboratory-based diagnosis of scabies: a review of the current status. Trans R Soc Trop Med Hyg 2021; traa094.
[http://dx.doi.org/10.1093/trstmh/trab049] [PMID: 33763705]

[10]   Arora P, Rudnicka L, Sar-Pomian M, *et al.* Scabies: A comprehensive review and current perspectives. Dermatol Ther 2020; 33(4): e13746.

[http://dx.doi.org/10.1111/dth.13746] [PMID: 32484302]

[11] Engelman D, Yoshizumi J, Hay RJ, *et al*. The 2020 international alliance for the control of scabies consensus criteria for the diagnosis of scabies. Br J Dermatol 2020; 183(5): 808-20.
[http://dx.doi.org/10.1111/bjd.18943] [PMID: 32034956]

[12] Sánchez-Borges M, González-Aveledo L, Capriles-Hulett A, Caballero-Fonseca F. Scabies, crusted (Norwegian) scabies and the diagnosis of mite sensitisation. Allergol Immunopathol (Madr) 2018; 46(3): 276-80.
[http://dx.doi.org/10.1016/j.aller.2017.05.006] [PMID: 29279260]

[13] Heukelbach J, Feldmeier H. Scabies. Lancet 2006; 367(9524): 1767-74.
[http://dx.doi.org/10.1016/S0140-6736(06)68772-2] [PMID: 16731272]

[14] Banerji A. Scabies. Paediatr Child Health 2015; 20(7): 395-8.
[http://dx.doi.org/10.1093/pch/20.7.395] [PMID: 26527041]

[15] Arlian LG, Morgan MS. A review of *Sarcoptes scabiei*: past, present and future. Parasit Vectors 2017; 10(1): 297.
[http://dx.doi.org/10.1186/s13071-017-2234-1] [PMID: 28633664]

[16] Engelman D, Cantey PT, Marks M, *et al*. The public health control of scabies: priorities for research and action. Lancet 2019; 394(10192): 81-92.
[http://dx.doi.org/10.1016/S0140-6736(19)31136-5] [PMID: 31178154]

[17] Vasanwala FF, Ong CY, Aw CWD, How CH. Management of scabies. Singapore Med J 2019; 60(6): 281-5.
[http://dx.doi.org/10.11622/smedj.2019058] [PMID: 31243462]

[18] Rinaldi G, Porter K. Mass drug administration for endemic scabies: a systematic review. Trop Dis Travel Med Vaccines 2021; 7(1): 21.
[http://dx.doi.org/10.1186/s40794-021-00143-5] [PMID: 34193305]

[19] Akram M, Riaz M, Noreen S, *et al*. Therapeutic potential of medicinal plants for the management of scabies. Dermatol Ther 2020; 33(1): e13186.
[http://dx.doi.org/10.1111/dth.13186] [PMID: 31830356]

[20] Khuda F, Iqbal Z, Khan A, *et al*. Report: Antibacterial and antifungal activities of leaf extract of *Achyranthes aspera* (Amaranthaceae) from Pakistan. Pak J Pharm Sci 2015; 28(5): 1797-800.https://pubmed.ncbi.nlm.nih.gov/26408900/
[PMID: 26408900]

[21] https://apps.who.int/iris/handle/10665/43034

[22] Ekor M. The growing use of herbal medicines: issues relating to adverse reactions and challenges in monitoring safety. Front Pharmacol 2014; 4: 177.
[http://dx.doi.org/10.3389/fphar.2013.00177] [PMID: 24454289]

[23] Wachtel-Galor S, Benzie IFF. Herbal Medicine: An Introduction to Its History, Usage, Regulation, Current Trends, and Research Needs.Herbal Medicine: Biomolecular and Clinical Aspects. 2nd ed. Boca Raton, FL: CRC Press/Taylor & Francis 2011; pp. 1-23.
https://www.ncbi.nlm.nih.gov/books/NBK92773/

[24] Klein-Junior LC, de Souza MR, Viaene J, *et al*. Quality Control of Herbal Medicines: From Traditional Techniques to State-of-the-art Approaches. Planta Med 2021; 87(12/13): 964-88.
[http://dx.doi.org/10.1055/a-1529-8339] [PMID: 34412146]

[25] Sofowora A, Ogunbodede E, Onayade A. The role and place of medicinal plants in the strategies for disease prevention. Afr J Tradit Complement Altern Med 2013; 10(5): 210-29.
[http://dx.doi.org/10.4314/ajtcam.v10i5.2] [PMID: 24311829]

[26] Tungmunnithum D, Thongboonyou A, Pholboon A, Yangsabai A. Flavonoids and Other Phenolic Compounds from Medicinal Plants for Pharmaceutical and Medical Aspects: An Overview. Medicines

(Basel) 2018; 5(3): 93.
[http://dx.doi.org/10.3390/medicines5030093] [PMID: 30149600]

[27]   Altaf MM, Khan MSA, Ahmad I. Diversity of Bioactive Compounds and Their Therapeutic
       Potential.New Look to Phytomedicine. Cambridge, MA, USA: Academic Press 2019; pp. 15-34.
       [http://dx.doi.org/10.1016/B978-0-12-814619-4.00002-1]

[28]   Bandaranayake MW. Quality control, screening, toxicity, and regulation of herbal drugs. Modern
       Phytomedicine Turning Medicinal Plants into Drugs KGaA. Weinheim: WILEY-VCH Verlag GmbH
       & Co. 2006; pp. 25-57.
       [http://dx.doi.org/10.1002/9783527609987.ch2]

[29]   World Health Organization: Traditional, Complementary and Integrative Medicine. Available from:
       www.who.int/health-topics/traditional-complementary-and-integrative-medicine#tab=tab_1 (Accessed
       on 24 August 2021).

[30]   Ceuterick M, Vandebroek I. Identity in a medicine cabinet: Discursive positions of Andean migrants
       towards their use of herbal remedies in the United Kingdom. Soc Sci Med 2017; 177: 43-51.
       [http://dx.doi.org/10.1016/j.socscimed.2017.01.026] [PMID: 28157568]

[31]   Sathasivampillai SV, Rajamanoharan PRS, Munday M, Heinrich M. Plants used to treat diabetes in Sri
       Lankan Siddha Medicine – An ethnopharmacological review of historical and modern sources. J
       Ethnopharmacol 2017; 198: 531-99.
       [http://dx.doi.org/10.1016/j.jep.2016.07.053] [PMID: 27448453]

[32]   Pan SY, Litscher G, Gao SH, *et al.* Historical perspective of traditional indigenous medical practices:
       the current renaissance and conservation of herbal resources. Evid Based Complement Alternat Med
       2014; 2014: 1-20.
       [http://dx.doi.org/10.1155/2014/525340] [PMID: 24872833]

[33]   Liu Y, Hu R, Shen S, *et al.* Plant diversity in herbal tea and its traditional knowledge in Qingtian
       County, Zhejiang Province, China. Plant Divers 2020; 42(6): 464-72.
       [http://dx.doi.org/10.1016/j.pld.2020.12.002] [PMID: 33733014]

[34]   Haustein UF. 1991.https://pubmed.ncbi.nlm.nih.gov/2010292/

[35]   Budhiraja SS, Cullum ME, Sioutis SS, Evangelista L, Habanova ST. Biological activity of Melaleuca
       alternifolia (tea tree) oil component, terpinen-4-ol, in human myelocytic cell line HL-60. J
       Manipulative Physiol Ther 1999; 22(7): 447-53.
       [http://dx.doi.org/10.1016/S0161-4754(99)70033-3] [PMID: 10519561]

[36]   Cox SD, Mann CM, Markham JL. Interactions between components of the essential oil of *Melaleuca
       alternifolia.* J Appl Microbiol 2001; 91(3): 492-7.
       [http://dx.doi.org/10.1046/j.1365-2672.2001.01406.x] [PMID: 11556915]

[37]   Surjushe A, Vasani R, Saple DG. *Aloe vera*: A short review. Indian J Dermatol 2008; 53(4): 163-6.
       [http://dx.doi.org/10.4103/0019-5154.44785] [PMID: 19882025]

[38]   Oyelami OA, Onayemi A, Oyedeji OA, Adeyemi LA. Preliminary study of effectiveness of *Aloe vera*
       in scabies treatment. Phytother Res 2009; 23(10): 1482-4.
       [http://dx.doi.org/10.1002/ptr.2614] [PMID: 19274696]

[39]   Abdel-Ghaffar F, Sobhy HM, Al-Quraishy S, Semmler M. Field study on the efficacy of an extract of
       neem seed (Mite -Stop®) against the red mite *Dermanyssus gallinae* naturally infecting poultry in
       Egypt. Parasitol Res 2008; 103(3): 481-5.
       [http://dx.doi.org/10.1007/s00436-008-0965-9] [PMID: 18481087]

[40]   Husni P, Dewi MK, Putriana NA, Hendriani R. *In-Vivo* effectiveness of 5% *Azadirachta indica* oil
       cream as anti-scabies. Pharmacol Clin Pharm Res 2019; 4(1): 10-5.
       [http://dx.doi.org/10.15416/pcpr.v4i1.21388]

[41]   Chen Z, Deng Y, Yin Z, *et al.* Studies on the acaricidal mechanism of the active components from
       neem (*Azadirachta indica*) oil against *Sarcoptes scabiei* var. cuniculi. Vet Parasitol 2014; 204(3-4):

323-9.
[http://dx.doi.org/10.1016/j.vetpar.2014.05.040] [PMID: 24974121]

[42] Seddiek SA, Khater HF, El-Shorbagy MM, Ali AM. The acaricidal efficacy of aqueous neem extract and ivermectin against *Sarcoptes scabiei* var. cuniculi in experimentally infested rabbits. Parasitol Res 2013; 112(6): 2319-30.
[http://dx.doi.org/10.1007/s00436-013-3395-2] [PMID: 23572045]

[43] Pasipanodya CN, Tekedza TT, Chatiza FP, Gororo E. Efficacy of neem (*Azadirachta indica*) aqueous fruit extracts against *Sarcoptes scabiei* var. suis in grower pigs. Trop Anim Health Prod 2021; 53(1): 135.
[http://dx.doi.org/10.1007/s11250-020-02545-7] [PMID: 33483804]

[44] Chen XL, Dodd G, Thomas S, *et al.* Activation of Nrf2/ARE pathway protects endothelial cells from oxidant injury and inhibits inflammatory gene expression. Am J Physiol Heart Circ Physiol 2006; 290(5): H1862-70.
[http://dx.doi.org/10.1152/ajpheart.00651.2005] [PMID: 16339837]

[45] Nieto G, Ros G, Castillo J. Antioxidant and antimicrobial properties of rosemary (*Rosmarinus officinalis*, L.): a review. Medicines (Basel) 2018; 5(3): 98.
[http://dx.doi.org/10.3390/medicines5030098] [PMID: 30181448]

[46] Zakaria ZA, Abdul Rahim MH, Roosli RAJ, *et al.* Antinociceptive activity of methanolic extract of *Clinacanthus nutans* leaves: possible mechanisms of action involved. Pain Res Manag 2018; 2018: 9536406.
[http://dx.doi.org/10.1155/2018/9536406] [PMID: 29686743]

[47] Hempenstall K, Nurmikko TJ, Johnson RW, A'Hern RP, Rice ASC. Analgesic therapy in postherpetic neuralgia: a quantitative systematic review. PLoS Med 2005; 2(7): e164.
[http://dx.doi.org/10.1371/journal.pmed.0020164] [PMID: 16013891]

[48] Suroowan S, Javeed F, Ahmad M, *et al.* Ethnoveterinary health management practices using medicinal plants in South Asia – a review. Vet Res Commun 2017; 41(2): 147-68.
[http://dx.doi.org/10.1007/s11259-017-9683-z] [PMID: 28405866]

[49] Jiang H, Wang J, Song L, *et al.* GC×GC-TOFMS analysis of essential oils composition from leaves, twigs and seeds of *Cinnamomum camphora* L. presl and their insecticidal and repellent activities. Molecules 2016; 21(4): 423.
[http://dx.doi.org/10.3390/molecules21040423] [PMID: 27043503]

[50] Nong X, Fang CL, Wang JH, *et al.* Acaricidal activity of extract from *Eupatorium adenophorum* against the Psoroptes cuniculi and *Sarcoptes scabiei in vitro.* Vet Parasitol 2012; 187(1-2): 345-9.
[http://dx.doi.org/10.1016/j.vetpar.2011.12.015] [PMID: 22244533]

[51] Gu X, Fang C, Yang G, *et al.* Acaricidal properties of an *Ailanthus altissima* bark extract against Psoroptes cuniculi and *Sarcoptes scabiei* var. cuniculi *in vitro.* Exp Appl Acarol 2014; 62(2): 225-32.
[http://dx.doi.org/10.1007/s10493-013-9736-0] [PMID: 24052400]

[52] Hanifah AL, Awang SH, Ming HT, Abidin SZ, Omar MH. Acaricidal activity of *Cymbopogon citratus* and *Azadirachta indica* against house dust mites. Asian Pac J Trop Biomed 2011; 1(5): 365-9.
[http://dx.doi.org/10.1016/S2221-1691(11)60081-6] [PMID: 23569794]

[53] Li M, Liu B, Bernigaud C, Fischer K, Guillot J, Fang F. Lemongrass (*Cymbopogon citratus*) oil: A promising miticidal and ovicidal agent against *Sarcoptes scabiei.* PLoS Negl Trop Dis 2020; 14(4): e0008225.
[http://dx.doi.org/10.1371/journal.pntd.0008225] [PMID: 32251453]

[54] Morsy TA, Rahem MA, el-Sharkawy EM, Shatat MA. *Eucalyptus globulus* (camphor oil) against the zoonotic scabies, *Sarcoptes scabiei.* J Egypt Soc Parasitol 2003; 33(1): 47-53.
[PMID: 12739800]

[55] Charles V, Charles SX. The use and efficacy of *Azadirachta indica* ADR ('Neem') and *Curcuma*

longa ('Turmeric') in scabies. A pilot study. Trop Geogr Med 1992; 44(1-2): 178-81.
[PMID: 1496714]

[56]   Topno SC, Sinha M. Study of medicinal plants used to heal skin diseases by tribes of west Singhbhum district of Jharkhand (India). J Pharmacogn Phytochem 2018; 7(1): 371-6.

[57]   Kamkar Asl M, Nazariborun A, Hosseini M. Analgesic effect of the aqueous and ethanolic extracts of clove. Avicenna J Phytomed 2013; 3(2): 186-92.
[PMID: 25050273]

[58]   Thomas J, Carson CF, Peterson GM, *et al.* Therapeutic potential of tea tree oil for scabies. Am J Trop Med Hyg 2016; 94(2): 258-66.
[http://dx.doi.org/10.4269/ajtmh.14-0515] [PMID: 26787146]

[59]   Mounsey KE, Holt DC, McCarthy J, Currie BJ, Walton SF. Scabies: molecular perspectives and therapeutic implications in the face of emerging drug resistance. Future Microbiol 2008; 3(1): 57-66.
[http://dx.doi.org/10.2217/17460913.3.1.57] [PMID: 18230034]

[60]   Walton SF, McKinnon M, Pizzutto S, Dougall A, Williams E, Currie BJ. Acaricidal activity of *Melaleuca alternifolia* (tea tree) oil: *in vitro* sensitivity of *Sarcoptes scabiei* var hominis to terpinenol. Arch Dermatol 2004; 140(5): 563-6.
[http://dx.doi.org/10.1001/archderm.140.5.563] [PMID: 15148100]

[61]   Zulkarnain I, Agusni RI, Hidayati AN. Comparison of tea tree oil 5% cream, tea tree oil 5%+permethrin 5% cream, and permethrine 5% cream in child scabies. Int J Clin Exp Med 2019; 4(6): 87-93.
[http://dx.doi.org/10.11648/j.ijcems.20180406.12]

[62]   Saravanan SKS, Velpandian V, Musthafa MD, *et al.* Clinical evaluation of thelkodukku chooranam (*Heliotropium indicum*) in the treatment of scabies. Int J Health Sci Res 2014; 4(1): 140-8.

[63]   Sharma B, Vasudeva N, Sharma S. Anti-scabies and mosquito repellent activity of *Crinum asiaticum* Linn. leaves extracts. Res J Pharm Technol 2020; 13(2): 895-900.
[http://dx.doi.org/10.5958/0974-360X.2020.00169.9]

[64]   Oladimeji FA, Orafidiya OO, Ogunniyi TAB, Adewunmi TA. Pediculocidal and scabicidal properties of *Lippia multiflora* essential oil. J Ethnopharmacol 2000; 72(1-2): 305-11.
[http://dx.doi.org/10.1016/S0378-8741(00)00229-4] [PMID: 10967487]

[65]   Samba N, Aitfella-Lahlou R, Nelo M, *et al.* Chemical composition and antibacterial activity of *Lippia multiflora* moldenke essential oil from different regions of angola. Molecules 2020; 26(1): 155.
[http://dx.doi.org/10.3390/molecules26010155] [PMID: 33396345]

[66]   Oladimeji FA, Orafidiya LO, Ogunniyi TAB, *et al.* A comparative study of the scabicidal activities of formulations of essential oil of *Lippia multiflora* Moldenke and benzyl benzoate emulsion BP. Int J Aromatherapy 2005; 15(2): 87-93.
[http://dx.doi.org/10.1016/j.ijat.2005.03.005]

[67]   Ullah N, Akhtar R, Lateef M, Jan SU, Zahid B, Durrani UF. Factors affecting the prevalence of ticks in cattle and acaricidal activity of *Nicotiana tabacum* extracts. J Hell Vet Med Soc 2019; 70(1): 1381-6.
[http://dx.doi.org/10.12681/jhvms.20343]

[68]   Castillo AL, Osi MO, Ramos JDA, De Francia JL, Dujunco MU, Quilala PF. Efficacy and safety of *Tinospora cordifolia* lotion in *Sarcoptes scabiei* var hominis-infected pediatric patients: A single blind, randomized controlled trial. J Pharmacol Pharmacother 2013; 4(1): 39-46.
[http://dx.doi.org/10.4103/0976-500X.107668] [PMID: 23662023]

[69]   Thomas CC, Miller EE. Rotenone in the treatment of scabies. a new, nonodorous, nonirritating form of treatment. preliminary report. Am J Med Sci 1940; 199(5): 670-4.
[http://dx.doi.org/10.1097/00000441-194005000-00011]

[70]   Singalavanija S, Limpongsanurak W, Soponsakunkul S. A comparative study between 10 per cent

sulfur ointment and 0.3 per cent gamma benzene hexachloride gel in the treatment of scabies in children. J Med Assoc Thai 2003; 86(3) (Suppl. 3): S531-6.
[PMID: 14700144]

[71]   Rais N, Ved A, Ahmad R, *et al.* Potential of s-allyl cysteine, a major bioactive component of garlic, as hypoglycemic and hypolipidemic agent. Curr Res Diabetes Obes J 2021; 14(4): 555895.
[http://dx.doi.org/10.19080/CRDOJ.2021.14.555895]

[72]   Abebe D, Ayehu A. Medicinal plants and enigmatic health practices of northern Ethiopia. Agri Inf Syst 1993; 13: 45-50.

[73]   Asres K. Alkaloids and flavonoids from the species of Leguminosae. PhD Thesis. 1986; pp. 56-60.

[74]   Abate G. Etse Debdabe (Ethiopian Traditional Medicine). Addis Ababa: Addis Ababa University 1989; pp. 34-40.

[75]   Seebaluck R, Gurib-Fakim A, Mahomoodally F. Medicinal plants from the genus Acalypha (Euphorbiaceae)–a review of their ethnopharmacology and phytochemistry. J Ethnopharmacol 2015; 159: 137-57.
[http://dx.doi.org/10.1016/j.jep.2014.10.040] [PMID: 25446604]

[76]   Rahmatullah M, Das A, Mollik M, *et al.* An ethnomedicinal survey of Dhamrai sub-district in Dhaka district, Bangladesh. Am Eurasian J Sust Agri 2009; 3(4): 881-8.

[77]   Acharya K, Kaphle K. Ethnomedicinal plants used by yak herders for management of health disorders. J Intercult Ethnopharmacol 2015; 4(4): 270-6.
[http://dx.doi.org/10.5455/jice.20151101093353] [PMID: 26649231]

[78]   Hossan MS, Hanif A, Khan M, *et al.* Ethnobotanical survey of the Tripura tribe of Bangladesh. Am Eurasian J Sustain Agric 2009; 3(2): 253-61.

[79]   Vaidyanathan D, Senthilkumar M, Basha M. Studies on ethnomedicinal plants used by malayali tribals in Kolli hills of eastern ghats, Tamilnadu, India. Asian J Plant Sci Res 2013; 3(6): 29-45.

[80]   Rahmatullah M, Ferdausi D, Mollik A, Jahan R, Chowdhury MH, Haque WM. A survey of medicinal plants used by kavirajes of chalna area, Khulna district, Bangladesh. Afr J Tradit Complement Altern Med 2010; 7(2): 91-7.
[http://dx.doi.org/10.4314/ajtcam.v7i2.50859] [PMID: 21304618]

[81]   De Britto J, Mahesh R. Evolutionary medicine of Kani tribal's botanical knowledge in Agasthiayamalai biosphere reserve, South India. Ethnobotanical Leaflets 2007; 7(1): 31-40.

[82]   Harsha VH, Hebbar SS, Shripathi V, Hegde GR. Ethnomedicobotany of Uttara Kannada District in Karnataka, India—plants in treatment of skin diseases. J Ethnopharmacol 2003; 84(1): 37-40.
[http://dx.doi.org/10.1016/S0378-8741(02)00261-1] [PMID: 12499074]

[83]   Zakaria Z, Mat A, Sulaiman M, *et al.* The *In-vitro* antibacterial activity of methanol and ethanol extracts of *Carica papaya* flowers and *Mangifera indica* leaves. J Pharmacol Toxicol 2006; 1(3): 278-83.
[http://dx.doi.org/10.3923/jpt.2006.278.283]

[84]   Goyer C, Vachon J, Beaulieu C. Pathogenicity of *Streptomyces scabies* mutants altered in thaxtomin a production. Phytopathology 1998; 88(5): 442-5.
[http://dx.doi.org/10.1094/PHYTO.1998.88.5.442] [PMID: 18944924]

[85]   Dimri U, Sharma MC. Effects of sarcoptic mange and its control with oil of *Cedrus deodara, Pongamia glabra, Jatropha curcas* and benzyl benzoate, both with and without ascorbic acid on growing sheep: epidemiology; assessment of clinical, haematological, cell-mediated humoral immune responses and pathology. J Vet Med A Physiol Pathol Clin Med 2004; 51(2): 71-8.
[http://dx.doi.org/10.1111/j.1439-0442.2004.00601.x] [PMID: 15153076]

[86]   Saha M, Sarker D, Kar P, Gupta P, Sen A. Indigenous knowledge of plants in local healthcare management practices by tribal people of Malda district, India. J Intercult Ethnopharmacol 2014; 3(4):

179-85.
[http://dx.doi.org/10.5455/jice.20140630022609] [PMID: 26401370]

[87]   Jeruto P, Arama PF, Anyango B, Maroa G. Phytochemical screening and antibacterial investigations of crude methanol extracts of *Senna didymobotrya* (Fresen.) H. S. Irwin & Barneby. J Appl Biosci 2017; 114(1): 11357-67.
[http://dx.doi.org/10.4314/jab.v114i1.9]

[88]   Njoroge GN, Bussmann RW. Ethnotherapeautic management of skin diseases among the Kikuyus of Central Kenya. J Ethnopharmacol 2007; 111(2): 303-7.
[http://dx.doi.org/10.1016/j.jep.2006.11.025] [PMID: 17207950]

[89]   Akubue PI, Mittal GC, Aguwa CN. Preliminary pharmacological study of some Nigerian medicinal plants. 1. J Ethnopharmacol 1983; 8(1): 53-63.
[http://dx.doi.org/10.1016/0378-8741(83)90089-2] [PMID: 6632937]

[90]   Ajose FOA. Some Nigerian plants of dermatologic importance. Int J Dermatol 2007; 46(s1) (Suppl. 1): 48-55.
[http://dx.doi.org/10.1111/j.1365-4632.2007.03466.x] [PMID: 17919209]

[91]   Heyndrickx G, Brioen P, Van Puyvelde L. Study of Rwandese medicinal plants used in the treatment of scabies. J Ethnopharmacol 1992; 35(3): 259-62.
[http://dx.doi.org/10.1016/0378-8741(92)90022-J] [PMID: 1548897]

[92]   Ravindranath N, Venkataiah B, Ramesh C, Jayaprakash P, Das B. Jatrophenone, a novel macrocyclic bioactive diterpene from *Jatropha gossypifolia.* Chem Pharm Bull (Tokyo) 2003; 51(7): 870-1.
[http://dx.doi.org/10.1248/cpb.51.870] [PMID: 12843600]

[93]   Félix-Silva J, Giordani RB, Silva-Jr AA, Zucolotto SM, Fernandes-Pedrosa MF. *Jatropha gossypiifolia* L. (Euphorbiaceae): a review of traditional uses, phytochemistry, pharmacology, and toxicology of this medicinal plant. Evid Based Complement Alternat Med 2014; 2014: 1-32.
[http://dx.doi.org/10.1155/2014/369204] [PMID: 25002902]

[94]   Eisenberg DM, Kessler RC, Foster C, Norlock FE, Calkins DR, Delbanco TL. Unconventional medicine in the United States. Prevalence, costs, and patterns of use. N Engl J Med 1993; 328(4): 246-52.
[http://dx.doi.org/10.1056/NEJM199301283280406] [PMID: 8418405]

[95]   Ahmad S, Parveen A, Parveen B, Parveen R. Challenges and guidelines for clinical trial of herbal drugs. J Pharm Bioallied Sci 2015; 7(4): 329-33.
[http://dx.doi.org/10.4103/0975-7406.168035] [PMID: 26681895]

[96]   Thadanipon K, Anothaisintawee T, Rattanasiri S, Thakkinstian A, Attia J. Efficacy and safety of antiscabietic agents: A systematic review and network meta-analysis of randomized controlled trials. J Am Acad Dermatol 2019; 80(5): 1435-44.
[http://dx.doi.org/10.1016/j.jaad.2019.01.004] [PMID: 30654070]

[97]   Campbell JJ, Paulson CP, Nashelsky J. Clinical Inquiry: What is the most effective treatment for scabies? J Fam Pract 2017; 66(8): E11-2.
[PMID: 28783773]

[98]   Atanasov AG, Waltenberger B, Pferschy-Wenzig EM, *et al.* Discovery and resupply of pharmacologically active plant-derived natural products: A review. Biotechnol Adv 2015; 33(8): 1582-614.
[http://dx.doi.org/10.1016/j.biotechadv.2015.08.001] [PMID: 26281720]

[99]   Harvey AL, Edrada-Ebel R, Quinn RJ. The re-emergence of natural products for drug discovery in the genomics era. Nat Rev Drug Discov 2015; 14(2): 111-29.
[http://dx.doi.org/10.1038/nrd4510] [PMID: 25614221]

[100]   Atanasov AG, Zotchev SB, Dirsch VM, Supuran CT. Natural products in drug discovery: advances and opportunities. Nat Rev Drug Discov 2021; 20(3): 200-16.

[http://dx.doi.org/10.1038/s41573-020-00114-z] [PMID: 33510482]

[101] https://www.who.int/news-room/fact-sheets/detail/scabies

[102] Swe PM, Reynolds SL, Fischer K. Parasitic scabies mites and associated bacteria joining forces against host complement defence. Parasite Immunol 2014; 36(11): 585-93.
[http://dx.doi.org/10.1111/pim.12133] [PMID: 25081184]

[103] Available from: https://www.cdc.gov/parasites/scabies/epi.html (Access on 25/08/2021).

[104] Hay RJ. Scabies and pyodermas - diagnosis and treatment. Dermatol Ther 2009; 22(6): 466-74.
[http://dx.doi.org/10.1111/j.1529-8019.2009.01270.x] [PMID: 19889132]

[105] Nigussie G. A review on traditionally used medicinal plants for scabies therapy in Ethiopia. Advances in Traditional Medicine 2021; 21(2): 199-208. [ADTM].
[http://dx.doi.org/10.1007/s13596-020-00453-7]

[106] Petrovska B. Historical review of medicinal plants' usage. Pharmacogn Rev 2012; 6(11): 1-5.
[http://dx.doi.org/10.4103/0973-7847.95849] [PMID: 22654398]

[107] Zhang J, Onakpoya IJ, Posadzki P, Eddouks M. The safety of herbal medicine: from prejudice to evidence. Evid Based Complement Alternat Med 2015; 2015: 1-3.
[http://dx.doi.org/10.1155/2015/316706] [PMID: 25838831]

CHAPTER 6

Back to the Roots: Natural Cosmetics and their Future Applications

Olayinka Oderinde[1,*], Onome Ejeromedoghene[2], Kingsley Igenepo John[3], Abimbola Koforowola Onasanya[4], Muyideen Olaitan Bamidele[1] and **Adegboyega Ayo Ogunbela[4]**

[1] *Department of Chemistry, Faculty of Natural and Applied Sciences, Lead City University, Ibadan, Nigeria*

[2] *School of Chemistry and Chemical Engineering, Southeast University, Jiulonghu Campus, Nanjing 211189, PR China*

[3] *Lab of Department of Pure and Applied Chemistry, College of Natural Sciences, Veritas University, Abuja, PMB 5171, Abuja, Nigeria*

[4] *Forestry Research Institute of Nigeria (FRIN), Jericho, PMB 5054, Ibadan, Nigeria*

Abstract: Numerous concerns have been raised on the side effects of the prolonged usage of synthetic compounds in cosmetics production, including skin damage due to inflammations, rashes, and itching, just to mention a few. These skin side effects have been reported to be linked to the break-down of homeostasis of the repair system against deoxyribonucleic acid (DNA) and tissue destruction. These can lead to accelerated aging, melanogenesis, and cell growth senescence or even cause cancer of the skin. Efforts to overcome these problems associated with synthetic cosmetics have led to the use of natural cosmetics of plant and animal origin. Natural cosmetics have been found to contain essential oils and other extracts that can alleviate or inhibit skin-associated problems, such as eczema, allergy, acne, dryness, and discoloration, while also containing anti-aging, anti-tyrosinase, antioxidants, and anti-inflammatory substances. In this chapter, some cosmetics products from plants (herbs) and animal extraction are highlighted alongside their applications in skin care. At the same time, also, the future perspectives and recommendations of these natural extracts are proffered.

Keywords: Cosmetics , Anti-microbials, Antioxidants, Anti-ageing, Collagen, Cosmeceutics, Microalgae, Natural clay, Plant, UV-protection.

---

* **Corresponding author Olayinka Oderinde:** Department of Chemistry, Faculty of Natural and Applied Sciences, Lead City University, Ibadan, Nigeria; Tel: +234-8032801872; E-mail: yinkaoderinde@yahoo.com

Heba Abd El-Sattar El-Nashar, Mohamed El-Shazly & Nouran Mohammed Fahmy (Eds.)

INTRODUCTION

Cosmetics are regarded as any substance or preparation intended to be placed in contact with the various outer parts of the human body or even with the tooth whitening and the mucous membranes of the oral cavity with a view, exclusively or mainly, to clean, perfume, change their appearance and/or correct body odors and/or protect or keep them in good condition. Cleansing shampoos, perfumes, skin moisturizers, whitening creams, hair colors, and other constituent elements meant for use in cosmetic applications are included as cosmetics. By this definition, cosmetics are often used to take care of body parts, but their usage alone does not benefit users [1 - 4]. For more than two decades, the research and development in the cosmetic industry are becoming huge. These have resulted in an extensive range of skincare products that treat signs of aging, inflammation, and other skin disease-related issues. The end-users of these cosmetics are now more oblivious about their appearance, thereby making efforts to accept the new societal paradigm shift, which has led to the present greater demand for natural cosmetics [5]. The recent paradigm shift and growth in the demand for cosmetics of natural component extraction have activated the search for plant extracts containing extraordinary sources of bioactive compounds, as these natural cosmetics have been perceived to be healthy for the skin [6]. This has brought about the development of cosmeceuticals, which combine the esthetical properties of a cosmetic with the efficacy of a dermatological drug [7].

In recent times, natural sources-based cosmetic ingredients are topping the list of newly-launched cosmeceutical products, chiefly due to the end-user acceptance of outstanding efficiency and reduction in side effects as several firms are actively involved in the evaluation of the efficacy of an identified natural product or discovery of a novel molecule from various natural sources [8]. This is in addition to the several reported side effects of synthetic chemicals used in the formulation of synthetic-based cosmetics [9 - 11]. Of the several sources of natural products for cosmetic production, herbs- and marine-algae-derived materials are highly valued ingredients, while animal-derived materials are under stringent monitoring due to animal rights regulations.

Natural ingredients in cosmetics play significant roles such as anti-inflammatory, anti-aging, anti-tumor, antioxidant, *etc.* For instance, *astaxanthin* from *Phaffia rhodozyma, Thraustochytrids,* and *Rhotorula spp.* is an antioxidant, while purified hyaluronic acid from *S. thermophilus* is used for anti-aging [12]. Several plants (herbs) have reportedly been utilized for cosmetics formulations. For example, the natural cosmeceutical potentials (antioxidant, anti-enzymatic, antimicrobial, anti-inflammatory, and photoprotection potential) of *Grateloupia turuturu* were reported [13], while Pipattanamomgkol *et al.* [14] also revealed the hair dyeing ability of *Cleistocalyx nervosum var. paniala* fruit. The extracted product was incorporated into the stable base of hair coloring spray and was found to be efficiently stained, with persisting ability even after five-cycle washing. Furthermore, the extracts from *Zingiber cassumunar Roxb.* rhizome was also researched for cosmetic potentials by Li *et al.* [15]. The team investigated the 1,1-diphenyl-2-picrylhydrazyl (DPPH) radical scavenging, HDFa collagen secretion promotion, tyrosinase inhibition, and NO generation inhibition activities of the extract and reported that *Z. cassumunar* possessed remarkable HDFa collagen secretion promotion and tyrosinase inhibition activities. The antioxidant and cytotoxicity of extracts from alfalfa herb and *Medicago sativa L.* were also reported by Zagórska-Dziok and coworkers [16]. A higher inhibitory effect on free radicals existing in the outer environment of the fibroblasts and keratinocytes cells was reported by the team, while a reduction in the intracellular reactive oxygen species (ROS) level was observed, which may have a potential contribution to the reduction of the cellular oxidative stress. More also, the anti-aging, skin-whitening, and antibacterial potentials of *Rosa chinensis* cv. 'JinBian' extracts were evaluated [17]. The study revealed that all the isolated compounds exhibited moderate to remarkable high antioxidant, anti-bacterial, and tyrosinase inhibitory activities, making *R. chinensis* a potential for cosmetic formulation. Additionally, herbal (black) soap made from non-timber forest- (NTFPs) and agro-processing waste products (APWPs), and some value-addition products (VAPs) have been reported [18]. This "black" soap is most widely used by locals in Southwest Nigeria for cosmetics, medicinal and cultural purposes. The herbal (black) soap was produced from saponified freshly-cultivated palm oil (palm kernel oil) mixed with some dried cocoa pods, cassava peels, palm oil bunches and lye. Further analysis revealed that the conductivity ranges from 18,200-47,150 (µS/cm), indicating the extent of dissolved ions in the soap materials, which then permeate into the skin and nourish it when used. Locally, this soap has been used in curing skin diseases such as ringworm, eczema, prosiasi, and wounds, as well as being used as an anti-fibroid drug when formulated with other local materials. Other plants reported for cosmeceutical applications include *Trichilia catigua* [19], *Anthriscus cerefolium,* and *Anthriscus sylvestris* [20], *Achillea biebersteinii* Afan [21], *Achillea millefolium* L [22], *Spirulina, Palmaria Palmata, Cichorium Intybus,* and *Medicago Sativa* [23] *Thunbergia laurifolia* Lindl [24], *Vitis vinifera* L, *Dirmophandra mollis* Benth, *Ruta graveolens* L, and *Ginkgo biloba* L [25], *Allium fistulosum* [26], Arabica coffee cherry [27], *Aloe vera* (L.) [28 - 30], amongst several others.

The several compounds of terpenoids, phenolics, polyphenolics, vitamins, selenium, polysaccharides, and volatile organic compounds found in several mushroom species (*Lentinula edodes, Ganoderma lucidum, Sparassis latifolia, Grifola frondose, Wolfiporia extensa*, just to mention a few, have also been reported to reveal remarkable anti-aging, antioxidant, anti-wrinkle, skin whitening and immunity-boosting effects, which make them be potentials in cosmetics products formulation [31 - 37]. For example, the natural cosmetic potentials of some mushroom species of *Agaricus bisporus*, *Lentinula edodes*, and *Pleurotus ostreatus* extracts have been evaluated and confirmed for their anti-inflammatory, anti-bacterial, antioxidant, and anti-tyrosinase activities [34, 38]. Interestingly, quite a number of reviews have been written showing the documentation on the utilization of herbal plants in the local production of cosmetics. For example, Wathoni *et al.* [39] published a review of several herbal-based cosmetics in Indonesia with different ingredients (*Solanum lycopersicum*, *Syzygium cumini*, *Eleutherine Americana Merr*, *Muntingia calabura*, *Murraya paniculate*, *Curcuma Domestica. Val.*, *Cananga odorata, etc.*) for varying usage on skin. Ndhlovu *et al.* [1] also wrote a comprehensive review of plants (*Acanthospermum hispidum DC*, *Adansonia digitata L*, *Aloe aageodonta L.*, *Brackenridgea zanguebarica Oliv.*, *Cannabis sativa L*, just to mention a few.) used for cosmetic and cosmeceutical purposes among women in Vhembe District Municipality in South Africa. In addition, Sagbo and Mbeng [40] analyzed 105 plant species (70 of the species for skin care) used by the Eastern Cape Province of South Africa. More also, Othman *et al.* [41] also published ten commonly used plants for cosmetic purposes in Malaysia, while Mahomoodally and Ramjuttun [3], reported a quantitative survey of twenty-nine (29) herbs belonging to twenty-one (21) families having twenty-nine (29) different cosmetic applications.

Algae (macroalgae and microalgae) which are aquatic photosynthetic organisms have caught the attention of cosmetic producers, as their metabolic products are known for their skin benefits, including UV radiation protection, rough texture prevention, wrinkles, and skin flaccidity. Their antioxidant compounds also inhibit skin aging [42]. The extract of marine algae, *Fucus vesiculosus*, is very active to reduce the appearance of dark circles in the skin beneath the eye. This is done by stimulating the heme oxygenase 1 (HO-1), which will, in turn, stimulate the scavenging of heme, thereby reducing the appearance of dark circles [43]. Also, *Ecklonia cava* is a perennial brown macroalga that contains phlorotannins, including eckol and dieckol. Both *E. cava* extract and dieckol have been reported to inhibit the expression of the *COX-1*, *COX-2*, *mPGES-1*, and *mPGES-2* genes involved in PGE_2 synthesis. In a three-dimensional reconstructed skin model, dieckol also debilitated the morphological changes induced by particulate matter. Eckol, on the other hand, decreases the reactive oxygen species (ROS) levels, in addition to inhibiting oxidative damage to lipids, proteins, and DNA in particulate matter-exposed HaCaT keratinocytes, and enervate PM-induced cell apoptosis by modulating MAP kinase signaling pathways [44 - 47]. Carotenes accumulated in microalgae have also been found to prevent over-reduction of the photosynthetic electron transport chain and the formation of excess ROS. They also provide protection due to their antioxidant activity, protecting the body from damaging free radicals, shielding the skin from UV radiation effects, ameliorating macular degeneration, and enhancing the immune system [48 - 50]. Mycosporine-like amino acids (MAAs) and scytone-min (Scy) are also important photoprotectants present in algae, with great efficacy to protect from harmful UV radiation (photoaging) and other ROS-associated disorder [51]. Furthermore, algal oil and sterols have been associated with restoring the water-lipid mantle of the skin, and also as potential agents for the treatment of atherosclerosis alongside having anti-tumor and anti-inflammatory effects, respectively [52, 53]. Several other biologically active compounds extracted from algae have been reviewed extensively and reported elsewhere [3, 54 - 57].

NATURAL-BASED COSMETICS

Natural ingredients used in cosmetic products can be extracted from plants and animals or by recombinant protein production systems, including yeast, bacteria, cells, or artificial fibrils [58]. A general overview of the oil extract and non-oil extract of natural ingredients in cosmetics, natural pigments in cosmetics, and natural clays is herein presented in this section.

Oil Extracts

Natural-based cosmetics can be derived from various oil extracts of plants and animals and are very useful as antioxidants, anti-aging, anti-inflammatory, *etc.*, agents in cosmetics. Essential oils contain volatile and liquid aromatic compounds, including terpenoids, benzenoids, fatty acid derivatives, and alcohols, and those extracted from plants have been used in the preparation of cosmetics, especially in perfumery, hair care, inhalation, baths, massages, and steam treatments. Additionally, some of them have been reported to exhibit different medicinal and cosmetic properties [59]. For example, coconut oil, which has been used in the manufacturing of marine soaps [60], is also an essential element for hair conditioners, shampoos, and shower gels, with remarkable usage as an emollient, anti-skin infections, anti-aging, anti-redness, preventing dry skin and loss of protein from hair [61]. Also, olive oil, which has shown potency for anti-inflammatory and anti-oxidating effects, its application has been reported to face and hand lightening and hair growth stimulation, while prolonged usage prevents sweat, alopecia, scabies and dandruff. The presence of vitamins and high concentrations of squalene, phytosterols, and tocopherols, as well as linoleic derivatives, gives its potential emollient and protective properties for the epidermis [62]. More also, the presence of linolenic acid in basil oil enhances its inhibition of the arachidonate metabolism pathways of lipoxygenase and cyclooxygenase, thereby preventing aging [61]. Other oils including pumpkin oil (for treating herpes lesions, pimples, and blackheads, with other applications in sprains and pulled ligaments) [61], calendula (for treating radiation dermatitis) [60], Jojoba oil (for white skin replenishment and natural pH restoration), carrot seed oil (for rejuvenating and anti-aging), eucalyptus oil (for hair nutrition and darkening) [61], *Salvia officinalis* essential oil (antioxidant and antimicrobial properties) [63], *Ferulago angulate* essential oil (antioxidant and antimicrobial properties) [64], pomelo peel essential oil (antioxidant and anti-melanogenic effects) [65], *Etlingera elatior* essential oil (photoprotective and antioxidant) [66], *Origanum vulgare L.* essential oil (anti-skin aging) [67], have been reported, amongst several others. Furthermore, a review of oil extracts and compositions alongside cosmeceutical properties from some plants has been written by Moore *et al.* [68].

Non-Oil Extracts

The largest group of non-oil extracts are biological surfactants. Surface-active chemicals generated from microorganisms such as yeast, fungus, and bacteria are known as bio-surfactants. Bio-surfactants are unique among natural surfactants because of their microbial origin and have gained significant attention due to their benefits over synthetic surfactants, including lower toxicity, higher biodegradability, excellent environmental compatibility, and a wide range of biological activities [69]. Bio-surfactants have been a popular choice in producing cosmetic and medicinal goods due to their potential to reduce interfacial/surface tension [70]. Based on their molecular weight, bio-surfactants are divided into two categories. Bio-surfactants with low molecular weight are effective at reducing surface and interfacial tension. Bio-surfactants with high molecular weight are more effective as emulsion stabilizers. Polymeric bio-surfactants, glycolipids: lipopeptides and lipoproteins, fatty acids, phospholipids, and neutral lipids, and particulate bio-surfactants are the five major categories of bio-surfactants [70]. Bio-surfactants are produced by microorganisms to increase cell mobility, offer nutrients, and aid in environmental growth. *Rhamnolipids*, a form of bio-surfactant produced by *Pseudomonas spp.*, are an example of this type of bio-surfactant [71]. Other microbes, such as *Arthrobacter spp.*, *Mycobacterium spp.*, and *Rhodococcus erythropolis*, modify their cell wall structure by generating lipopolysaccharides surfactants or nonionic *trehalose corynomycolates* [71]. A certain number of these surfactants are now available for commercial use. As a case study, "Saponin", a class of water-soluble high molecular weight glycosidic surfactant extracted from plants and animals, is now registered with the International Nomenclature of Cosmetic Ingredients (INCI) and commercially available for use [71].

Extracts from species such as *Agrimonia pilosa* (*A. pilosa)*, *Houttuynia cordata*, and *Licorice (Glycyrrhiza uralensis)*, have also been associated with skin barrier restoration, anti-inflammation, alleviated atopic dermatitis, anti-aging, respectively [12, 72, 73]. For over a century in Asia, *Paeonia lactiflora* extract has been proven to help with various skin irritations and skin damage caused by ROS in a previously reported study [74]. Some of these plant extracts have been commercialized. The first plant cell extract to be commercialized was *Malus Domestica* and named PhytoCELLTECH by Mibelle Biochemistry Company. Its effect on human skin cells was also investigated by this company [75]. The core of an endangered Swiss apple species, the *Uttwiler Spätlauber*, was used to create PhytoCELLTECH *Malus Domestica*, which can be preserved for a long time without fading or losing flavor. Apple cell culture extracts derived from the *Malus Domestica* cultivar *Uttwiler Spätlauber* which protects skin cells, have been patented [75]. One of the most common animal extract sources is collagen. Collagen has sparked a lot of interest in the cosmetic industry because of its availability, strength, and direct relationship with skin aging [58]. Collagen fibers in the body are known to be damaged over time, losing thickness and strength, linked to skin aging. Therefore, cosmetic manufacturers incorporate collagen extracts to correct or replace damaged collagen, which improves users' youthfulness and well-being. Collagen extracts are formulated in creams, nutritional supplements, vascular and heart restoration, skin replacement, and soft skin augmentation. Collagen extract from marine fish for cosmetic formulation has been researched by Alves *et al.* [76]. The team analysed collagen extract from salmon and codfish skins and revealed that the Type I collagen was of high purity and demonstrated a good water retention capacity, hence suitable for applications as a dermal moisturizer. Also, lecithin extracts (phosphatidylcholine and phosphatidylethanolamine) and lecithin-derived composites from marine animals (including salmon, squids, krill, and water fleas) have also been identified due to their high content of ω-3 fatty acids, hence providing anti-inflammatory and immunological properties [77 - 80]. Moreover, extracts from other plant sources that have been linked to remarkable cosmeceutical properties include cucumber- and lemon extracts for hyperpigmentation treatment [81]; garlic extract for controlling dandruff [82]; *Morinda citrifolia* L for wrinkles and protection of the skin from erythema caused by ultraviolet light, as well as anti-inflammatory activity in acne [83]; black tea, telang flower as secang wood extracts can functionell as possessing the antioxidants potential which can inhibit UV radiation to the skin [84]; methanolic extract of *Pradosia mutisii* have been associated with anti-photoaging and anti-melanogenic properties *via* mitogen-activated protein kinase regulation [85], just to mention a few.

Natural Pigments for Cosmetics

Pigments are organic or inorganic chemicals used to color foods, textiles, cosmetics, and pharmaceuticals [86]. The toxicity and carcinogenicity of synthetic pigments have a significant setback to their continuous use. Thus, friendly natural pigments that can substitute synthetic ones are now the focus of researchers. Anthocyanins, carotenoids, betalains, and chlorophylls are just a few of the components that make up plant pigments [87]. Plant pigments are divided into fat-soluble pigments found in the plastid of plant protoplasm (protoplasts) and water-soluble pigments found in the cell sap. Anthoxanthins and anthocyanins are fat-soluble pigments, while chlorophylls and carotenoids are water-soluble pigments. Anthocyanins occur in all tissues of higher plants, providing color in all parts of plants, and can range in hue from red to blue depending on the pH [87]. Because of their ability to endure harsh climatic conditions, microalgae are a vital source of natural pigments used in cosmetics products. They are accessible all year and easy to extract [88]. Due to the entire microalgae biomass incorporation challenge into cosmetic formulations, innovative extraction and purification procedures have been developed to explore its potential in cosmetics. Common traditional microalgae species extracted and applied in cosmetic formulations include *Dunaliella, Chlorella, Haematococcus, and Arthrospira* [56]. Table **1** summarizes microalgae pigment used in cosmetics obtainable in the market [88].

Table 1. Microalgae and their pigments used in commercialized cosmetic products [88].

Cosmetics	Microalgae	Pigment	Dealer
Dermochlorella®D	*Chlorella Vulgaris*	Carotenoids	Codif Recherche and Nature (France) (CODIF 2020)
Megassane®	*Phaeodactylum tricornutum*	NI*	Soliance (France) (GIVAUDAN 2020)
Astapure®-Ctive	*Haematococcus pluvialis*	Astaxanthin	Algatech (Israel) (ALGATECH 2020)
Linablue®	*Arthrospira spp.*	Phycocyanin	Dainippon Ink and Chemicals Inc. (Japan) (DIC 2020)
Pepha®-Ctive	*Dunaliella salina*	β-Carotene	Pentapharm Ltd. (Switzerland) (DSM 2020)

NI*: no information.

Natural Clays

Natural clays are microscopic (< 2 µm) finely ground rocky materials consisting of one or several clay minerals with fewer other types of minerals or organic substances. Natural clay minerals are widely used in cosmetic products due to their high specific surface area, optimum rheological characteristics, and outstanding ion exchangeability [89]. The high cation-exchange capacity allows them to be organophilized to enhance their properties. This mineral product has also found its use in dermo-cosmetics applications, which predates history [90]. For applications of cosmetics formulations, natural clay should be innocuous, stable, chemically inert, and display a safe microbiological activity following the limit endorsed in the international Pharmacopoeia Standards. Kaolinite, talc, smectites, and fibrous clays are the most common clay minerals used in the cosmetics industry [91]. Natural clays are usually employed without applying any enrichment process, though sometimes there may be a need to remove some associated minerals that may lead to an overshoot of the pharmacopoeia requirements [92]. Clays have been found to be effective poultices in treating cutaneous inflammatory processes such as seborrhoeic dermatitis, psoriasis, chronic eczemas, or acne while it assists in the removal of skin oiliness and toxins, in addition to covering up skin maculae and patches [93, 94]. Also, due to their iridescence and high reflectance, clay cosmeceuticals have been used in makeup production and skin brightener in moisturizing creams [95], while their high refraction index and optimal light dispersion properties have made them useful as sunscreen [89, 96]. More also, some clay types also produce biogenic silica, which provides silicon, essential for collagen fibers synthesis, which helps in the treatment of osteo-articular and muscular-skeletal infections [97, 98]. Hoang-Minh *et al.* [99] have reported clays as protectants against UV radiation in the range of 250–400 nm. The team revealed that the UV-transmission values of some studied clay-cream samples were higher than those of the commercial sun cream Ladival® allerg 20, while Madikizela *et al.* [100] confirmed that cosmetic products manufactured from natural clay material have high sun protection factors (SPF) values, hence shield the skin from the damage of UV. On the other hand, Williams and Haydel [101] and Lafi and Al-Dulaimy [102] have both reported the antiseptic and disinfectant activities of clays against pathogenic bacteria, including *Mycobacterium ulcers, E. coli, S. typhimurium, P. aeruginosa,* and *M. marinum* [101] and *P. aeruginosa* and *S. aureus* [102]. Furthermore, da Silva Favero *et al.* [103] carried out extensive work on Melo bentonite clay as a suspensor agent in cosmetics, which was reported to be very efficient, while Bergamaschi *et al.* [104] reported the Spa Mud (from B.I.O.C.E.)–Italy for skin applications. The team, after making comparisons with industrially optimized mud, concluded that despite the high concentration of some heavy metals (*e.g.*, nickel) detected, there are no adverse effects, such as intolerance or allergy associated with the Spa bath.

TYPES OF NATURAL PRODUCTS-BASED COSMETICS

Skin Care Cosmetics

The human skin appears to be the largest organ and outer covering of the body, which protects the body against environmental factors and chemical compounds in cosmetic products [105]. Different chemical formulations in skin care cosmetic products have the potential to cause acute skin irritation or corrosion when it is not in coherence with the body system. More so, long-time use of synthetic chemicals-based skin care products could result in contact dermatitis, allergic contact dermatitis, phototoxic and photo-allergic reactions, amongst others [106]. Therefore, this must be assessed in order to protect the general users of such cosmetic products [107]. Nevertheless, the significant uprising in the consciousness of end users with regards to the components in skin care and beauty products has led to an increasing demand for natural products-based cosmetics. For example, Kamaruzaman and Mohamad [108] extracted water-soluble elastin powder from poultry skin and incorporated it into the moisturizer formulation system to promote better skin elasticity. In another study, Sim and Nyam [109] prepared a natural cosmetic prototype using *H. cannabinus* L. (Kenaf) leaves extract (KLE) as skin whitening and anti-aging agents. It was reported that the KLE lotion containing 15% kenaf seed oil and 0.1% w/w KLE yields the best physico-microbiological stability, without any toxicity on human cells. In a comparative study, Kozlowska *et al.* [110] showed that peeling products (exfoliators) containing natural biopolymers, sodium alginate and sodium alginate with starch beads had no skin irritation, redness, itching, or dryness compared to synthetic microbeads, and could be employed as abrasive ingredients in developing skin care cosmetic recipe. Although hyaluronic acid is considered among the best natural moisturizing substance, Chen *et al.* [111] revealed that quaternized carboxymethyl chitosan (QCMC)/organic montmorillonite nanocomposite (QCOM) displayed better moisture-adsorption and retention behaviors as well as good UV-protection ability. In the investigations of Almendinger *et al.* [112], it was reported that malt and beer-related by-products are biological sources of constituents for skin whitening cosmeceutical products with high antioxidant properties. Meanwhile, Barreto *et al.* [113] identified the polysaccharide-enriched fraction (EF) from the by-product of *Agave sisalana* as a promising moisturizing cosmetic raw material and nanoemulsion with no cytotoxic or phototoxic effects.

Hair Care Cosmetics

Human hair is very vital in reflecting the physical state and appearance of an individual. Primarily, the human hair contains fiber (~50–100 µm in diameter) comprising different layers of cellular structure such as the cuticle (the outer component responsible for the aesthetic properties of the hair), the cortex (the inner component comprising of biopolymeric keratin filaments held by disulfide and hydrogen bonds and is responsible for in the mechanical properties of the hair), and in some cases the medulla in the central region of the hair [114 - 116]. Hair treatment using synthetic chemical treatments like thioglycolate, ammonium persulfate, and hydrogen peroxide, *etc.* for coloring, permanent waving, bleaching, and straightening can cause scalp burn and hair damage due to peptide bonds breakage by using such treatment chemicals [117, 118].

Howbeit, natural products provide a broad source of cosmetic materials for hair care which serves as a source of food for hair growth, structure maintenance, and hair moisturizing agent. Fernández-Peña *et al.* [119] designed an eco-friendly hair washing formulation based on pseudo-binary mixtures of different glycolipids as biosurfactants for the adsorption of hair-conditioning polymer. The mixture of poly(diallyl-dimethylammonium chloride) and short alkyl chains glycolipids displayed improved adsorption efficiency and hydration than their conventional sulfate-based surfactant counterparts. In an experimental study, Sho *et al.* [120] showed that sweet potato *shochu* oil could increase human follicle dermal papilla cells in an upregulated expression of vascular endothelial growth factor in a concentration-dependent manner, which is an indication of the hair growth and restoration properties of *shochu* oil; meanwhile, Tinoco *et al.* [121] prepared keratin-based particles by high pressure homogenization of keratin and silk fibroin that was able to recover and improve the mechanical properties and smoothness of virgin and overbleached hair up to 40%. More so, the human eye γD-crystallin, a protein from the superfamily, has been reported as a good hair-strengthening agent that can bind to the damaged hair and penetrate the cortex for recovery of damaged hair [122]. Similarly, Tinoco *et al.* [123] demonstrated that the conjugation of γD-crystallin with a keratin-based peptide possesses a high capacity to protect human hair against thermal damage.

Furthermore, natural products containing protein based-particles also render numerous advantages towards the encapsulation and the delivery of sweet-smelling fragrances to human hair [124]. Based on these, Tinoco *et al.* [125] designed a new system based on Keratin:Zein particles with high potential for developing personal hair cosmetic products and promising capacity to improve hair's mechanical properties and hydration degree. Meanwhile, for hair dyeing products, Boga *et al.* [126] explored some natural organic products like anthocyanins from mulberry fruits and alizarin for red shades, anthocyanin-blue and curcumin for blue and yellow, respectively, and *p*-benzoquinone and juglone for brown coloration.

Additionally, considering that hair shampoo often contains a number of surfactants, there is typically a primary surfactant that does most of the foaming and cleaning. Many natural surfactants that apply in shampoo making consist of saponins, found in plant species including soap bark, soapwort, sarsaparilla, pawpaw, and ivy, *etc.*, and have been used for the treatment of hair infections like lice [127, 128]. Saikia [129] reported the high promising benefits of introducing *Dillenia indica* seed sap as a component of hair conditioner, shaving cream, hair gel, shampoo, hair coloring gel ingredients, *etc.* In the same vein, the natural pigments extracted from six species of Thai plants revealed excellent coloration ability, morphologically-smooth hair surface, high-affinity interaction, and color-fastness shampoo products and hair dyes [130].

Nail Polish Cosmetics

Nail polish cosmetics are cosmetic products popularly known as nail enamel, lacquer, or varnish that are often used for coloring, beautification, and protection of the human nail, which is considered a continuously growing structure composed of keratin, water, minerals, and cholesterol [131]. Basically, nail polishes are a composite mixture of film former, thermoplastic resin, plasticizer, solvent-extender, pigment and sometimes suspending agent in variable proportions [132]. These components are majorly volatile organic compounds (VOCs) like acetone, ethyl and *n*-butyl acetate, toluene, and formaldehyde, *etc.* which have been detected and quantified in nail salons, where they are emitted from nail care products, including nail polish remover [133]. Long-term exposure to these compounds is widely associated with pulmonary health effects, cancer, neurological issues, and reproductive complications, especially in women. Also, excess use of acetone as nail polish remover causes nail brittleness, prone to peeling, splitting, and breaking [9 - 11].

Although, not many studies have been performed on the use of natural products extracts as a recipe for the production of nail polish, however, nitrocellulose, the primary film former in lacquers, can be obtained from cotton or wood chips as a naturally-derived polymer produced by nitrating cellulose [134]. Also, sugarcane (*Saccharum officinarum* L.), one of the most profound crops widely used to produce ethanol and sugar, is also known to be very rich in multifunctional byproducts like bagasse and straw, which have been utilized in the production of paints, varnishes, polishes [135]. More so, the dehydrated and brittle-looking nail beds due to acetone and other synthetic compound-based nail polish remover can be overcome with the use of natural nail polish remover (Table **2**) [136].

Table 2. The functions of some natural products used as nail polish remover.

Natural Nail Polish Remover	Function
Essential lemon grass oil	Protects the nails against fungal and microbial infection
Lavender essential oil	Maintains moisture in nail beds
Avocado oil	Boost the health of nails and cuticles
Soy-based infused with argan oil and Vitamins A, C, and E	Boost the health of nails
Tocopherol and *Aloe vera* gel	For nail smoothing and moisture retaining
Horsetail extract	Strengthen nails
Lemon and vinegar	Dissolve stray color from the nails
Rosemary	Protects the nails against bacterial infection
Equisetum (horsetail) arvense extract	Protects the nails against inflammation
Rosa rubiginosa seed oil	For the regeneration of damaged nails

Perfumes

Perfumes are sweet-smelling cosmetic products that give one an attractive smell, boost confidence and are mood enhancers. Perfumes are a complex mixture of synthetic or natural (*e.g.*, essential oils) ingredients such as aldehydes, alcohols, lactones, esters, and terpene derivatives [137, 138].

Many plants and their volatile compounds have been utilized as the major sources of natural fragrances for perfumes and cosmetics over the years. Natural fragrances are complex fragrance compounds made exclusively from natural aromatics, such as essential oils, oleoresins, distillates, fractions, concretes, absolutes, *etc.*, without causing any skin irritation [139]. For example, the peels and skin of citrus fruits including lemon (*Citrus limon*), bitter orange (*Citrus aurantium*), berkane clementine, (*Citrus clementina*) and navel, a species of orange (*Citrus sinensis*) contain bioethanol and bioactive essential oils suitable for perfume making [140, 141]. Similarly, the essential oil obtained from the peel of lime fruit is very rich in bicyclic hydrocarbons, and aldehydes, especially citral, while the reverse is true for the distillate from crushed lime fruit but contains a high amount of terpene alcohols; and finds a wide application as a fragrance in cosmetics, and as flavoring agent [142, 143]. Also, lemongrass, a common plant in Southeast Asia, has a yellowish color and mixed fragrance of citrus, grass, and lemon and is used in the cosmetic industries and perfumery [144]. In addition, Peppermint (*Mentha piperita* Linn.) and spearmint (*Mentha spicata*) belonging to the Lamiaceae family plants possesses a strong aroma of sweet character with a sharp menthol undertone [145].

Moreover, the essential oils of basil are well known for their aromatherapy. For instance, Linalool, which exists as two optical isomers, such as (R)-(−) (form has a flowery-fresh, lavender-like note reminiscent of lily of the valley) and (S)-(+)-isomer (exhibits sweet, floral with the citricnote), has been reported as an odorant having a pleasant odor, with an average odor threshold of 3.2 ng/L [146 - 148]. Furthermore, the aromatic medicinal plant *Eucalyptus* and its essential oils have enjoyed multi-purpose functional applications in cosmetic, perfume, anesthetic, antiseptic, deodorant, and disinfectant production [149–151].

Lipstick Cosmetics

Lipsticks are basically cosmetic products used to beautify the lips by changing the natural colors or to moisturize them [152]. Lipsticks also provide a certain degree of protection against environmental hazards such as harsh weather conditions and UV radiation. The major component in lipsticks is wax, oil, and coloring agents, as well as some minor constituents like antioxidants, preservatives, and perfumes [153]. The first lipstick products were made from ocher nuggets by cave dwellers, however, in Paris in 1884, lipstick products were made with a castor oil-beeswax-deer tallow mixture. For the production of lipsticks, mixtures of waxes of plant origin (*e.g.*, carnauba, candelilla), animal (*e.g.*, beeswax), mineral (*e.g.*, ozokerite, paraffin), and synthetic materials (*e.g.*, polyethylene, which prevent oil drying) are mainly used in different quantitative ratios [154, 155].

Body Soap Cosmetics

Soaps are surface-active agents whose structural features consist of hydrophobic and hydrophilic groups, and are prepared by the saponification reaction, characterized by alkaline hydrolysis of triglycerides from fats and oils [156]. Over the years, many commercial soaps producers traditionally use synthetic chemicals like triclosan and parabens to impart anti-bacterial properties and preservatives into the soap formulation [157 - 159], as well as the addition of butylhydroxyanisol and butylated hydroxytoluene for antioxidant properties [160]. However, these chemical compounds have been characterized by numerous skin allergies and carcinogenic properties. Hence, replacing these toxic chemicals with naturally-sourced antimicrobial agents and antioxidants derived from green sources is presently undergoing intense research and development in the soap industry.

The green chemistry approach towards the production of soaps from natural ingredients like seed oils has gained tremendous attention due to their biodegradability, skin adaptability, eco-friendliness, and wide range ability to inhibit the growth of disease pathogens, scavenging of free radicals in the body, mild on cells owing to their antibacterial, antiseptic and antioxidant properties

(Table **3**) [161, 162]. More so, natural products have also been explored to possess characteristic aromas, garnished with essential minerals and vitamins, providing anti-aging and skincare effects when added to the recipe for soap making [163, 164]. In addition, traditional African black soap (also known as herbal soaps) is made from the ashes obtained from agricultural waste and oil extracted from vegetable matter containing no preservatives, color enhancers, or soap-enhancing agents [165]. These soaps contain natural nutrients like Vitamin E that keep the skin healthy, glowing, and beautiful [166].

Table 3. Different types of soaps produced from natural product extracts and some seed oils.

Natural Extract	Function of Extract	Type of Soap	Refs.
Millet stalks and palm oil	Add hardness to soap and produce stable creamy leather	Bathing soap	[170]
Neem oil to Shea butter oil	Antibacterial properties	Antiseptic soap	[171]
Almond shells and orange essential oil	Exfoliating agent	Artisanal soap	[172]
Citrus sinensis seed oil, natural honey, *Ocimum gratissimum* leaves extract, *Moringa oleifera* seed oil, and coconut oil	Antioxidant, antimicrobial, and fragrance properties	Medicinal soap	[173]
Egg yolk tempera	Soap binder	Metal soap	[174]
Ganoderma lucidum and coconut oil	Antibacterial and antioxidant activity	Transparent soap	[175]
Noni (*Morinda citrifolia* L.) fruit, yam (*Pachyrizus erosus*) root, rose (*Rosa damascena*) petal, and betel (*Piper betle* L.) leaf extracts	Antimicrobial property	Herbal transparent soaps	[176]
Fig extract	Antimicrobial and antifungal ability	Fig solid soap	[177]
Cymbopogon citratus, *Cymbopogon martini*, *Eucalyptus globules*, *A. indica* and *Ocimum sanctum* plant oils	Antimicrobial and antifungal properties	Medicated soap and shampoo	[178]
Date fruit syrup waste extract	Bactericidal and antioxidant additive activity	Antibacterial soap	[179]

In a study, Atolani *et al.* [167] utilized *Vitellaria paradoxa, Daniellia oliveri, and Elaeis guineensis* as sources of oil or fat for saponification with *Moringa oleifera* seed oil and leaf extract as antimicrobial agents, as well as *Ocimum basilicum* as a source of fragrance and antiseptic agent for the production of antiseptic soaps. Also, Ogunsuyi and Akinnawo [168] prepared black soap from purified palm bunch ash-derived alkali and coconut oil with comparatively improved physicochemical qualities than its conventional black soap counterparts. More so, Zauro *et al.* [169] showed that the combination of shea butter oil, palm kernel oil, and plantain peels displayed improved hardness, moisture, and foaming stability than soaps produced with the individual oils separately.

Facial Makeup Cosmetics

Facial makeup is cosmetics applied to the face for beautification. Many women consider it as a tool to even skin color, modify skin color, or contribute to smoothing out the skin surface [180]. Facial makeup materials consist of different formulations comprising of powder, foundations, colorants, and pigments, which are produced from varieties of precursor materials. It is often arduous to clean facial makeup using mere detergents since they contain solid and oily materials that require physical force to rub on the skin to dissolve them before rinsing the face. This rubbing of the skin often causes irritation and barrier perturbation [181].

Currently, commercially available makeup removers are emulsions produced from mineral oil, water, and surfactants [182]. For skin cleansing, many formulations of surfactants often result in decreased natural moisturizing factor, intercellular lipids dissolution and weakening of the permeability barrier function of stratum corneum, as well as causing irritation and corneocyte retention [181, 183]. Therefore, in addition to the incorporation of natural extracts in the preparation of facial makeup, makeup cleansing oils containing natural extracts are becoming popular for makeup removers [184]. They consist of oil-based materials and surfactants from plants, that can cause the dispersion, or dissolution of oily cosmetics, which can thereafter be rinsed easily with water. For example, castor oil extracts from *Ricinus communis* seeds are unique for their high ricinoleate content [185]; and a C-12 hydroxy group that makes it more polar than other vegetable oils; thereby conferring a hydrophilic property towards the removal of emulsion [186, 187]. Based on this information, Pakkang *et al.* [188] successfully prepared water-in-oil (w/o) microemulsion from mixtures of castor oil and sunflower oil as a makeup remover with high transparency of emulsion and cleansing efficiency, which could be traced to the hydrophilicity of the surfactant and castor oil. Also, Kim *et al.* [189] developed an emulsifying w/o microemulsion cleansing agent with good wettability containing a mixture of a spontaneous emulsifier, cosurfactant, and oil, and solubilizing the mixture during the addition of water for the removal of oil makeup cosmetics.

Eye Cosmetics

Though not much investigation has been carried out on natural product extracts for eye cosmetics, it is noteworthy that different types of eye cosmetic products have been produced for the decoration and beautification of the eyes. In the past, a mixture of charcoal and Kohl with animal fat were used to make an ointment for darkening the lashes and eyelids in ancient Egypt. In the 19th century, women use lamp black and soot collected over a candle flame to darken their lashes [190]. The majority of the women who uses eye cosmetic products make use of mascara (available as a water-based emulsion), eyeshadows (available as creams, sticks, and liquids), and eyeliners (available in liquid form and wood or mechanical pencils), which typically contains waxes, polymers, colors, and pigments that can be obtained from several natural sources.

CONCLUSION AND FUTURE PERSPECTIVES

Several pieces of research have been done on naturally-derived cosmetics and derivatives, with remarkable advantages in external applications, as against the several demerits associated with synthetic materials presently used in the cosmetics industry. While some of these researches have been reportedly documented, many of the formulation and production of the cosmetics are still being carried out and yet undocumented at the local and primitive levels, especially in developing countries, indicating that there is still a lot to do to maximize the huge economic potential in the industry. Natural plants are numerous, renewable, cheap, easily accessible, and contain several cosmeceutical and medicinal properties. Some black soaps are even orally taken for many curative purposes in different parts of the world. More so, secondary metabolites (oil and non-oil) extracted from numerous plant species have been reported with remarkable biological effects, showing prolific antibiotic, antifungal, antioxidant, and anti-inflammatory potentials in several cosmetic products. However, many of these locally-used cosmetics are not labelled with required mixtures and doses, while many were not determined clinically in randomized controlled trials to simultaneously monitor and ascertain any hazardous effects. Also, increasing industrialization and climate change have been pushing most of these natural plants into extinction. The stringent monitoring and protection of animals by rights regulations have caused limited works to be performed on animal-derived materials for the production of cosmetic materials, however, animal waste materials can be efficiently explored and screened as additives for cosmetic products. In addition, a surfactant is a very crucial recipe in cosmetic formulation, therefore, extensive research on natural surfactants for nail polish, eye, and facial makeup cosmetics will open many avenues in the cosmetic industry.

Furthermore, synergistic and effective collaboration with diverse professionals, including chemists and chemical engineers, microbiologists and conservationists, should be forged to explore the research relationship among these professions towards sustaining the green environment.

REFERENCES

[1] Ndhlovu PT, Mooki O, Otang Mbeng W, Aremu AO. Plant species used for cosmetic and cosmeceutical purposes by the Vhavenda women in Vhembe District Municipality, Limpopo, South Africa. S Afr J Bot 2019; 122: 422-31.
[http://dx.doi.org/10.1016/j.sajb.2019.03.036]

[2] Mohd-Nasir H, Mohd-Setapar SH. Natural ingredients in cosmetics from malaysian plants: a review. Sains Malays 2018; 47(5): 951-9.
[http://dx.doi.org/10.17576/jsm-2018-4705-10]

[3] Mahomoodally MF, Ramjuttun P. A quantitative ethnobotanical survey of phytocosmetics used in the tropical island of Mauritius. J Ethnopharmacol 2016; 193: 45-59.
[http://dx.doi.org/10.1016/j.jep.2016.07.039] [PMID: 27422163]

[4] European Union. Cosmetics Info. Cosmetic Regulation in the European Union. 2016.

[5] Rodrigues F, LuzCádiz-Gurrea M de la, Nunes MA, *et al.* Cosmetics. In: Galanakis CM, Ed. Polyphenols: Properties, Recovery, and Applications. Woodhead Publishing Limited; 2018. pp. 1–35.

[6] Nizioł-Łukaszewska Z. Extracts of cherry and sweet cherry fruit as active ingredients of body wash formulations. Not Bot Horti Agrobot Cluj-Napoca 2018; 47(1): 100-7.
[http://dx.doi.org/10.15835/nbha47111212]

[7] Espinosa-Leal C, Garcia-Lara S. Current methods for the discovery of new active ingredients from natural products for cosmeceutical applications. Planta Med 2019; 85(7): 535-51.
[http://dx.doi.org/10.1055/a-0857-6633] [PMID: 30925621]

[8] Akhtar MS, Practices HC. Natural Bio-active Compounds. Natural Bio-active Compounds 2019; Vol. 2.

[9] Alford KL, Kumar N. Pulmonary health effects of indoor volatile organic compounds - a meta-analysis. Int J Environ Res Public Health 2021; 18(4): 1578.
[http://dx.doi.org/10.3390/ijerph18041578] [PMID: 33562372]

[10] Lamplugh A, Harries M, Xiang F, Trinh J, Hecobian A, Montoya LD. Occupational exposure to volatile organic compounds and health risks in Colorado nail salons. Environ Pollut 2019; 249: 518-26.
[http://dx.doi.org/10.1016/j.envpol.2019.03.086] [PMID: 30933751]

[11] Reinecke JK, Hinshaw MA. Nail health in women. Int J Womens Dermatol 2020; 6(2): 73-9.
[http://dx.doi.org/10.1016/j.ijwd.2020.01.006] [PMID: 32258335]

[12] Lee KH, Lee JP, Kim W. Effects of a complex mixture prepared from agrimonia, houttuynia, licorice, peony, and phellodendron on human skin cells. Sci Rep 2020; 10(1): 22132.
[http://dx.doi.org/10.1038/s41598-020-79301-2] [PMID: 33335246]

[13] Félix C, Félix R, Carmona AM, *et al.* Cosmeceutical potential of grateloupia turuturu: Using low-cost extraction methodologies to obtain added-value extracts. Appl Sci (Basel) 2021; 11(4): 1650.
[http://dx.doi.org/10.3390/app11041650]

[14] Pipattanamomgkol P, Lourith N, Kanlayavattanakul M. The natural approach to hair dyeing product with Cleistocalyx nervosum var. paniala. Sustain Chem Pharm 2018; 8: 88-93.
[http://dx.doi.org/10.1016/j.scp.2018.04.001]

[15] Li MX, Bai X, Ma YP, *et al.* Cosmetic potentials of extracts and compounds from Zingiber cassumunar Roxb. rhizome. Ind Crops Prod 2019; 141: 111764.
[http://dx.doi.org/10.1016/j.indcrop.2019.111764]

[16] Zagórska-Dziok M, Ziemlewska A, Nizioł-Łukaszewska Z, Bujak T. Antioxidant activity and cytotoxicity of *Medicago sativa* L. seeds and herb extract on skin cells. Biores Open Access 2020; 9(1): 229-42.
[http://dx.doi.org/10.1089/biores.2020.0015] [PMID: 33117615]

[17]   Li MX, Xie J, Bai X, Du ZZ. Anti-aging potential, anti-tyrosinase and antibacterial activities of extracts and compounds isolated from *Rosa chinensis* cv. 'JinBian'. Ind Crops Prod 2021; 159: 113059.
[http://dx.doi.org/10.1016/j.indcrop.2020.113059]

[18]   Oluwalana EOA. Effects of Physico-chemical attributes of forest-based herbal soap on human skin in southwestern Nigeria. IOP Conf Ser Earth Environ Sci 2018; 173(1): 012035.
[http://dx.doi.org/10.1088/1755-1315/173/1/012035]

[19]   Longhini R, Lonni AASG, Sereia AL, Krzyzaniak LM, Lopes GC, Mello JCP. *Trichilia catigua*: therapeutic and cosmetic values. Rev Bras Farmacogn 2017; 27(2): 254-71.
[http://dx.doi.org/10.1016/j.bjp.2016.10.005]

[20]   Lajayer HL, Norouzi R, Shahi-Gharahlar A. Essential oil components, phenolic content and antioxidant activity of *Anthriscus cerefolium* and *Anthriscus sylvestris* from Iran. J Hortic Postharvest Res 2020; 3(2): 355-66.

[21]   Gaweł-Bęben K, Strzępek-Gomółka M, Czop M, Sakipova Z, Głowniak K, Kukula-Koch W. *Achillea millefolium L.* and *Achillea biebersteinii* Afan. hydroglycolic extracts-bioactive ingredients for cosmetic use. Molecules 2020; 25(15): 3368.
[http://dx.doi.org/10.3390/molecules25153368] [PMID: 32722270]

[22]   Becker LC, Bergfeld WF, Belsito DV, *et al.* Safety Assessment of *Achillea millefolium* as Used in Cosmetics. Int J Toxicol 2016; 35(3_suppl) (Suppl.): 5S-15S.
[http://dx.doi.org/10.1177/1091581816677717] [PMID: 27913788]

[23]   Campos PMBGM, Benevenuto CG, Calixto LS, Melo MO, Pereira KC, Gaspar LR. *Spirulina, Palmaria Palmata, Cichorium Intybus*, and *Medicago Sativa* extracts in cosmetic formulations: an integrated approach of *in vitro* toxicity and *in vivo* acceptability studies. Cutan Ocul Toxicol 2019; 38(4): 322-9.
[http://dx.doi.org/10.1080/15569527.2019.1579224] [PMID: 30821523]

[24]   Chaiyana W, Chansakaow S, Intasai N, *et al.* Chemical constituents, antioxidant, Anti-MMPs, and anti-hyaluronidase activities of thunbergia laurifolia lindl. Leaf extracts for skin aging and skin damage prevention. Molecules 2020; 25(8): 1923.
[http://dx.doi.org/10.3390/molecules25081923] [PMID: 32326348]

[25]   Cefali LC, Ataide JA, Fernandes AR, *et al.* Evaluation of *in vitro* solar protection factor (SPF), antioxidant activity, and cell viability of mixed vegetable extracts from *Dirmophandra mollis* Benth, *Ginkgo biloba* L., *Ruta graveolens* L., and *Vitis vinifera* L. Plants 2019; 8(11): 453.
[http://dx.doi.org/10.3390/plants8110453] [PMID: 31717792]

[26]   Chen LH, Chen IC, Chen PY, Huang PH. Efficacy of green onion root extract in cosmetics and skin care products. Biosci J 2019; 35(4): 1276-89.
[http://dx.doi.org/10.14393/BJ-v35n4a2019-45086]

[27]   Kiattisin K, Intasai N, Nitthikan N, *et al.* Antioxidant, anti-tyrosinase, anti-aging potentials and safety of arabica coffee cherry extract. Warasan Khana Witthayasat Maha Witthayalai Chiang Mai 2019; 46(5): 930-45.

[28]   Hęś M, Dziedzic K, Górecka D, Jędrusek-Golińska A, Gujska E. *Aloe vera* (L.) webb.: natural sources of antioxidants – a review. Plant Foods Hum Nutr 2019; 74(3): 255-65.
[http://dx.doi.org/10.1007/s11130-019-00747-5] [PMID: 31209704]

[29]   Kupnik K, Primožič M, Knez Ž, Leitgeb M. Antimicrobial efficiency of *Aloe arborescens* and *Aloe barbadensis* natural and commercial products. Plants 2021; 10(1): 92.
[http://dx.doi.org/10.3390/plants10010092] [PMID: 33466284]

[30]   Sacan O, Akev N, Yanardag R. *In vitro* inhibitory effect of *Aloe vera* (L.) Burm. f. leaf extracts on the activity of some enzymes and antioxidant activity. Indian J Biochem Biophys 2017; 54(1–2): 82-9.

[31]   Taofiq O, González-Paramás AM, Martins A, Barreiro MF, Ferreira ICFR. Mushrooms extracts and

compounds in cosmetics, cosmeceuticals and nutricosmetics - a review. Ind Crops Prod 2016; 90: 38-48.
[http://dx.doi.org/10.1016/j.indcrop.2016.06.012]

[32]   Taofiq O, Heleno SA, Calhelha RC, *et al.* Mushroom-based cosmeceutical ingredients: Microencapsulation and *in vitro* release profile. Ind Crops Prod 2018; 124: 44-52.
[http://dx.doi.org/10.1016/j.indcrop.2018.07.057]

[33]   Wu Y, Choi MH, Li J, Yang H, Shin HJ. Mushroom cosmetics: The present and future. Cosmetics 2016; 3(3): 22.
[http://dx.doi.org/10.3390/cosmetics3030022]

[34]   Taofiq O, Rodrigues F, Barros L, Barreiro MF, Ferreira ICFR, Oliveira MBPP. Mushroom ethanolic extracts as cosmeceuticals ingredients: Safety and *ex vivo* skin permeation studies. Food Chem Toxicol 2019; 127(March): 228-36.
[http://dx.doi.org/10.1016/j.fct.2019.03.045] [PMID: 30922966]

[35]   Liu W, Wang M, Xu S, Gao C, Liu J. Inhibitory effects of shell of *Camellia oleifera Abel* extract on mushroom tyrosinase and human skin melanin. J Cosmet Dermatol 2019; 18(6): 1955-60.
[http://dx.doi.org/10.1111/jocd.12921] [PMID: 31033161]

[36]   Wu Z, Zhang M, Yang H, Zhou H, Yang H. Production, physico-chemical characterization and antioxidant activity of natural melanin from submerged cultures of the mushroom *Auricularia auricula*. Food Biosci 2018; 26: 49-56.
[http://dx.doi.org/10.1016/j.fbio.2018.09.008]

[37]   Sharpe E, Farragher-Gnadt AP, Igbanugo M, *et al.* Comparison of antioxidant activity and extraction techniques for commercially and laboratory prepared extracts from six mushroom species. J Agric Food Res 2021; 4: 100130.
[http://dx.doi.org/10.1016/j.jafr.2021.100130]

[38]   Taofiq O, Heleno S, Calhelha R, *et al.* Development of Mushroom-Based cosmeceutical formulations with Anti-Inflammatory, Anti-Tyrosinase, antioxidant, and antibacterial properties. Molecules 2016; 21(10): 1372.
[http://dx.doi.org/10.3390/molecules21101372] [PMID: 27754433]

[39]   Wathoni N, Haerani A, Yuniarsih N, Haryanti R. A review on herbal cosmetics in Indonesia. Int J Appl Pharm 2018; 10(5): 13-6.
[http://dx.doi.org/10.22159/ijap.2018v10i5.28102]

[40]   Sagbo I, Mbeng W. Plants used for cosmetics in the Eastern Cape Province of South Africa: a case study of skin care. Pharmacogn Rev 2018; 12(24): 139.
[http://dx.doi.org/10.4103/phrev.phrev_9_18]

[41]   Shazalyana Azman NF, Masitah I, Shankar M, *et al.* Ten commonly available medicinal plants in malaysia used for cosmetic formulations – a review. Int J Res Pharm Sci 2020; 11(2): 1716-28.
[http://dx.doi.org/10.26452/ijrps.v11i2.2073]

[42]   Ariede MB, Candido TM, Jacome ALM, Velasco MVR, de Carvalho JCM, Baby AR. Cosmetic attributes of algae - a review. Algal Res 2017; 25: 483-7.
[http://dx.doi.org/10.1016/j.algal.2017.05.019]

[43]   Sun Y, Chavan M. Heme oxygenase stimulation by Fucus water extract. Vol. 2. US Patent No.: US9603790B2, 2017.

[44]   Boo YC. Can plant phenolic compounds protect the skin from airborne particulate matter? Antioxidants 2019; 8(9): 379.
[http://dx.doi.org/10.3390/antiox8090379] [PMID: 31500121]

[45]   Lee J won, Seok JK, Boo YC. Ecklonia cava Extract and Dieckol Attenuate Cellular Lipid Peroxidation in Keratinocytes Exposed to PM10. In: Sacchetti G, Ed.; Evidence-Based Complement Altern Med 2018; 2018: 8248323.

[46]   Zhen AX, Hyun YJ, Piao MJ, *et al.* Eckol inhibits particulate matter 2.5-induced skin keratinocyte damage *via* mapk signaling pathway. Mar Drugs 2019; 17(8): 444.
[http://dx.doi.org/10.3390/md17080444]

[47]   Zhen AX, Piao MJ, Hyun YJ, *et al.* Diphlorethohydroxycarmalol attenuates fine particulate matter-induced subcellular skin dysfunction. Mar Drugs 2019; 17(2): 95.
[http://dx.doi.org/10.3390/md17020095]

[48]   Henríquez V, Escobar C, Galarza J, Gimpel J. Carotenoids in Microalgae. In: Stange C, Ed. Carotenoids in Nature. Cham: Springer International Publishing 2016; pp. 219-37.
[http://dx.doi.org/10.1007/978-3-319-39126-7_8]

[49]   Fassett RG, Coombes JS. Astaxanthin: a potential therapeutic agent in cardiovascular disease. Mar Drugs 2011; 9(3): 447-65.
[http://dx.doi.org/10.3390/md9030447] [PMID: 21556169]

[50]   Oren A. A hundred years of Dunaliella research: 1905–2005. Saline Syst 2005; 1(1): 2-2.
[http://dx.doi.org/10.1186/1746-1448-1-2] [PMID: 16176593]

[51]   Rastogi RP, Sonani RR, Madamwar D. UV Photoprotectants From Algae—Synthesis and Bio-Functionalities. Algal Green Chemistry. Elsevier 2017; pp. 17-38.
[http://dx.doi.org/10.1016/B978-0-444-63784-0.00002-3]

[52]   Puchkova TV, Khapchaeva SA, Zotov VS, Lukyanov AA, Solovchenko AE. Marine and freshwater microalgae as a sustainable source of cosmeceuticals. Marine Biol J 2021; 6(1): 67-81.
[http://dx.doi.org/10.21072/mbj.2021.06.1.06]

[53]   Malcata FX, Sousa Pinto I, Guedes AC, Eds. Marine Macro- and Microalgae First. Boca Raton, FL: CRC Press 2018.
[http://dx.doi.org/10.1201/9781315119441]

[54]   Ibrahim M, Salman M, Kamal S, *et al.* Algae-Based Biologically Active Compounds. Algae Based Polymers, Blends, and Composites: Chemistry Biotechnology and Materials Science. Elsevier Inc. 2017; pp. 155-271.
[http://dx.doi.org/10.1016/B978-0-12-812360-7.00006-9]

[55]   Priyan Shanura Fernando I, Kim KN, Kim D, Jeon YJ. Algal polysaccharides: potential bioactive substances for cosmeceutical applications. Crit Rev Biotechnol 2019; 39(1): 99-113.
[http://dx.doi.org/10.1080/07388551.2018.1503995] [PMID: 31690134]

[56]   Mourelle M, Gómez C, Legido J. The potential use of marine microalgae and cyanobacteria in cosmetics and thalassotherapy. Cosmetics 2017; 4(4): 46.
[http://dx.doi.org/10.3390/cosmetics4040046]

[57]   Hu Y, Zeng H, Huang J, Jiang L, Chen J, Zeng Q. Traditional asian herbs in skin whitening: the current development and limitations. Front Pharmacol 2020; 11: 982.
[http://dx.doi.org/10.3389/fphar.2020.00982] [PMID: 32733239]

[58]   Avila Rodríguez MI, Rodríguez Barroso LG, Sánchez ML. Collagen: a review on its sources and potential cosmetic applications. J Cosmet Dermatol 2018; 17(1): 20-6.
[http://dx.doi.org/10.1111/jocd.12450] [PMID: 29144022]

[59]   Reddy DN. Essential Oils Extracted from Medicinal Plants and Their Applications. In: Akhtar MS, Swamy MK, Sinniah UR, Eds. Natural Bio-active Compounds. Singapore: Springer Singapore 2019; pp. 237-83.
[http://dx.doi.org/10.1007/978-981-13-7154-7_9]

[60]   Sumit K, Vivek S, Sujata S, Ashish B. Herbal cosmetics: used for skin and hair. Inven J 2012; 2012(4): 1-7.

[61]   Venkatachalam D, Thavamani S, Varghese V, Vinod KR. Review on herabal cosmetics in skin care. Indo Am J Pharm Sci 2019; 06(1): 781-9.

[62]   Gorini I, Iorio S, Ciliberti R, Licata M, Armocida G. Olive oil in pharmacological and cosmetic traditions. J Cosmet Dermatol 2019; 18(5): 1575-9.
[http://dx.doi.org/10.1111/jocd.12838] [PMID: 30618094]

[63]   Khedher MRB, Khedher SB, Chaieb I, Tounsi S, Hammami M. Chemical composition and biological activities of Salvia officinalis essential oil from Tunisia. EXCLI J 2017; 16: 160-73.
[PMID: 28507464]

[64]   Ghasemi Pirbalouti A, Izadi A, Malek Poor F, Hamedi B. Chemical composition, antioxidant and antibacterial activities of essential oils from *Ferulago angulata*. Pharm Biol 2016; 54(11): 2515-20.
[http://dx.doi.org/10.3109/13880209.2016.1162816] [PMID: 27102982]

[65]   He W, Li X, Peng Y, He X, Pan S. Anti-oxidant and anti-melanogenic properties of essential oil from peel of Pomelo cv. Guan XI. Molecules 2019; 24(2): 242.
[http://dx.doi.org/10.3390/molecules24020242] [PMID: 30634693]

[66]   Khor PY, Na'im Mohamed FS, Ramli I, *et al.* Phytochemical, antioxidant and photo-protective activity study of bunga kantan (Etlingera elatior) essential oil. J Appl Pharm Sci 2017; 7(8): 209-13.

[67]   Laothaweerungsawat N, Sirithunyalug J, Chaiyana W. Chemical compositions and anti-skin-ageing activities of *Origanum vulgare* L. essential oil from tropical and mediterranean region. Molecules 2020; 25(5): 1101.
[http://dx.doi.org/10.3390/molecules25051101] [PMID: 32121614]

[68]   Moore EM, Wagner C, Komarnytsky S. The enigma of bioactivity and toxicity of botanical oils for skin care. Front Pharmacol 2020; 11: 785.
[http://dx.doi.org/10.3389/fphar.2020.00785] [PMID: 32547393]

[69]   Lukic M, Pantelic I, Savic S. An overview of novel surfactants for formulation of cosmetics with certain emphasis on acidic active substances. Tenside Surfactants Deterg 2016; 53(1): 7-19.
[http://dx.doi.org/10.3139/113.110405]

[70]   Bhattacharya B, Ghosh TK, Das N. Application of bio-surfactants in cosmetics and pharmaceutical industry. Sch Acad J Pharm 2017; 6(7): 320-9.

[71]   Ahmadi-Ashtiani HR, Baldisserotto A, Cesa E, *et al.* Microbial biosurfactants as key multifunctional ingredients for sustainable cosmetics. Cosmetics 2020; 7(2): 46.
[http://dx.doi.org/10.3390/cosmetics7020046]

[72]   Wang L, Zhang K, Han S, *et al.* Constituents isolated from the leaves of *Glycyrrhiza uralansis* and their anti-inflammatory activities on LPS-induced RAW264.7 cells. Molecules 2019; 24(10): 1923.
[http://dx.doi.org/10.3390/molecules24101923] [PMID: 31109095]

[73]   Aipire A, Yuan P, Aimaier A, *et al.* Preparation, characterization, and immuno-enhancing activity of polysaccharides from *Glycyrrhiza uralensis*. Biomolecules 2020; 10(1): 159.
[http://dx.doi.org/10.3390/biom10010159] [PMID: 31963790]

[74]   Yu C, Fan X, Li Z, Liu X, Wang G. Efficacy and safety of total glucosides of paeony combined with acitretin in the treatment of moderate-to-severe plaque psoriasis: a double-blind, randomised, placebo-controlled trial. Eur J Dermatol 2017; 27(2): 150-4.
[http://dx.doi.org/10.1684/ejd.2016.2946] [PMID: 28400341]

[75]   Eibl R. Plant cell culture technology in the cosmetics and food industries: current state and future trends. Appl Microbiol Biotechnol 2018; 102(20): 8661-75.
[http://dx.doi.org/10.1007/s00253-018-9279-8] [PMID: 30099571]

[76]   Alves A, Marques A, Martins E, Silva T, Reis R. Cosmetic potential of Marine fish skin collagen. Cosmetics 2017; 4(4): 39.
[http://dx.doi.org/10.3390/cosmetics4040039]

[77]   Alhajj MJ, Montero N, Yarce CJ, Salamanca CH. Lecithins from vegetable, land, and marine animal sources and their potential applications for cosmetic, food, and pharmaceutical sectors. Cosmetics

2020; 7(4): 87.
[http://dx.doi.org/10.3390/cosmetics7040087]

[78]   Schneider M. Marine phospholipids and their applications: next-generation omega-3 lipids. In: De Meester F, Watson RR, Zibadi S, Eds. Omega-6/3 Fatty Acids. Totowa, NJ: Humana Press 2013; pp. 297-308.
[http://dx.doi.org/10.1007/978-1-62703-215-5_15]

[79]   Lordan R, Tsoupras A, Zabetakis I. Phospholipids of animal and marine origin: structure, function, and anti-inflammatory properties. Molecules 2017; 22(11): 1964.
[http://dx.doi.org/10.3390/molecules22111964] [PMID: 29135918]

[80]   Lordan R, Redfern S, Tsoupras A, Zabetakis I. Inflammation and cardiovascular disease: are marine phospholipids the answer? Food Funct 2020; 11(4): 2861-85.
[http://dx.doi.org/10.1039/C9FO01742A] [PMID: 32270798]

[81]   Gökdoğan O. Determination of input-output energy and economic analysis of lavender production in Turkey. Int J Agric Biol Eng 2016; 9(3): 154-61.

[82]   Kaur A, Singh TG, Dhiman S, Arora S, Babbar R. Novel herbs used in cosmetics for skin and hair care: a review. Plant Arch 2020; 20: 3784-93.

[83]   Abou Assi R, Darwis Y, Abdulbaqi IM, khan AA, Vuanghao L, Laghari MH. Morinda citrifolia (Noni): a comprehensive review on its industrial uses, pharmacological activities, and clinical trials. Arab J Chem 2017; 10(5): 691-707.
[http://dx.doi.org/10.1016/j.arabjc.2015.06.018]

[84]   Rini AT, Anggraini T, Ritonga NB. Making skin lotion from virgin coconut oil with adding several natural plants extract as a skin protector. IOP Conf Ser Earth Environ Sci 2020; 515(1): 012031.
[http://dx.doi.org/10.1088/1755-1315/515/1/012031]

[85]   Lorz L, Yoo B, Kim MY, Cho J. Anti-wrinkling and anti-melanogenic effect of pradosia mutisii methanol extract. Int J Mol Sci 2019; 20(5): 1043.
[http://dx.doi.org/10.3390/ijms20051043] [PMID: 30818884]

[86]   Sharmila G, Muthukumaran C, Suriya E, *et al.* Ultrasound aided extraction of yellow pigment from Tecoma castanifolia floral petals: Optimization by response surface method and evaluation of the antioxidant activity. Ind Crops Prod 2019; 130(January): 467-77.
[http://dx.doi.org/10.1016/j.indcrop.2019.01.008]

[87]   Boo HO, Hwang SJ, Bae CS, Park SH, Heo BG, Gorinstein S. Extraction and characterization of some natural plant pigments. Ind Crops Prod 2012; 40(1): 129-35.
[http://dx.doi.org/10.1016/j.indcrop.2012.02.042]

[88]   Morocho-Jácome AL, Ruscinc N, Martinez RM, *et al.* (Bio)Technological aspects of microalgae pigments for cosmetics. Appl Microbiol Biotechnol 2020; 104(22): 9513-22.
[http://dx.doi.org/10.1007/s00253-020-10936-x] [PMID: 33015721]

[89]   Mattioli M, Giardini L, Roselli C, Desideri D. Mineralogical characterization of commercial clays used in cosmetics and possible risk for health. Appl Clay Sci 2016; 119: 449-54.
[http://dx.doi.org/10.1016/j.clay.2015.10.023]

[90]   Moraes JDD, Bertolino SRA, Cuffini SL, Ducart DF, Bretzke PE, Leonardi GR. Clay minerals: Properties and applications to dermocosmetic products and perspectives of natural raw materials for therapeutic purposes - a review. Int J Pharm 2017; 534(1-2): 213-9.
[http://dx.doi.org/10.1016/j.ijpharm.2017.10.031] [PMID: 29038067]

[91]   Khurana IS, Kaur S, Kaur H, Khurana RK. Multifaceted role of clay minerals in pharmaceuticals. Future Sci OA, 2015; 1(3).
[http://dx.doi.org/10.4155/fso.15.6]

[92]   Silva-Valenzuela MG, Chambi-Peralta MM, Sayeg IJ, de Souza Carvalho FM, Wang SH, Valenzuela-Díaz FR. Enrichment of clay from Vitoria da Conquista (Brazil) for applications in cosmetics. Appl

Clay Sci 2018; 155: 111-9.
[http://dx.doi.org/10.1016/j.clay.2018.01.011]

[93]   Gubitosa J, Rizzi V, Fini P, Cosma P. Hair care cosmetics: from traditional shampoo to solid clay and herbal shampoo, a review. Cosmetics 2019; 6(1): 13.
[http://dx.doi.org/10.3390/cosmetics6010013]

[94]   Viseras C, Aguzzi C, Cerezo P, Lopezgalindo A. Uses of clay minerals in semisolid health care and therapeutic products. Appl Clay Sci 2007; 36(1-3): 37-50.
[http://dx.doi.org/10.1016/j.clay.2006.07.006]

[95]   Carretero MI, Pozo M. Clay and non-clay minerals in the pharmaceutical and cosmetic industries, Part II. Active ingredients. Appl Clay Sci 2010; 47(3-4): 171-81.
[http://dx.doi.org/10.1016/j.clay.2009.10.016]

[96]   Ghadiri M, Chrzanowski W, Rohanizadeh R. Biomedical applications of cationic clay minerals. RSC Adv 2015; 5(37): 29467-81.
[http://dx.doi.org/10.1039/C4RA16945J]

[97]   Gomes C, Silva J. Minerals and clay minerals in medical geology. Appl Clay Sci 2007; 36(1-3): 4-21.
[http://dx.doi.org/10.1016/j.clay.2006.08.006]

[98]   Valenti DMZ, Silva J, Teodoro WR, Velosa AP, Mello SBV. Effect of topical clay application on the synthesis of collagen in skin: an experimental study. Clin Exp Dermatol 2012; 37(2): 164-8.
[http://dx.doi.org/10.1111/j.1365-2230.2011.04216.x] [PMID: 22340693]

[99]   Hoang-Minh T, Le TL, Kasbohm J, Gieré R. UV-protection characteristics of some clays. Appl Clay Sci 2010; 48(3): 349-57.
[http://dx.doi.org/10.1016/j.clay.2010.01.005]

[100]   Madikizela LM, Nkwentsha N, Mlunguza NY, Mdluli PS. Physicochemical characterization and *in vitro* evaluation of the sun protection factor of cosmetic products made from natural clay material. S Afr J Chem 2017; 70: 113-9.
[http://dx.doi.org/10.17159/0379-4350/2017/v70a016]

[101]   Williams LB, Haydel SE. Evaluation of the medicinal use of clay minerals as antibacterial agents. Int Geol Rev 2010; 52(7-8): 745-70.
[http://dx.doi.org/10.1080/00206811003679737] [PMID: 20640226]

[102]   Lafi S, Al-Dulaimy M. Antibacterial effect of some mineral clays *in vitro.* Egypt Acad J Biol Sci G Microbiol 2011; 3(1): 75-81.
[http://dx.doi.org/10.21608/eajbsg.2011.16697]

[103]   da Silva Favero J, dos Santos V, Weiss-Angeli V, *et al.* Evaluation and characterization of Melo Bentonite clay for cosmetic applications. Appl Clay Sci 2019; 175(175): 40-6.
[http://dx.doi.org/10.1016/j.clay.2019.04.004]

[104]   Bergamaschi B, Marzola L, Radice M, *et al.* Comparative study of spa mud from "bacino idrominerario omogeneo dei colli euganei (B.i.o.c.e.)–italy" and industrially optimized mud for skin applications. Life (Basel) 2020; 10(6): 78.
[http://dx.doi.org/10.3390/life10060078] [PMID: 32466481]

[105]   Riviere JE, Monteiro-Riviere NA. Dermal exposure and absorption of chemicals and nanomaterials. Compr Toxicol, 2nd edn. 2010; Vols. 1-14: pp. 111–22.
[http://dx.doi.org/10.1016/B978-0-08-046884-6.00105-6]

[106]   Mukherjee PK, Maity N, Nema NK, Sarkar BK. Bioactive compounds from natural resources against skin aging. Phytomedicine 2011; 19(1): 64-73.
[http://dx.doi.org/10.1016/j.phymed.2011.10.003] [PMID: 22115797]

[107]   Kose O, Erkekoglu P, Sabuncuoglu S, Kocer-Gumusel B. Evaluation of skin irritation potentials of different cosmetic products in Turkish market by reconstructed human epidermis model. Regul Toxicol Pharmacol 2018; 98(May): 268-73.

[http://dx.doi.org/10.1016/j.yrtph.2018.08.010] [PMID: 30138660]

[108]   Kamaruzaman N, Yusop SM. Determination of stability of cosmetic formulations incorporated with water-soluble elastin isolated from poultry. J King Saud Univ Sci 2021; 33(6): 101519.
[http://dx.doi.org/10.1016/j.jksus.2021.101519]

[109]   Sim YY, Nyam KL. Application of Hibiscus cannabinus L. (kenaf) leaves extract as skin whitening and anti-aging agents in natural cosmetic prototype. Ind Crops Prod 2021; 167(1): 113491.
[http://dx.doi.org/10.1016/j.indcrop.2021.113491]

[110]   Kozlowska J, Prus W, Stachowiak N. Microparticles based on natural and synthetic polymers for cosmetic applications. Int J Biol Macromol 2019; 129(129): 952-6.
[http://dx.doi.org/10.1016/j.ijbiomac.2019.02.091] [PMID: 30776440]

[111]   Chen K, Guo B, Luo J. Quaternized carboxymethyl chitosan/organic montmorillonite nanocomposite as a novel cosmetic ingredient against skin aging. Carbohydr Polym 2017; 173: 100-6.
[http://dx.doi.org/10.1016/j.carbpol.2017.05.088] [PMID: 28732847]

[112]   Almendinger M, Rohn S, Pleissner D. Malt and beer-related by-products as potential antioxidant skin-lightening agents for cosmetics. Sustain Chem Pharm 2020; 17(March): 100282.
[http://dx.doi.org/10.1016/j.scp.2020.100282]

[113]   Barreto SMAG, Maia MS, Benicá AM, *et al.* Evaluation of *in vitro* and *in vivo* safety of the by-product of Agave sisalana as a new cosmetic raw material: Development and clinical evaluation of a nanoemulsion to improve skin moisturizing. Ind Crops Prod 2017; 108(July): 470-9.
[http://dx.doi.org/10.1016/j.indcrop.2017.06.064]

[114]   Yu Y, Yang W, Wang B, Meyers MA. Structure and mechanical behavior of human hair. Mater Sci Eng C 2017; 73: 152-63.
[http://dx.doi.org/10.1016/j.msec.2016.12.008] [PMID: 28183593]

[115]   McKittrick J, Chen PY, Bodde SG, Yang W, Novitskaya EE, Meyers MA. The structure, functions, and mechanical properties of keratin. J Miner Met Mater Soc 2012; 64(4): 449-68.
[http://dx.doi.org/10.1007/s11837-012-0302-8]

[116]   Thieulin C, Vargiolu R, Zahouani H. Effects of cosmetic treatments on the morphology, biotribology and sensorial properties of a single human hair fiber. Wear 2019; 426–427: 186-94.
[http://dx.doi.org/10.1016/j.wear.2019.01.065]

[117]   Pienpinijtham P, Thammacharoen C, Naranitad S, Ekgasit S. Analysis of cosmetic residues on a single human hair by ATR FT-IR microspectroscopy. Spectrochim Acta A Mol Biomol Spectrosc 2018; 197: 230-6.
[http://dx.doi.org/10.1016/j.saa.2018.01.084] [PMID: 29496404]

[118]   Jeong MS, Lee CM, Jeong WJ, Kim SJ, Lee KY. Significant damage of the skin and hair following hair bleaching. J Dermatol 2010; 37(10): 882-7.
[http://dx.doi.org/10.1111/j.1346-8138.2010.00916.x] [PMID: 20860738]

[119]   Fernández-Peña L, Guzmán E, Leonforte F, *et al.* Effect of molecular structure of eco-friendly glycolipid biosurfactants on the adsorption of hair-care conditioning polymers. Colloids Surfaces B Biointerfaces 2020; 185: 110578.
[http://dx.doi.org/10.1016/j.colsurfb.2019.110578]

[120]   Sho C, Kawano K, Kurata R, Yoshimoto M, Okuno H. Hair growth-promoting activity of components derived from sweet potato shochu. J Biosci Bioeng 2021; 131(4): 405-11.
[http://dx.doi.org/10.1016/j.jbiosc.2020.12.004] [PMID: 33431342]

[121]   Tinoco A, Gonçalves J, Silva C, *et al.* Keratin-based particles for protection and restoration of hair properties. 2018.
[http://dx.doi.org/10.1111/ics.12483]

[122]   Ribeiro A, Matamá T, Cruz CF, Gomes AC, Cavaco-Paulo AM. Potential of human γD-crystallin for hair damage repair: insights into the mechanical properties and biocompatibility. Int J Cosmet Sci

2013; 35(5): 458-66.
[http://dx.doi.org/10.1111/ics.12065] [PMID: 23651449]

[123] Tinoco A, Gonçalves J, Silva C, Cavaco-Paulo A, Ribeiro A. Crystallin fusion proteins improve the thermal properties of hair. Front Bioeng Biotechnol 2019; 7(OCT): 298.
[http://dx.doi.org/10.3389/fbioe.2019.00298] [PMID: 31709253]

[124] Sansukcharearnpon A, Wanichwecharungruang S, Leepipatpaiboon N, Kerdchaoen T, Arayachukeat S. High loading fragrance encapsulation based on a polymer-blend: Preparation and release behavior. Int J Pharm 2010; 391(1-2): 267-73.
[http://dx.doi.org/10.1016/j.ijpharm.2010.02.020] [PMID: 20170720]

[125] Tinoco A, Gonçalves F, Costa AF, Freitas DS, Cavaco-Paulo A, Ribeiro A. Keratin:Zein particles as vehicles for fragrance release on hair. Ind Crops Prod 2020; 2021: 159.

[126] Boga C, Delpivo C, Ballarin B, *et al*. Investigation on the dyeing power of some organic natural compounds for a green approach to hair dyeing. Dyes Pigments 2013; 97(1): 9-18.
[http://dx.doi.org/10.1016/j.dyepig.2012.11.020]

[127] Cornwell PA. A review of shampoo surfactant technology: consumer benefits, raw materials and recent developments. Int J Cosmet Sci 2018; 40(1): 16-30.
[http://dx.doi.org/10.1111/ics.12439] [PMID: 29095493]

[128] Luengo GS, Fameau AL, Léonforte F, Greaves AJ. Surface science of cosmetic substrates, cleansing actives and formulations. Adv Colloid Interface Sci 2021; 290: 102383.
[http://dx.doi.org/10.1016/j.cis.2021.102383] [PMID: 33690071]

[129] Saikia JP. Hair waving natural product: Dillenia indica seed sap. Colloids Surf B Biointerfaces 2013; 102: 905-7.
[http://dx.doi.org/10.1016/j.colsurfb.2012.10.008] [PMID: 23124020]

[130] Boonsong P, Laohakunjit N, Kerdchoechuen O. Natural pigments from six species of Thai plants extracted by water for hair dyeing product application. J Clean Prod 2012; 37: 93-106.
[http://dx.doi.org/10.1016/j.jclepro.2012.06.013]

[131] Wollina U, Abdel-Naser MB. Drug reactions affecting hair and nails. Clin Dermatol 2020; 38(6): 693-701.
[http://dx.doi.org/10.1016/j.clindermatol.2020.06.009] [PMID: 33341202]

[132] Arora H, Tosti A. Safety and efficacy of nail products. Cosmetics 2017; 4(3): 24.
[http://dx.doi.org/10.3390/cosmetics4030024]

[133] Lamplugh A, Harries M, Nguyen A, Montoya LD. VOC emissions from nail salon products and their effective removal using affordable adsorbents and synthetic jets. Build Environ 2020; 168(September 2019): 106499.
[http://dx.doi.org/10.1016/j.buildenv.2019.106499]

[134] Francisco F. Raw Materials in the Production of Nail Polish. Design life-cycle, 2016. Available from:http://www.designlife-cycle.com/nail-polish

[135] Carvalho MJ, Oliveira AL, Pedrosa SS, Pintado M, Madureira AR. Potential of sugarcane extracts as cosmetic and skincare ingredients. Ind Crops Prod. 2021; 169(November 2020): 113625.
[http://dx.doi.org/10.1016/j.indcrop.2021.113625]

[136] Lapidos R. 6 Natural Nail Polish Removers That Will Keep Your Tips Super Soft and Healthy. Well+Good LLC. 2020. Available from: https://www.wellandgood.com/pedicure-art-ideas/

[137] Villatoro C, Vera L, Gygax H. Comparative study of odours present in twin fragrances by GC-sniffing-ToFMS. Chem Eng Trans 2016; 54: 133-8.

[138] Jarboui A, Marx ÍMG, Veloso ACA, *et al*. An electronic tongue as a classifier tool for assessing perfume olfactory family and storage time-period. talanta 2020; 208(June 2019): 120364.
[http://dx.doi.org/10.1016/j.talanta.2019.120364]

[139] Vijaya N, Umamathi T, Baby AG, *et al.* Nanomaterials in fragrance products. Nanocosmetics 2020; pp. 247-65.

[140] Brahmi F, Mokhtari O, Legssyer B, *et al.* Chemical and biological characterization of essential oils extracted from citrus fruits peels. Mater Today Proc 2021; 45: 7794-9.
[http://dx.doi.org/10.1016/j.matpr.2021.03.587]

[141] Widmer W, Zhou W, Grohmann K. Pretreatment effects on orange processing waste for making ethanol by simultaneous saccharification and fermentation. Bioresour Technol 2010; 101(14): 5242-9.
[http://dx.doi.org/10.1016/j.biortech.2009.12.038] [PMID: 20189803]

[142] Lawal OA, Ogunwande IA, Owolabi MS, *et al.* Comparative analysis of essential oils of citrus aurantifolia swingle and citrus reticulata blanco, from two different localities of lagos state, nigeria. Am J Essent Oils Nat Prod 2014; 2(2): 8-12.

[143] Jakab E, Blazsó M, Barta-Rajnai E, *et al.* Thermo-oxidative decomposition of lime, bergamot and cardamom essential oils. J Anal Appl Pyrolysis 2018; 134(May): 552-61.
[http://dx.doi.org/10.1016/j.jaap.2018.08.003]

[144] Tovar LP, Pinto GMF, Wolf-Maciel MR, Batistella CB, Maciel-Filho R. Short-path-distillation process of lemongrass essential oil: Physicochemical characterization and assessment quality of the distillate and the residue products. Ind Eng Chem Res 2011; 50(13): 8185-94.
[http://dx.doi.org/10.1021/ie101503n]

[145] Ali B, Al-Wabel NA, Shams S, Ahamad A, Khan SA, Anwar F. Essential oils used in aromatherapy: a systemic review. Asian Pac J Trop Biomed 2015; 5(8): 601-11.
[http://dx.doi.org/10.1016/j.apjtb.2015.05.007]

[146] Elsharif SA, Banerjee A, Buettner A. Structure-odor relationships of linalool, linalyl acetate and their corresponding oxygenated derivatives. Front Chem 2015; 3(oct): 57.
[http://dx.doi.org/10.3389/fchem.2015.00057] [PMID: 26501053]

[147] Aprotosoaie AC, Hǎncianu M, Costache II, Miron A. Linalool: a review on a key odorant molecule with valuable biological properties. Flavour Fragrance J 2014; 29(4): 193-219.
[http://dx.doi.org/10.1002/ffj.3197]

[148] Maurya R, Gupta P, Chanotiya CS, *et al.* Investigation of monoterpenoids rich essential oils of two *Ocimum basilicum* L. varieties at different agro-climatic conditions in India. Acta Ecol Sin 2022; 42(2): 1-10.
[http://dx.doi.org/10.1016/j.chnaes.2020.11.002]

[149] Bachir RG, Benali M. Antibacterial activity of the essential oils from the leaves of Eucalyptus globulus against *Escherichia coli* and *Staphylococcus aureus*. Asian Pac J Trop Biomed 2012; 2(9): 739-42.
[http://dx.doi.org/10.1016/S2221-1691(12)60220-2] [PMID: 23570005]

[150] Goldbeck JC, do Nascimento JE, Jacob RG, Fiorentini ÂM, da Silva WP. Bioactivity of essential oils from Eucalyptus globulus and Eucalyptus urograndis against planktonic cells and biofilms of Streptococcus mutans. Ind Crops Prod 2014; 60: 304-9.
[http://dx.doi.org/10.1016/j.indcrop.2014.05.030]

[151] Limam H, Ben Jemaa M, Tammar S, *et al.* Variation in chemical profile of leaves essential oils from thirteen *Tunisian eucalyptus* species and evaluation of their antioxidant and antibacterial properties. Ind Crops Prod 2020; 158(November): 112964.
[http://dx.doi.org/10.1016/j.indcrop.2020.112964]

[152] Tinas H, Ozbek N, Akman S. Method development for the determination of cadmium in lipsticks directly by solid sampling high-resolution continuum source graphite furnace atomic absorption spectrometry. Microchem J 2018; 138: 316-20.
[http://dx.doi.org/10.1016/j.microc.2018.01.031]

[153] López-López M, Özbek N, García-Ruiz C. Confocal Raman spectroscopy to trace lipstick with their

smudges on different surfaces. Talanta 2014; 123: 135-9.
[http://dx.doi.org/10.1016/j.talanta.2014.02.025] [PMID: 24725875]

[154] Gładysz M, Król M, Kościelniak P. Current analytical methodologies used for examination of lipsticks and its traces for forensic purposes. Microchem J 2021; 164(January): 106002.
[http://dx.doi.org/10.1016/j.microc.2021.106002]

[155] Heusèle C, Cantin H, Bonté F. Lips and Lipstick. In: Draelos ZD, Ed. Cosmetic Dermatology: Products and Procedures. 2nd Edition. John Wiley & Sons, Ltd.; 2016. pp. 193–8.

[156] Solaiman DKY, Ashby RD, Erhan SZ. Soaps. Bailey's Ind Oil Fat Prod 2020; pp. 1-16.

[157] Han X, Tan Z, Huang Z, *et al.* Nondestructive detection of triclosan in antibacterial hand soaps using digitally labelled Raman spectroscopy. Anal Methods 2017; 9(24): 3720-6.
[http://dx.doi.org/10.1039/C7AY00118E]

[158] Chen MJ, Liu YT, Lin CW, Ponnusamy VK, Jen JF. Rapid determination of triclosan in personal care products using new in-tube based ultrasound-assisted salt-induced liquid–liquid microextraction coupled with high performance liquid chromatography-ultraviolet detection. Anal Chim Acta 2013; 767(1): 81-7.
[http://dx.doi.org/10.1016/j.aca.2013.01.014] [PMID: 23452790]

[159] Garner N, Siol A, Eilks I. Parabens as preservatives in personal care products. Chem Act 2014; (December): 38-43.

[160] Salam DA, Suidan MT, Venosa AD. Effect of butylated hydroxytoluene (BHT) on the aerobic biodegradation of a model vegetable oil in aquatic media. Environ Sci Technol 2012; 46(12): 6798-805.
[http://dx.doi.org/10.1021/es2046712] [PMID: 22680298]

[161] Zubair MF, Atolani O, Ibrahim SO, *et al.* Chemical and biological evaluations of potent antiseptic cosmetic products obtained from Momordica charantia seed oil. Sustain Chem Pharm 2018; 9(May): 35-41.
[http://dx.doi.org/10.1016/j.scp.2018.05.005]

[162] Anastas P, Eghbali N. Green chemistry: principles and practice. Chem Soc Rev 2010; 39(1): 301-12.
[http://dx.doi.org/10.1039/B918763B] [PMID: 20023854]

[163] Cavalcanti RN, Forster-Carneiro T, Gomes MTMS, Rostagno MA, Prado JM, Meireles MAA. Uses and applications of extracts from natural sources. RSC Green Chem 2013; 1-57.

[164] Abdulkadir AG, Jimoh WLO. Comparative analysis of physico-chemical properties of extracted and collected palm oil and tallow. ChemSearch J 2013; 4(2): 44-54.

[165] Ogunbiyi A, Enechukwu NA. African black soap: physiochemical, phytochemical properties, and uses. Dermatol Ther (Heidelb) 2020; 2021: 1-7.

[166] Joshi LS, Pawar HA. Herbal cosmetics and cosmeceuticals: an overview. Nat Prod Chem Res 2015; 3(2)

[167] Atolani O, Olabiyi ET, Issa AA, *et al.* Green synthesis and characterisation of natural antiseptic soaps from the oils of underutilised tropical seed. Sustain Chem Pharm 2016; 4: 32-9.
[http://dx.doi.org/10.1016/j.scp.2016.07.006]

[168] Ogunsuyi HO, Akinnawo CA. Quality assessment of soaps produced from palm bunch ash-derived alkali and coconut oil. J Appl Sci Environ Manag 2012; 16(4).

[169] Zauro SA, Abdullahi MT, Aliyu A, Muhammad A, Abubakar I, Sani YM. Production and analysis of soap using locally available raw-materials. Appl Chem 2016; 96(7): 41479-83.

[170] Atiku F, Fakai I, Warra A, Birnin-yauri A, Musa M. Production of soap using locally available alkaline extract from millet stalk: a study on physical and chemical properties of soap. Int J Adv Res Chem Sci 2014; 1(7): 1-7.

[171] Ameh AO, Muhammad JA, Audu HG. Synthesis and characterization of antiseptic soap from neem oil and shea butter oil. Afr J Biotechnol 2013; 12(29): 4656-62.

[172] Félix S, Araújo J, Pires AM, Sousa AC. Soap production: a green prospective. Waste Manag 2017; 66: 190-5.
[http://dx.doi.org/10.1016/j.wasman.2017.04.036] [PMID: 28455208]

[173] Atolani O, Adamu N, Oguntoye OS, *et al.* Chemical characterization, antioxidant, cytotoxicity, Anti-*Toxoplasma gondii* and antimicrobial potentials of the *Citrus sinensis* seed oil for sustainable cosmeceutical production. Heliyon 2020; 6(2): e03399.
[http://dx.doi.org/10.1016/j.heliyon.2020.e03399] [PMID: 32099925]

[174] Švarcová S, Kočí E, Plocek J, Zhankina A, Hradilová J, Bezdička P. Saponification in egg yolk-based tempera paintings with lead-tin yellow type I. J Cult Herit 2019; 38: 8-19.
[http://dx.doi.org/10.1016/j.culher.2018.12.004]

[175] Hayati SN, Rosyida VT, Darsih C, *et al.* Physicochemical properties, antimicrobial and antioxidant activity of ganoderma transparent soap. IOP Conf Ser Earth Environ Sci 2020; 462(1): 012047.
[http://dx.doi.org/10.1088/1755-1315/462/1/012047]

[176] Rosyida VT, Nisa K, Hayati SN, *et al.* Physicochemical properties of noni fruit, yam root, rose petal, and betel leaf transparent soap and their antimicrobial activities. IOP Conf Ser Earth Environ Sci 2019; 251(1): 012024.
[http://dx.doi.org/10.1088/1755-1315/251/1/012024]

[177] Ryu SR. A study on the elucidation of antimicrobial activity of separated fig component and the preparation of fig soap. J Korean Appl Sci Technol 2015; 32(4): 669-84.
[http://dx.doi.org/10.12925/jkocs.2015.32.4.669]

[178] Bansod SD, Bawaskar MS, Gade AK, Rai MK. Development of shampoo, soap and ointment formulated by green synthesised silver nanoparticles functionalised with antimicrobial plants oils in veterinary dermatology: treatment and prevention strategies. IET Nanobiotechnol 2015; 9(4): 165-71.
[http://dx.doi.org/10.1049/iet-nbt.2014.0042] [PMID: 26224344]

[179] Rambabu K, Edathil AA, Nirmala GS, *et al.* Date-fruit syrup waste extract as a natural additive for soap production with enhanced antioxidant and antibacterial activity. Environ Technol Innov 2020; 20: 101153.
[http://dx.doi.org/10.1016/j.eti.2020.101153]

[180] Guichard S, Roulier V. Colored Facial Cosmetics. In: Draelos ZD, Ed. Cosmetic Dermatology: Products and Procedures. Blackwell Publishing Ltd. 2010; pp. 167-75.

[181] Hosokawa K, Taima H, Kikuchi M, Tsuda H, Numano K, Takagi Y. Rubbing the skin when removing makeup cosmetics is a major factor that worsens skin conditions in atopic dermatitis patients. J Cosmet Dermatol 2021; 20(6): 1915-22.
[http://dx.doi.org/10.1111/jocd.13777] [PMID: 33040474]

[182] Chularojanamontri L, Tuchinda P, Kulthanan K, Pongparit K. Moisturizers for acne: what are their constituents? J Clin Aesthet Dermatol 2014; 7(5): 36-44.
[PMID: 24847408]

[183] Watanabe K, Matsuo A, Inoue H, Adachi K, Noda A. Innovation in the key performance of a cleansing oil by controlling the phase sequence of the surfactant system. J Soc Cosmet Chem Japan 2012; 46(4): 287-94.
[http://dx.doi.org/10.5107/sccj.46.287]

[184] Draelos ZD. The science behind skin care: Cleansers. J Cosmet Dermatol 2018; 17(1): 8-14.
[http://dx.doi.org/10.1111/jocd.12469] [PMID: 29231284]

[185] Ayuba L, Agboire S, Gana AK, *et al.* Efficacy of castor oil in the control of throat, skin and enteric bacteria. Adv Food Sci Eng 2017; 1(3): 95-9.

[186] Salimon J, Nallathamby N, Salih N, Abdullah BM. Synthesis and physical properties of estolide ester using saturated Fatty Acid and ricinoleic Acid. J Autom Methods Manag Chem 2011; 2011: 1-4.
[http://dx.doi.org/10.1155/2011/263624] [PMID: 22007150]

[187] Shombe GB, Mubofu EB, Mlowe S, Revaprasadu N. Synthesis and characterization of castor oil and ricinoleic acid capped CdS nanoparticles using single source precursors. Mater Sci Semicond Process 2016; 43: 230-7.
[http://dx.doi.org/10.1016/j.mssp.2015.11.011]

[188] Pakkang N, Uraki Y, Koda K, Nithitanakul M, Charoensaeng A. Preparation of water-in-oil microemulsion from the mixtures of castor oil and sunflower oil as makeup remover. J Surfactants Deterg 2018; 21(6): 809-16.
[http://dx.doi.org/10.1002/jsde.12189]

[189] Kim EJ, Kong BJ, Kwon SS, Jang HN, Park SN. Preparation and characterization of W/O microemulsion for removal of oily make-up cosmetics. Int J Cosmet Sci 2014; 36(6): 606-12.
[http://dx.doi.org/10.1111/ics.12163] [PMID: 25234159]

[190] Vickery SA, Wyatt P, Gilley J. Eye cosmetics. Cosmet Dermatology Prod Proced 2010; pp. 190-6.

CHAPTER 7

Natural Products and Nanoparticles in Skin Delivery

Adeola Ahmed Ibikunle[1,*] and **Nurudeen Olanrewaju Sanyaolu**[1]

[1] Department of Chemical Sciences, Olabisi Onabanjo University, Ago-Iwoye, Nigeria

Abstract: Some synthetic drugs are usually associated with side effects, while natural products may be characterized by poor solubility and/or stability. The application of nanoparticles, cutting across all human utilities with drug development is no exception. Skin disease treatment is one aspect of medicine that is so distinct in the sense that treatment usually involves topical application involving eventual absorption onto the skin surface. The use of nanoparticles has proven to be an effective way to solve the issues with the use of natural products in skin care and treatment. This effectiveness has been shown to be due to efficacy in the properties of these natural products, including solubility, stability, permeability, toxicity, side effects, the release of active ingredients-and biocompatibility. This section examines the role of nanosized natural products in treating skin disorders.

Keywords: Skin treatment, Nanoparticles, Nanosized natural products, Skin disorder, Cosmetic dermatology.

INTRODUCTION

In the past, natural products derived from plants and animals were used for decoration and protection of the skin; *Impatiens balsaminal Linn* for the nail, indigo for the eyebrow, *etc.*, and some animal oils were used as skin moisturizers [1, 2]. There are both, deficiencies in action and difficulties in applications attached to natural products cosmetics. Chemical ingredients are less safer, contain less metal concentration, and are less affected by environmental factors than natural products cosmetics. Natural product cosmetics are prone to contamination, produce toxic compounds, and experience loss of value. There are no standardized quality control measures for natural products in cosmetics, and the ions, acids and mucopolysaccharides which may be present in natural products, make formulations inaccurate as they break down lotions and creams.

---

* **Corresponding author Adeola Ahmed Ibikunle:** Department of Chemical Sciences, Olabisi Onabanjo University, Ago-Iwoye, Nigeria; E-mail: adeola.ibikunle@oouagoiwoye.edu.ng

Heba Abd El-Sattar El-Nashar, Mohamed El-Shazly & Nouran Mohammed Fahmy (Eds.)

As a result, it is very essential to consider a clean production process and quality analysis for natural products.

In addition, some skin whitening products have low stability and slow efficacy, and there isthe formation of hazardous compounds due to the nature of the ingredients used whereas, natural products as active ingredients in a whitening agent are safe, mild, long-lasting and highly effective. A drug is composed of both the active ingredient and the vehicle, both of which determine its efficacy. If every other factor is constant, the use of natural materials in the drug delivery to the skin would facilitate product consistency and effective penetration through the skin [3]. The inclusion of natural products in drug formulations can be in a number of semi-solids, such as ointments, rubber plasters, and gel plasters (Fig. 1).

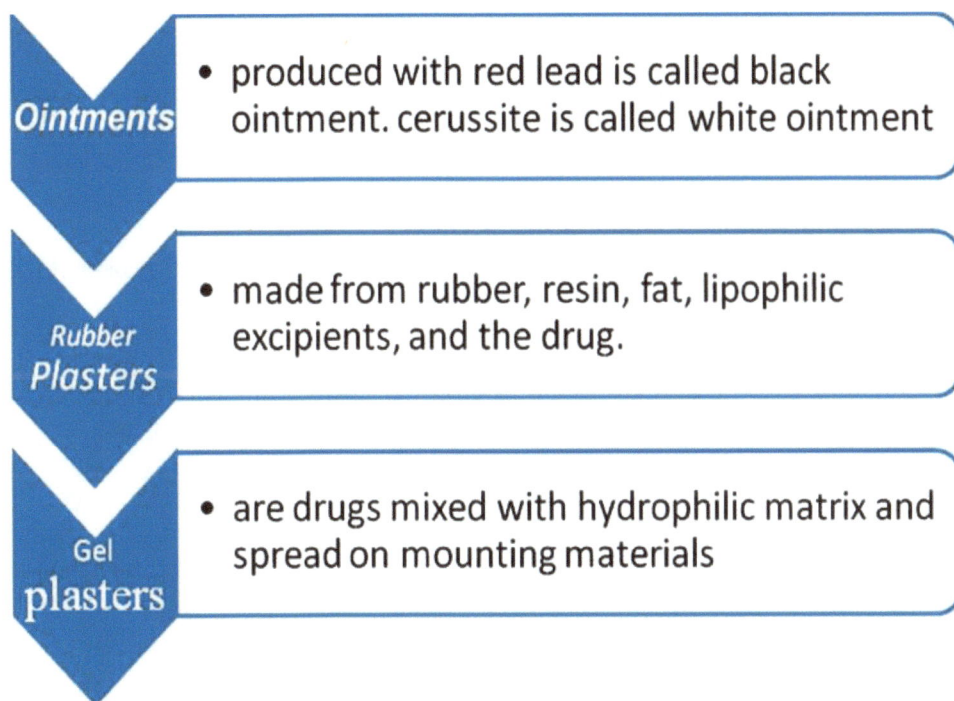

Ointments — produced with red lead is called black ointment. cerussite is called white ointment

Rubber Plasters — made from rubber, resin, fat, lipophilic excipients, and the drug.

Gel plasters — are drugs mixed with hydrophilic matrix and spread on mounting materials

Fig. (1). General compositions of some natural products in transdermal drugs.

Novel Applications in Natural Product Transdermal Delivery

The applications of natural products have been extensively developed to include the development of nanoemulsion, microneedles, lipid nanoparticles, dendrimers and liposomes (a class of delivery vectors). The introduction of novel technology like supercritical fluid extraction, microwave-assisted extraction and ultrasonic extraction coupled with nanosize drug delivery,has enhanced the persistent solubility and bioavailability issues attached to natural products. The nanoscaled size of the drug has improved the transdermal permeation of active ingredients in the drug compared to the conventional ones. Natural products are considered environmentally sustainable and ecologically friendly. Varieties of cosmetics products are composed of biosynthetic materials, which pose threats to the environment both at the manufacturing and disposal stages. The incorporation of cosmetic formulation agents innaturalproducts has brought a drastic decrease in the tonne of generated waste [4].

Natural products can also be used as potential antibacterial agents when incorporated into wound dressings [3, 5]. Most of these natural products are principal natural ingredients that are extracted from flowers, plants, seeds and roots. However, chemical instability and low bioavailability have been severely hampering the clinical application of most of them. In most cases, they can be easily oxidized, hydrolyzed, and polymerized by light, high temperature, and alkaline conditions due to their structural characteristics. The high polarity directly leads to the difficulty of transmembrane transport, resulting in low bioavailability. To address these problems, new drug delivery systems have been developed to improve the therapeutic efficacies of most lipid-based carriers, such as microemulsions, self-emulsifying systems, nanoparticles, chitosan, and the combination with other drugs, which may have a good application prospect [6].

Significance of Nanomaterials in Research

In recent times, nanotechnologyhas redirected and opened new fonts in major research in this modern society of ours. The classic top-down approach is already being put into extinction by the bottom-up approach from the ongoing miniaturization of processes at the nanoscale. Nanomaterials have found applications in plethoral of fields in science ranging from catalysis, medicine, sensing, and optoelectronics to mention but a few. Currently, the three main areas of development include: building specialized structures whose dimensions are controlled on a nanoscale; nanobiotechnology, *i.e.*, the manipulation of living systems using nanoscale engineering); and nanoelectronics involving the development of microelectronics for devices, such as radio frequency identification (Fig. **2**).

The production of materials at the nanoscale increases both the cost of production and improves the properties therein. In the areas of medicine and pharmaceutical industries, nanotechnological methods are under implementation but in the fields of biomedical and cosmetic fields, the enormous potentials are yet to be fully harnessed [6, 7].

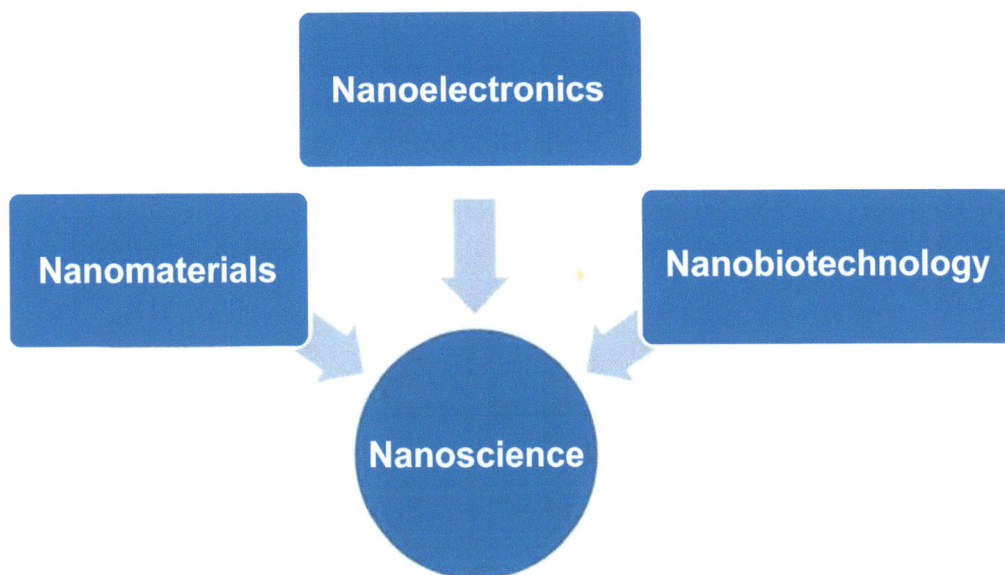

Fig. (2). The main areas of nanoscience.

Nanomaterials in Dermatology

Out of all the sense organs in the body, the largest is the skin, and it performs varying functions like protection of underlying organs, prevention of excessive water loss, provision of hydration and regulation of temperature [5, 8 - 10]. The functional as well as aesthetic roles played by the skin make its research domain very essential owing to the fact that its impairment could subject the underlying tissues to infiltration by bacteria. In addition, damage to the epithelium and the connecting structures on the skin would result in a reduction in the protective roles of the outer layer by exposing the nutrient-riched, warm and humid underlying environment to the development and growth of bacteria.

Nanomaterials and nanobiotechnology can easily change the mode of action or the mechanism of cosmetics and drug delivery. One of the applications of skin care creams is aimed at improving the skin barrier function towards skin diseases. The skin functions mainly in the protection of important organs like the liver, spleen, lung, heart liver and kidney from the external environment. It is as a result of this connectivity that the application of natural products on the skin is indirectly applied to these organs [1, 11 - 13].

Enactment of Law on Risk Assessment Analysis of Nanomaterials in Dermatology

There are hypothetical risks attached to the safety of the use of nanomaterials in dermatology; the methods of conventional toxicology are not adequate to give the best interpretation of the risk involved. The European Union is putting on frantic efforts at enacting laws for the use of nanomaterials in dermatology with the risk assessment being embarked on by many universities, government laboratories and industries in Europe [6].

Nanoparticles in Dermatology

By simple description, particles identified through their dimensions which are at least in one dimension and are smaller than 100 nm are ascribed to be nanoparticles [14], and natural products are ingredients derived from living organisms with applications over eons of years. Accordingly, particles with different morphologies from equi-axial shapes, whiskers, and nanotubes to nanorods need to be considered. Recently, Auffan *et al.* [15] reported that the sizes of nanoparticles have a great influence on their properties and suggested that the nanoparticles of diameter ≤ 30 nm are likely to possess unique properties and thus, they could be of great concern owing to their appearances. In this size range, there are unusual dramatic changes that hinge on the interfacial reactivity. The arrangement of the atoms are in such a way that less than 20% of the atoms are ubiquitous at the surface while the constituent atoms of nanoparticles in 10 nm has 35-40% of its atoms localized at the surface [10, 16, 17].

Different labile particles like micro or nanoemulsion can be produced from nanoparticles with diameters in the range of 50-5000 nm which can serve the dual purpose of protection against side reactions and as a carrier for easy penetration when used in skin treatment. The rate at which materials can penetrate the skin is a function of the size of the molecule thus nanotechnology research has been directed at developing a nanosize delivery system with varying sophistications [6]. To be specific, the use of nanoparticles broadens the horizon of the application of a wide range of beneficial ingredients to the skin. Among the dual principal approaches usually applied for the synthesis of nanoparticles; the bottom-up and the top-down method, the latter has a higher frequency in terms of usage in cosmetics in which structures of immense application are produced. Such structures include nanosomes, liposomes, cubosomes, and niosomes.

Sophisticated Applications of Nanoparticles in Skin Delivery

Nanoparticles have applications in cosmetics and pharmaceuticals ranging from the simplest to the most sophisticated form. Some of the sophisticated development of nanoparticles in pharmaceutical and cosmetic applications includes nanovesicles, solid lipid nanoparticles (SLN), UV filters titanium dioxide (TiO_2) and zinc oxide (ZnO), nanocapsules, and microcapsules [6]. The amphiphilic properties of vesicles are used in the skin delivery of both water-soluble and water-insoluble compounds in the presence of lipids and surfactants. The vesicles can be used as carriers, penetration enhancers, depots and site-limiting membranes in delivery systems. Solid lipid nanoparticles (SLN) are another sophisticated application of nanoparticles. Comparatively, the vesicle shows greater stability and increases skin hydration on the account of the formation of a nanolayer lipid film when in use. SLN are nanocarriers formed from lipids with a mean size in the range of 1000 nm. They are solids at room body temperature and emulsifiers are used in their formulation as stabilizers. SLN are advantaged on account that they function to protect drugs from the unfriendly environment and they can be produced en-mass, but the crystalline structure affects its drug loading capacity. However, both the vesicle and SLN are used in cosmetic emulsion, and their mean dimension is in the range of 100 nm.

The inorganic physical UV filters of titanium dioxide (TiO_2) and zinc oxide (ZnO), are another group of sophisticated applications of nanoparticles that are unfriendly to both water and oil (insoluble), and are usually regarded as sunscreen in the US, Japan and Germany. These minerals are used in transparent emulsion form with the dimension within the range 600-200 nm and this miniaturized nature accounts for its higher reflective index and its UVA and UVB filter properties. The microcapsule is another group of insoluble nanoparticles, compatible with different ingredients, and can protect against side reactions when used in cosmetic dermatology. Microcapsules have varying sizes; they are nanocapsules (size smaller than 1 μm) and macrocapsule (size larger than 1000 μm) in cosmetic dermatology [6].

Adverse Effects of Nanoparticles

The toxicological description of nanoparticles could be based on characteristics; shape, surface chemistry, size, crystallinity, charge, solubility, agglomeration/aggregation state and surface area [10, 14 - 18]. The mechanistic toxicological studies revealed that nanoparticles are predominant as causative agents of cell damage, inflammation, genotoxicity immune responses, *etc*. The route has been attributed to the generation of oxidative stress which acts as a precursor to the adverse effects aforementioned. The reactive strength and bioavailability of the nanoparticles governtheir physical and chemical properties and as such, are a strong determinant of the extent of the damage as well as the type of the damage. The versatility of nanoparticles has made some organisations invest heavily in research studies on nanoparticles. One such was carried out on

TiO_2 by the International Agency for Research on Cancer (IARC) and National Institute for Occupational Safety and Health labelling wherein TiO_2 was tagged as "possible carcinogenic to humans" and "occupational carcinogen" respectively making inference from the experimental report obtained from animal inhalation studies carried out [14].

The nanometer size level of nanoparticles is responsible for the high reactivity and overall, determines the physicochemical properties of nanoparticles. However, the size range is linked to undesirable properties, such as the induction of oxidative stress or cellular dysfunction caused by TiO_2.

CONCLUDING REMARKS

The numerous functions of the largest sense organ, the skin, make research on it to be inevitably attractive. Researches in this field are upsurging due to its high efficiency in taking care of the excesses of some of the synthetic materials in skin treatments. There have been a lot of efforts ongoing on skin treatments with natural products or biomaterials and this can be traced to the connectivity of the skin with the vital organs. These compounds are those obtained from living materials with microbes and plant inclusive. Some of the unique characteristics of natural products such as moisture content, high encapsulation, low-toxicity and biodegradability make them an excellent substitute for synthetic drugs which sufferfrom mild side effects. The use of natural materials in drug delivery to the skin would facilitate product efficiency and effective penetration through the skin among other advantages. The introduction of nanoparticles ensures greater encapsulation and modulation of the release of active ingredients and it is non-toxic. The advent of nanotechnology has led to the development of nanoparticles used as carriers in cosmetic dermatology with effective delivery at the target action site with adulteration of the active material. Thus, the use of nanoparticles has proven to be an effective way to solve the problemsassociated with the use of natural products in skin care and treatment.

REFERENCES

[1]   Cheng YC, Li TS, Su HL, Lee PC, Wang HMD. Transdermal delivery systems of natural products applied to skin therapy and care. Molecules 2020; 25(21): 5051.
[http://dx.doi.org/10.3390/molecules25215051] [PMID: 33143260]

[2]   Higgins S, Miller KA, Wojcik KY, *et al.* Phytochemicals and naturally occurring substances in the chemoprevention of skin cancer. Curr Dermatol Rep 2017; 6(3): 196-203.
[http://dx.doi.org/10.1007/s13671-017-0190-9]

[3]   Esposito E, Nastruzzi C, Sguizzato M, Cortesi R. Nanomedicines to treat skin pathologies with natural molecules. Curr Pharm Des 2019; 25(21): 2323-37.
[http://dx.doi.org/10.2174/1381612825666190709210703] [PMID: 31584367]

[4]   Ng S, Anuwi N, Tengku-Ahmad T. Topical lyogel containing xorticosteroid decreases IgE expression and enhances the therapeutic efficacy against atopic eczema. AAPS Pharm Sci Tech 2015; 16(3): 656-

63.
[http://dx.doi.org/10.1208/s12249-014-0248-y] [PMID: 25511806]

[5]   Negut I, Grumezescu V, Grumezescu A. Treatment strategies for infected wounds. Molecules 2018; 23(9): 2392.
[http://dx.doi.org/10.3390/molecules23092392] [PMID: 30231567]

[6]   Morganti P. Use and potential of nanotechnology in cosmetic dermatology. Clin Cosmet Investig Dermatol 2010; 3: 5-13.
[http://dx.doi.org/10.2147/CCID.S4506] [PMID: 21437055]

[7]   Bharali DJ, Siddiqui IA, Adhami VM, *et al.* Nanoparticle delivery of natural products in the prevention and treatment of cancers: current status and future prospects. Cancers (Basel) 2011; 3(4): 4024-45.
[http://dx.doi.org/10.3390/cancers3044024] [PMID: 24213123]

[8]   Norouzi M, Boroujeni SM, Omidvarkordshouli N, Soleimani M. Advances in skin regeneration: application of electrospun scaffolds. Adv Healthc Mater 2015; 4(8): 1114-33.
[http://dx.doi.org/10.1002/adhm.201500001] [PMID: 25721694]

[9]   Chua AWC, Khoo YC, Tan BK, Tan KC, Foo CL, Chong SJ. Skin tissue engineering advances in severe burns: review and therapeutic applications. Burns Trauma 2016; 4(3): s41038-016-0027-y.
[http://dx.doi.org/10.1186/s41038-016-0027-y] [PMID: 27574673]

[10]   Pivetta TP, Simões S, Araújo MM, Carvalho T, Arruda C, Marcato PD. Development of nanoparticles from natural lipids for topical delivery of thymol: Investigation of its anti-inflammatory properties. Colloids Surf B Biointerfaces 2018; 164: 281-90.
[http://dx.doi.org/10.1016/j.colsurfb.2018.01.053] [PMID: 29413607]

[11]   Souza C, de Freitas LAP, Maia Campos PMBG, Maria P, Gonçalves B, Campos M. Topical formulation containing beeswax-based nanoparticles improved *in vivo* skin barrier function. AAPS PharmSciTech 2017; 18(7): 2505-16.
[http://dx.doi.org/10.1208/s12249-017-0737-x] [PMID: 28213845]

[12]   Kheradmandnia S, Vasheghani-Farahani E, Nosrati M, Atyabi F. Preparation and characterization of ketoprofen-loaded solid lipid nanoparticles made from beeswax and carnauba wax. Nanomedicine 2010; 6(6): 753-9.
[http://dx.doi.org/10.1016/j.nano.2010.06.003] [PMID: 20599527]

[13]   Liu Y, Feng N. Nanocarriers for the delivery of active ingredients and fractions extracted from natural products used in traditional Chinese medicine (TCM). Adv Colloid Interface Sci 2015; 221: 60-76.
[http://dx.doi.org/10.1016/j.cis.2015.04.006] [PMID: 25999266]

[14]   Skocaj M, Filipic M, Petkovic J, Novak S. Titanium dioxide in our everyday life; is it safe? Radiol Oncol 2011; 45(4): 227-47.
[http://dx.doi.org/10.2478/v10019-011-0037-0] [PMID: 22933961]

[15]   Auffan M, Rose J, Bottero JY, Lowry GV, Jolivet JP, Wiesner MR. Towards a definition of inorganic nanoparticles from an environmental, health and safety perspective. Nat Nanotechnol 2009; 4(10): 634-41.
[http://dx.doi.org/10.1038/nnano.2009.242] [PMID: 19809453]

[16]   Gao S, Tian B, Han J, *et al.* Enhanced transdermal delivery of lornoxicam by nanostructured lipid carrier gels modified with polyarginine peptide for treatment of carrageenan-induced rat paw edema. Int J Nanomedicine 2019; 14: 6135-50.
[http://dx.doi.org/10.2147/IJN.S205295] [PMID: 31447556]

[17]   Agrawal YO, Mahajan UB, Mahajan HS, Ojha S. Methotrexate-loaded nanostructured lipid carrier gel alleviates imiquimod-induced psoriasis by moderating inflammation: formulation, optimization, characterization, *in-vitro* and *in-vivo* studies. Int J Nanomedicine 2020; 15: 4763-78.
[http://dx.doi.org/10.2147/IJN.S247007] [PMID: 32753865]

[18]   Müller R, Petersen R, Hommoss A, Pardeike J. Nanostructured lipid carriers (NLC) in cosmetic dermal products. Adv Drug Deliv Rev 2007; 59(6): 522-30.
[http://dx.doi.org/10.1016/j.addr.2007.04.012] [PMID: 17602783]

SUBJECT INDEX

A

V

Vascular 21, 70, 96, 100, 179
  endothelial growth factor (VEGF) 70, 96,
    100, 179
  thrombosis 21
Volatile organic compounds (VOCs) 171, 180

W

Water-binding capability 40
Wound healing 67, 69, 77, 80, 93, 94, 95, 96,
    97, 98, 99, 100, 101, 102, 103, 104, 105,
    106
  activity 77
  process 69, 80, 94
Wound infection 64
Wrinkle reduction 22